Facilitating the Genetic Couns

Patricia McCarthy Veach
Bonnie S. LeRoy · Nancy P. Callanan

Facilitating the Genetic Counseling Process

Practice-Based Skills

Second Edition

Springer

Patricia McCarthy Veach, Ph.D., L.P.
Department of Educational Psychology
University of Minnesota
Minneapolis, MN
USA

Nancy P. Callanan, M.S., C.G.C.
Genetic Counseling Program
University of North Carolina
Greensboro, NC
USA

Bonnie S. LeRoy, M.S., C.G.C., L.G.C.
Department of Genetics,
Cell Biology and Development
University of Minnesota
Minneapolis, MN
USA

ISBN 978-3-319-74798-9 ISBN 978-3-319-74799-6 (eBook)
https://doi.org/10.1007/978-3-319-74799-6

Library of Congress Control Number: 2018933097

Printed on acid-free paper

This Springer imprint is published by the registered company Springer International Publishing AG part of Springer Nature
The registered company address is: Gewerbestrasse 11, 6330 Cham, Switzerland

Preface

The genetic counseling landscape has changed dramatically in the 14 years since the initial publication of this book. During that time, genetic knowledge, tests, and technologies have burgeoned, often presenting patients and their family members with more options and increasingly difficult decisions. The sheer amount and type of available information and options further complicate decision-making processes. Now, perhaps more than ever, basic counseling skills are essential for providing genetic counseling services that facilitate patients' understanding, decision-making, coping, and adaptation to their genetic situation. Given their importance, basic skills remain the focus of the second edition of this book. We are excited, however, to frame the skills within a growing literature in the genetic counseling field that includes models of practice and research on genetic counseling processes and outcomes.

This book is intended to help genetic counseling students develop basic helping skills that form the foundation of effective genetic counseling relationships. These skills are integral to all aspects of a genetic counseling session, from obtaining history to providing information, to presenting options, facilitating decision-making, and providing anticipatory guidance and supportive counseling. They are essential for helping patients become educated so they can use genetic information to their benefit. In addition to a basic helping skills (microskills) focus, the content of this book promotes case conceptualization and self-reflective practice. A noteworthy feature is the inclusion of numerous structured activities and written exercises that provide opportunities for supervised practice in basic helping skills (which comprise the tools of interaction), self-reflection skills, and critical thinking skills necessary for making connections between basic skills and broader competencies. The exercises and activities are grounded in active and cooperative learning approaches that emphasize a high level of student participation and student responsibility for learning (Johnson et al. 1991). Students work together in learning activities that promote cooperation rather than competition. Furthermore, this approach facilitates student self-assessment of strengths and limitations. Note that many of the activities at the end of each chapter can be modified for use as a written exercise, and many of the exercises can be modified for use as an interactive activity.

The chapters address several of the psychosocial, practice-based competencies endorsed by the Accreditation Council for Genetic Counseling (2015) [see Appendix A for a list of the ACGC practice-based competencies for genetic counselors, including interpersonal psychosocial and counseling skills (Chaps. 2–11) and professional development (Chaps. 12–13).] The contents of this book will not fully prepare students to practice independently, but they will provide a skill base that deepens and broadens as students gain additional academic and clinical preparation. Although designed for use in a classroom setting, most of the materials, activities, and exercises can be adapted by clinical supervisors for use in the clinical setting.

This book edition contains a discussion of the Reciprocal-Engagement Model of genetic counseling practice (Chap. 2), expanded content on two basic counseling skills—advice and influencing skills (Chap. 10), new content on genetic counselor burnout and compassion fatigue (Chap. 12) and professional development and self-reflective practice (Chap. 13), genetic counseling examples/scenarios that reflect current testing and technologies, incorporation of genetic counseling research findings, additional activities and exercises in each chapter, and two role playing models for skills practice (Chap. 1). We deleted a chapter on using Internet resources as the current generation of students and practitioners are well-versed in Internet usage.

When revising this book, we drew upon numerous sources, including our combined professional experience as practitioners, educators, and researchers in the fields of genetic counseling and mental health counseling and from literature in genetic counseling and psychology. There are striking similarities between psychological counseling and genetic counseling, and many concepts are virtually interchangeable. Our goal, however, is not to train genetic counseling students to be psychotherapists. Therefore, examples provided to illustrate skills, concepts, and processes are always specific to the genetic counseling relationship. Furthermore, as genetic counseling is first and foremost a medically based health-care profession, important distinctions between mental health counseling and genetic counseling are highlighted throughout the book.

The content reflects a variety of theoretical orientations, including humanistic theories that stress the significance of helper genuineness, positive regard, respect, and nondirectiveness; psychodynamic theories that emphasize the strength and quality of the helper-patient working alliance and conscious and unconscious processes; and cognitive-behavioral theories that describe complex interactions of thoughts, feelings, and behaviors and the importance of defining patient concerns and goals in concrete, behavioral terms.

Our perspective is strongly influenced by our white, Western cultural backgrounds and by the tenets of traditional Western medicine. We attempt to broaden this perspective by including genetic counseling research on cultural variables and by pointing out limitations of certain concepts and techniques for patients whose cultural practices, beliefs, and worldviews differ from our own. Additionally, we include examples of patients with diverse backgrounds. It is important to keep in mind, however, that examples do not necessarily represent all cultural groups, nor do they apply to every member of a certain group.

While the focus of this book is on the genetic counseling skills relevant to patient interactions in face-to-face clinical settings, we recognize that an increasing number of genetic counselors are working in non-clinical settings, or they may be providing clinical services in expanded formats, such as telemedicine or web-based services. We believe these core skills are *transferrable* across all areas of genetic counseling practice. The unique combination of a health-care professional who is competent in the science of genetics *and* possesses communication and counseling skills is one of the major factors that has led to the tremendous growth of the genetic counseling profession over the past 50 years and will sustain this profession well into the future.

Format of the Book

We begin each chapter by stating general learning objectives. Then we define the skills, place them in a context (their function or purpose in genetic counseling), and provide illustrative examples. The reader may notice some redundancy in the examples (e.g., many involve prenatal genetic counseling situations, and Down syndrome, breast cancer, muscular dystrophy, and Huntington's disease are mentioned frequently). This redundancy is intentional as we wanted "basic" examples that students at all levels, including those with limited knowledge about genetic conditions, would be able to understand.

We conclude each chapter with structured activities and written exercises for skills practice. Structured activities can be done either before the written exercises to stimulate student thinking or after the written exercises to afford students the opportunity to consider how much they are comfortable sharing. Regardless of which exercises and activities are chosen, and whether they are done in writing or orally, *students need to be cautioned to select only those issues they are comfortable disclosing to others*. Instructors/supervisors should reinforce this point and always inform students in advance about the types of information they will be expected to share with others.

Closing Comments

We suggest you begin with the chapter "Guidelines for Users of the Book" as it "sets the stage" for the remaining chapters. We hope you find this book useful, and we welcome any comments or questions you might have about it. Our contact information is veach001@umn.edu, leroy001@umn.edu, and npcallan@uncg.edu.

References

Accreditation Council for Genetic Counseling. Practice based competencies for genetic counselors. 2015. http://gceducation.org/Documents/ACGC%20Core%20Competencies%20Brochure_15_Web.pdf. Accessed 18 Aug 2017.

Johnson DW, Johnson RT, Smith KA. Active learning: cooperation in the college classroom. Edina, MN: Interaction; 1991.

Minneapolis, MN, USA — Patricia McCarthy Veach
Minneapolis, MN, USA — Bonnie S. LeRoy
Greensboro, NC, USA — Nancy P. Callanan

Acknowledgments

The first edition of this book was supported by a grant from the Jane Engelberg Memorial Fellowship.

It was shaped by the expertise of several professionals from the genetic counseling field, bioethics, and adult learning. We would like to especially thank one of the original authors of this book, Dr. Dianne Bartels, whose knowledge and perspective are present in each chapter of the second edition.

Contents

Abbreviations

ACGC	Accreditation Council for Genetic Counseling
The ARC	The ARC of the United States
ASHG	American Society of Human Genetics
BRCA	Breast cancer
CEGRM	Colored Eco-Genetic Relationship Map
CF	Cystic fibrosis
cfDNA	Cell-free DNA
Co	Counselor
COE	Code of Ethics
Cl	Client
CMA	Chromosomal microarray analysis
DMD	Duchenne muscular dystrophy
EOFAD	Early-onset familial Alzheimer's disease
FAP	Familial adenomatous polyposis
GC	Genetic counselor
GLBT	Gay, lesbian, bi-sexual, transgender
HBOC	Hereditary breast and ovarian cancer
HD	Huntington's disease
IA	Intermediate allele
ID	Intellectual disabilities
ITM	Interactive Training Model
LGBT	Lesbian, gay, bi-sexual, transgender
MPSII	Hunter syndrome
NSGC	National Society of Genetic Counselors
OCD	Obsessive-compulsive disorder
Obs	Observer
Pt	Patient
REM	Reciprocal-Engagement Model
SDM	Shared decision-making
SMA	Spinal muscular atrophy
SUVQ	Schwartz Universal Values Questionnaire

TAGC	Transnational Alliance for Genetic Counseling
TS	Tuberous sclerosis
VUS	Variants of uncertain significance
WES	Whole exome sequencing

Chapter 1
Guidelines for Book Users: Instructors, Supervisors, and Students

Learning Objectives
1. Describe philosophical and pedagogical base of the book.
2. Identify common challenges in the development of basic helping skills.
3. Recommend strategies to facilitate teaching and learning of basic helping skills.

Helping skills are fun to teach and learn. Students are eager to acquire the techniques of their craft, and they appreciate the variety of activities involved in skills practice. At the same time, helping skills training poses unique challenges (e.g., distinguishing between similar types of counselor responses such as primary empathy and advanced empathy, managing student anxiety and resistance, and differentiating developmental issues from issues of skill deficiency). In this chapter, we provide a philosophical and pedagogical context for the contents of this book, discuss some of the challenges involved in helping skills development, and offer suggestions for teaching and learning helping skills. Suggestions include active learning techniques that are appropriate for helping skills training, tips for facilitating role-playing and feedback processes, and strategies for conducting discussions. We also offer suggestions about evaluation and student resistance, and we include activities for integrating student learning (see Appendices). Most of the suggestions can be adapted by clinical supervisors for use with supervisees. Many of these ideas have been shaped by the students and colleagues with whom we have worked over the last 30+ years. We are particularly grateful to the Center for Educational Innovation at the University of Minnesota.

P. McCarthy Veach et al., *Facilitating the Genetic Counseling Process*,
https://doi.org/10.1007/978-3-319-74799-6_1

1.1 Philosophical Underpinnings and General Learning Objectives

Extensive empirical evidence demonstrates that basic counseling skills (e.g., attending, reflecting) can be improved through microskills training (cf. Ridley and Mollen 2011). A major aim of this book is to develop student competencies with respect to both basic counseling skills (see Appendix 1 for a list of each basic skill and brief description) and selected key elements of genetic counseling (e.g., contracting, decision-making). The dual emphasis will help students learn how to adapt these *building blocks* for work with specific patients in specific genetic counseling situations and increase their appreciation for the complex *art and science* of genetic counseling.

Two general learning objectives involve students increasing their knowledge and skills and forming professional attitudes appropriate for clinical practice. They accomplish these objectives by personalizing the concepts, theories, and skills presented herein through firsthand experiences of sitting "hypothetically" in the genetic counselor's chair and through their involvement in an interactive supervision process (giving and receiving feedback). Another general learning objective is recognizing how basic skills fit within broader competencies; this objective is accomplished through structured activities and written assignments focusing on basic helping skills, case conceptualization, and self-reflection. Demonstration of the interrelatedness of basic skills and broader competencies early in students' professional training may prevent them from perceiving the competencies as overly simplistic and "siloed."

We want students to gain a realistic appreciation of the complexities of genetic counseling, build their self-confidence and self-awareness, and become more strategic in their conceptualization of patients and in their use of skills during genetic counseling sessions. In sum, we hope to increase students' ability to talk to, listen to, and understand people; know themselves; and appreciate what it means to be a professional.

1.1.1 Self-Reflective Practice

Numerous activities and exercises in this book require students to engage in introspection. Self-reflection is an intentional mental processing used primarily for complicated or uncertain situations or ideas in order to meet a particular objective (Lowe et al. 2007). Self-reflection has several potential benefits, including increasing the likelihood that professional education and training have a meaningful influence on one's behavior, thus helping practitioners continue to develop professionally (Lowe et al. 2007); allowing practitioners to better distinguish patients' concerns from their own (Silverman 2008); and promoting expression of empathy and perspective-taking. Theoretically, practitioners who are more aware of their own internal processes, life challenges, and personal strengths and limitations are better able to relate to those of their patients (Joireman et al. 2002). Self-reflection helps students acquire self-supervisory skills; create a conceptual map of the helping process (Bennett-Levy 2007); and develop cultural competency, as deep self-knowledge is considered an essential component of culturally competent practice. Ridley et al. (2011) cite several counseling/psychotherapy studies demonstrating that "Continuous self-reflection and self-awareness … are critical to quality therapeutic relationships and professional development" (p. 829). Evidence from the genetic counseling literature supports the necessity of self-reflection in genetic counselor professional development (e.g., Callanan and Redlinger-Grosse 2016; Miranda et al. 2016; Wells et al. 2016; Zahm et al. 2016).

1.1.2 General Principles for Maximizing Learning

The type of skills learning approach recommended in this book is quite novel for many students. As such, we find it helpful to set the stage for learning by sharing several principles with them:

- It is more important to *know what the questions are* than to feel confident you have all the answers. Questions demonstrate your critical thinking, willingness to seek consultation, and desire to find answers. Development of "self-supervision" skills is essential. As a professional, you must be able to critically evaluate and then modify your performance as necessary.
- You will be immersed in an *ethos of feedback*. Every feedback interaction should involve positive and corrective feedback, and you should strive to be open and willing to give and receive feedback in a respectful manner.
- We expect you to be open and willing to share personal reflections regarding your development as a genetic counselor.
- We encourage you to *try on for size* the various basic skills presented.
- We ask you to make efforts to become comfortable in the genetic counselor chair—sitting across from patients you do not know and engaging in interactions that are unpredictable.
- We encourage you to spend more time focusing on the patient(s), rather than on yourself.
- You should work to become proactive and strategic rather than reactive during counseling interchanges.
- We want you to try to speculate about what lies beneath the surface of genetic counseling interactions. Refrain from automatically taking either patient behaviors or your own actions and reactions at face value.
- We expect you to realize that at all times, you are held to a higher standard as a professional and to behave accordingly.

1.2 Active Learning Guidelines and Techniques

The primary pedagogical approach of this book is *active* and *cooperative* learning (cf. Johnson et al. 1991). Theory and research demonstrate students are not *passive receptacles* who learn best by accruing information delivered primarily through lectures (cf. Smith et al. 2013). Rather, they achieve superior learning through active engagement with course content. Furthermore, students do not develop clinical skills simply by reading and discussing them; clinical skill development requires supervised practice that includes focused feedback. Accordingly, this book is highly experiential, containing self-reflective activities and written exercises designed to give students opportunities for supervised practice.

In the following sections, we offer general suggestions for using an active learning approach, followed by examples of different types of active learning techniques.

1.2.1 General Suggestions

Get Started

- Describe the active learning philosophy and how it relates to your learning objectives. We include a description of active learning on our syllabus and discuss it during the first class period. For some students, this may be the first time they participate in a course that it is not primarily lecture-format.
- Begin the first class with an "icebreaker" active learning exercise. This sets the tone for the types of activities that will occur throughout the course. For example, in a "note cards" icebreaker exercise, students write down on index cards personal information such as their name, hometown, favorite book or movie, and one or two things they hope to learn from the course. Then they walk around and share their information with others in the class.

Build the Relationship

- You and your students should learn each other's names as quickly as possible if you don't already know them. You might use name tags and/or play a "name game" in which you go around the circle and each person says her or his first name and a self-descriptive adjective beginning with the first letter of her or his name (e.g., athletic Annie); the next person says her or his name and adjective and repeats the name and adjective of the previous person. Continue this way around the circle until the last person (perhaps the instructor) repeats everyone's name and adjective.
- Vary the way students join dyads, triads, and small groups so they have an opportunity to interact with everyone (e.g., count off; preassign; everyone who is at the

same table; let students pick a partner—especially appropriate early in the course and/or for activities where students might disclose more intimate information).

Stay Focused

- Give verbal and written directions for every activity (provide handouts, put directions on PowerPoint slides, and/or write them on the board).
- Ask a student to verbally summarize your directions for an activity.
- Earlier in the course you will need to provide more structure and instructions than you will later. During group activities, in particular, students may not naturally engage in necessary activities such as keeping time, recording group member ideas, and working to include everyone in the conversation. You should assign essential roles for small group discussions (e.g., go around the small group and say, "The person whose last name is the shortest will be the recorder, the person to her or his left is the timekeeper, the next person is the process observer, the next person is the divergent thinker, the next person is the facilitator, the next person is the reporter").
- Walk around during active learning exercises to get a feel for what is developing, to help keep students on task, and to clarify instructions. Inform students that you will be "listening in" throughout the course; they will quickly acclimate to having you walk around or sit in with them.
- Move people along, especially as individuals would rather talk than practice. For instance, try saying, "I know there is more we could discuss, but I want to be sure you all get a chance to practice the skills, so let's take one more comment before we move on."

Be Efficient

- For small group activities, specify the way roles are assigned so they are determined quickly (e.g., the recorder is the person wearing red, or the person with a birthday closest to that day, or the tallest person, etc.). Vary the role assignments so students have an opportunity to play them all.
- Avoid undue redundancy when debriefing an activity in which more than one small group discusses the same questions. An effective approach is to ask each group to give one idea or have each group give their answers to a different part of the question. Keep going around until all unique ideas have been expressed.
- When planning activities, be sure to allot time for instructions and for students to get into work groups. We provide time estimates for activities at the end of each chapter. The times will vary considerably, however, depending on (1) class size, (2) student verbosity, (3) the number and type of questions you use to process an activity, and (4) the complexity of the skill or concept on which an activity is based.

1.2.2 Tips for Instructors

The structured activities in this book emphasize self-reflection, discussion, and skills practice. To maximize learning processes and outcomes, we suggest the following:

Responding to Student Questions and Comments

- Occasionally when students ask you a question, redirect the question back to the group (e.g., "What are your thoughts about this?"), but only if you believe someone will have a good answer that you can summarize and/or expand upon.
- Be respectful yet selective in what you reinforce. Try to relate everyone's responses to the issues at hand. Repeat the most pertinent or useful comments in a summary statement.

Encouraging Student Participation

- Watch for nonverbal behaviors to "draw" individuals into the discussion, but invite rather than demand a response (e.g., "You look as if you might want to say something?").
- Be sensitive to individual differences. As you get to know your students, you will be able to tailor the ways in which you bring them into discussions. For example, if a student never volunteers and seems reluctant, occasionally invite this student to give a reaction first during a discussion. Or, if a student is verbose, ask for that student's feedback last.

Using Small Groups

- When using a small group format, four to five students per group are optimal for encouraging participation and generating quality discussion.
- To facilitate discussion, begin with questions anyone could answer, and then make them progressively difficult.

  Example: Begin a discussion about "relationships" by asking everyone to respond to the question, "What are they?" Then ask more specifically about what the "genetic counseling relationship" entails, the goal(s) of the relationship, and counselor and patient roles and responsibilities.

- To maximize small group discussion, first define and provide a brief overview of the concepts or terms that will be discussed. When processing the discussion, try to *tie together* student comments by summarizing major themes, issues, etc. Also, be prepared to correct any inaccurate information that may emerge.

Use Examples

- Provide as many examples as feasible when presenting material. Novices are extremely interested in seeing "what it looks like" and "how it's done." One technique is to refer students to places in the text where there is an example and ask them to generate several more. This will facilitate their learning and comprehension.
- Concrete examples are very helpful for illustrating concepts. When you able to, provide students with video and/or audio recordings and live demonstrations of genetic counseling (preferably by more than one genetic counselor). If possible, bring in volunteers to serve as genetic counselors and patients for some of the demonstrations.
- Make your examples basic enough that students do not need a lot of knowledge about the genetic condition. Provide them with some details about the condition so they can proceed with the activities.

Organize Class Sessions

- When preparing each class, prioritize activities so you know in advance which ones you will delete if you run over time.
- Arrange your class activities so they progress from easier to more challenging ones. You should also begin with less threatening activities (e.g., defining *defense mechanisms*) and then move to more threatening activities (e.g., discussing one's own defense mechanisms). When arranging activities, remember the more threatening an activity, the fewer people you may want to have listening to a student's disclosure (e.g., use a dyad format in which students select who they want as a partner). When processing a more threatening activity, don't ask for details, although students are free to offer them. For instance, in processing a defense mechanisms dyadic exercise, ask, "How was it to do this activity? What did you learn about the impact of defense mechanisms on genetic counseling?" Do not ask, "What defense mechanisms do you use?"
- Have on hand an assortment of role-play scenarios you could assign to students for role-play practice. Various exercises and activities in this book include scenarios that may be used for role-playing. You can also assign students the task of creating role-play scenarios. The objective is to give them practice in perspective-taking, thereby promoting empathy as well as practice in case conceptualization. For instance, a 24-year-old white male might create a scenario in which the patient is a 38-year-old Asian female with breast cancer, thus providing practice with cultural empathy (Ridley and Lingle 1996). Appendix 2 contains a description of a written exercise for developing genetic counseling role-plays. If you have students create scenarios, we recommend you review them in order to insure their appropriateness and accuracy.

- If feasible, use co-instructors (e.g., advanced genetic counseling students). They will provide different viewpoints, and you may have enough co-instructors to directly observe small groups of students when doing role-plays and engaging in other small group activities. Ideally there would be one instructor for each small group. Co-instructors can also serve as counselors and patients when demonstrating helping skills.

Demonstrate/Model

- One way individuals learn is by contrast. When time allows, model both low-level (poor) and high-level (good) helping skills, always beginning with low-level ones. Ask students to articulate the differences between the skills demonstrated in the two levels.
- Use processing questions after a counseling skills demonstration: What did you observe the counselor saying? Doing? What effect did it have on the patient? What did the patient say/do to give you that impression? Is the counselor's behavior desirable? Undesirable? What would you have done differently and why?
- You can set norms by going first to model how to do an activity.
- For individual skills demonstrations (which are typically briefer interactions of 10–15 min), we highly recommend using the same role-play/patient throughout the course. One option is to demonstrate portions of two genetic counseling sessions (an initial session at which genetic testing is discussed as an option the patient eventually decides to pursue and then a results discussion session in which the patient decides what she/he will do with the test results). This approach will allow you to demonstrate appropriate use of more advanced skills (e.g., confrontation, decision-making models) and will give students a concrete sense of how genetic counseling progresses.

Role-Play Formats

Role-playing is the primary learning activity for the skills described in this book. Despite their artificial nature, role-plays have been shown to be effective in increasing students' skills (cf. Duys and Hedstrom 2000). Ongoing support and guidance can occur through verbal and written feedback immediately after role-plays. There is no single way to conduct and process/debrief role-plays. We describe two possible formats in Appendix 3. In addition, we recommend the following:

- Organize students into role-play practice groups (change group composition frequently).
- Remind students of how much time they have for each role-play.
- Ask for volunteers to go first as the counselor and patient.

- Remind observers to take notes and to keep track of time.
- Have the counselor and patient position themselves as if it were an actual genetic counseling session (they may have to move chairs).
- Direct student counselors to focus on every skill they have covered so far and use them *as appropriate* (in other words, don't force a skill just for the sake of demonstrating it).
- Tell counselors they can call for a *time-out* during the role-play if they get stuck. The observer can also call a time-out if things seem to be bogged down. During the time-out, the counselor should talk about what she/he thinks is going on (what the patient has been saying, doing, feeling), and the counselor and observer can consult about ways for the counselor to proceed. The patient should be silent during the time-out. Then resume the role-play (it usually helps to have the patient begin). When there is a time-out, reduce the amount of feedback time at the end of that role-play.
- Debrief by having the observer share at least one positive and one corrective piece of feedback. Next ask the patient to provide feedback. As the students gain experience during the course, debriefing can begin with the counselor providing a self-critique and then proceeding to observer and patient feedback.
- Remind students that feedback should *focus on the counselor and not the patient!*
- Remind students to first focus their feedback on the skill for that class session and then provide feedback about skills that have been covered in previous class sessions. Try to minimize feedback on skills that have not been covered (this is especially likely to happen in early class sessions; for instance, students are practicing attending skills but their classmates will give them feedback about questioning skills).
- Some *patients* get caught up in role-plays and may become emotional. Let them regain composure before eliciting their feedback. Also, *depersonalize* feedback to the counselor that involves comments about the patient as some elements of the role-play are likely the student's real reactions and/or history. For instance, you could say, "Your use of open questions with this type of verbal patient was…." Or you could say, "When patients are highly defensive, it's a good idea to…." Avoid saying, "Joan was a highly defensive patient, so you should have…."
- Sit in and observe each student during role-plays as much as possible during the course.
- Once students have participated in a few role-plays and have a sense of their current skill level, you can invite them in advance of the role-play to identify specific skills for which they would like feedback (feedback is most effective when it is requested).
- If feasible, video record students during some role-plays. They will likely feel anxious about being recorded, but they will learn a great deal from seeing and hearing themselves. The recordings will also provide a concrete way to chart their progress.
- Be sure to give role-play observation notes to the counselor at the end of each role-play/class.

Critical Issues in Role-Playing and Debriefing

- Students prefer to *talk* rather than *do*. You can easily get off-schedule, talking about the skills and not having enough time to practice. Encourage students to practice.
- The counselor and/or patient get off track during the role-play. When this happens, the observer should call for a time-out.
- Time is running out. If you wish to limit discussion, have each observer and the patient give only one or two pieces of feedback to the counselor. The role-plays could also be shortened a couple of minutes.
- Students provide invalid and/or harsh feedback. Sit in on role-plays and model for students how to give feedback. If you openly disagree with a student's feedback while sitting in on a role-play, be tactful (e.g., "I think I had a different reaction to the counselor's approach to this patient. I think this shows how different patients might react differently to the same counselor behavior"). Another option is to ask the other students in the group (either the patient or the observers) if they had a similar reaction to that of the feedback giver.
- The counselor is defensive. Remember to use basic helping skills—a little empathy goes a long way! Also, put feedback into a *context* for the student (e.g., "This is something most beginners do," "This isn't a big deal," or "With practice, you'll improve on that behavior"). Role-playing is a threatening activity, so expect some anxiety. In our course evaluations, students often tell us it's the activity they *dreaded* the most, but they also found it to be one of the activities from which they learned the most (they respond similarly to self-critiqued, audio- or video-recorded role-play assignments). Also, the most experienced students are often the most nervous about role-playing. Perhaps they believe more is expected of them.
- Students hear discrepant feedback. Student will likely hear contradictory feedback from different observers, and they may become frustrated or confused by this. We tell our students to listen for the *themes* in the feedback they receive. One isolated comment that they were too directive may not be as valid as several comments from different sources. Contradictory feedback may be particularly troublesome for some students who are looking for formulas or the *right way* to do things.
- Students complain about using made-up material during role-plays. Some students complain about the artificial nature of simulated role-plays (e.g., it's not how a session would really happen; they couldn't *get into* the role because they knew it wasn't real). We acknowledge that there is a certain degree of artificiality. We also talk about how practice is important (e.g., student nurses administer shots to each other before they do so with actual patients) and encourage students to try for as much realism as possible. Furthermore, we believe once students get over some of their initial anxiety about being observed, they *settle into* role-playing. We also point out that it's very difficult to construct and act out an entirely hypothetical role. The role-player will project her or his own feelings, thoughts, and attitudes into the role.
- Prior to beginning role-play practice, we recommend addressing student anxiety about engaging in role-plays and feedback by reviewing common student concerns and ways to respond to their concerns (see Appendix 4).

Providing Feedback

- Provide a balance of positive and corrective feedback. It can help to begin with positive comments. Next move to corrective comments, being certain to always suggest what the student might try in order to improve. Try the *sandwich technique*, that is, tell the student what she/he did well, next suggest areas to work on, and finish with a reiteration of what she/he did well.
- Ask students to self-evaluate.
- When students give each other feedback, tell them to talk directly to the person receiving the feedback and not to the instructor.
- When giving feedback, students may go to extremes—only talking about the positive aspects of another student's role-play (e.g., "You did everything just great!") or *hammering* another student with a laundry list of everything the student did wrong. We recommend that you discuss giving and receiving feedback at the beginning of the course and use feedback exercises (described in Appendix 5) to allow students to practice their feedback skills.

1.2.3 Selected Active Learning Techniques

Active Learning Exercises

The following list contains a sampling of different types of active learning exercises that might be appropriate for your setting and learning objectives:

- Survey the Class: "How many of you agree with the author's point of view? How many disagree?" Have students raise their hands.
- Random Calling: For larger classes, randomly call on individual students or dyads (e.g., write the name of each student on Popsicle sticks. Randomly draw a stick from a container and call on that student).
- Bean Counters: In small groups, everyone receives three beans or three poker chips, and each time a person speaks, she/he throws a bean into a bowl or box. When a person's beans are gone, then she/he can no longer speak.
- Speaking Stick: Based on Native American practice, the stick is passed among the group members. Whoever has the stick is the only one allowed to speak.
- Margin-It: Students write down answers to questions in their notebook margins. This is a safe, anonymous way to check themselves out on what they know. After doing this, the instructor provides the answer or asks volunteers to share what they wrote.
- Think-Pair-Share: This is a dyadic activity. Students first think about a question, concept, etc. Next, they find a partner, and the dyad shares responses with each other. To process, you could go around and ask each dyad to share one idea until the concept or question has been fully explored. One variation is to have students write down their response before talking with a partner (e.g., "Write down everything that you know about empathy"). Another variation is to have one dyad join another dyad for "Round 2." The resulting *quad* shares their responses to the question.

- In Class Writing: Give students 1–5 min to "Take a stance," "Defend a position," or "Formulate a response to the following patient statement…." Then ask students to discuss what they wrote with a dyad partner, small group, or the whole class.
- Data Interpretation: Instruct dyads or small groups to read and interpret graphs, tables, or charts. For example, they could read a table of data about risk for a particular genetic condition, interpret the data, and formulate a way to explain this risk to a patient.
- Laundry List: Students raise every question they have about a topic (e.g., touching patients, nondirectiveness, self-disclosing with patients), while you list their questions on the board or overhead. Then proceed to address each question (using whatever format is appropriate—lecture, in-class writing, dyads, etc.).
- 10–20-Minute Press Conference: Students write down anonymous questions about topics covered in the course so far. Collect their questions, shuffle them, and redistribute them (give one question to each student). Then student volunteers read any interesting questions, and you attempt to answer them. We have used this format at the end of a course. By then students are quite comfortable raising complex issues and sensitive topics. This technique should also work well earlier in a course. This exercise is particularly effective if your course format includes co-instructors—students can hear differing opinions to the same question. One caveat: Tell students the questions should be about course content and not format (we discourage questions such as "Why is assignment #1 worth so many points?" That type of question is more appropriate for course/instructor evaluations).
- Student Originated Cases: Assign students the task of finding challenging genetic counseling situations in the literature and then bringing them to class to work on in groups (e.g., strategizing how to respond, role-playing the situations, discussing them).
- Dialogue Journals: Students pair off and respond to each other's journal entries for 5 min of each class session. These dyads remain intact for the whole course. You can assign them journal topics to discuss or leave it fairly open-ended. Require the journal entries to be focused on the course content. You should periodically collect the journals and informally look at them. We also suggest providing some examples of journal entries to give students a sense of the expected length, scope, and topics.
- Matching and Milling: Give each student a paper with a piece of information written on it (different information for each student), and then have them move around the room comparing their information with the other students' information. Their task is to figure out how the pieces fit together. For instance, you could give each student pieces of a patient's family history, including some relevant and nonrelevant information. The students' task would be to figure out the patient's risk. Next, groups of four to five students could brainstorm and then role-play how to convey this risk information to the patient.

Example: Construct a complicated family history for cancer. Assign some class members to portray the family (each student has a couple of pieces of information about the family history); assign other members to be the genetic counselors who are responsible for gathering information by asking the right questions of the family members. Have the genetic counselors first brainstorm how to counsel the family and then engage in a role-play in which they conduct a *team* counseling session with the family.

- Clustering: This is a more structured form of brainstorming in which you begin by writing a term in the middle of the board (e.g., risk, patient anger, confrontation). Using this word as a focus, students brainstorm associated words, phrases, and ideas that you write in a circle around the term. Next you could ask students to identify themes they see in the words that are written around the circle, and/or you could give an "impromptu" lecture in which you connect the various words. You could follow this activity with a laundry list exercise, in which students generate every question they have about the concept (see earlier description of this technique).

1.3 Grading and Evaluation

1.3.1 General Criteria: Written Assignments

- Make your evaluation criteria explicit. For example, we tell students our evaluation of assignments is based on the quality of information, coherence, consistency, and degree of self-reflection. It is not based on whether we agree with a student's opinions or, for instance, on whether we like her or his motives for being a genetic counselor. We also stress that we are looking for improvement in basic helping skills by the end of the course and encourage students to take risks and make mistakes in order to develop their skills. We also indicate that we value self-awareness of one's strengths and weaknesses as opposed to perfection.
- Tie your feedback to your course objectives (Flash et al. 1995).
- Provide samples of good assignments (more feasible once you've taught the course once) that you have obtained from other students (with their written permission and after you have submitted their final course grade). Always remove the student's name and any identifying information from a sample assignment.
- If you assign points for each major section of an assignment, state the number of points the student received for each major section and explain why points were deducted. Regardless of whether you assign points, provide one or two general reasons for the grade they receive, especially if it is less than full credit.
- Provide behavioral feedback, and try to balance positive and corrective comments. Suggest how the student might improve the next assignment (decide if you will allow students to revise and resubmit assignments). Raise rhetorical questions throughout an assignment to encourage further reflection.

- Give students an opportunity to use feedback to improve their performance (e.g., on large assignments, allow them to submit drafts before a final product is due) (Flash et al. 1995).
- Give clear, specific feedback that offers guidance on how to improve.
- Remind students to address all aspects of the assignment. We spell out each part of an assignment and state the maximum number of points that can be obtained for each section.
- Although the emphasis of this book is basic helping skills, you will simultaneously need to evaluate and correct *technical* or *content* errors regarding genetic conditions, information, etc. Emphasize to students that on more objective tasks (e.g., calculating a risk rate), accuracy is important. For assignments requiring self-reflection (e.g., personal values, philosophy of genetic counseling, etc.), look for evidence that the student has personalized her or his response and is not merely quoting others' ideas. Encourage students to provide specific examples from their own experience.
- Suggest to students that they read their answers aloud in exercises requiring them to formulate actual counselor responses. We don't speak the way we write. Saying them aloud will help students formulate more *natural* responses.
- Evaluate frequently. Frequent feedback provides multiple pieces of data, increases student comfort with the process, allows you and your students to assess how they are doing, stimulates ideas for rectifying problems, and prompts students to keep up with the material.
- Give students periodic opportunities to tell you what they believe they are learning. For instance, use journaling [written or audio recorded (see Parikh et al. (2012) for an example of recorded journaling)], self-reflection papers, and *1-minute papers* (Davis et al. 1983). For a 1-minute paper, at the end of a class session, ask students to spend 1 min anonymously writing about one or two of the most important things they learned that day and one or two things about which they have further questions. Collect and review their papers and clarify any questions/confusion in a subsequent class period.
- Try to get a feel for the overall quality of an assignment when determining the final grade.
- As you get to know students, grade with their backgrounds in mind. For instance, we expect more mature and complete products from students who are older and have previous experience in a human service profession; we recognize that students for whom English is a second language may have some grammatical and spelling difficulties; etc.

1.3.2 Evaluating Role-Plays

Methods for evaluating helping skills are highly subjective. Nevertheless, it is important to be as clear and consistent as you can in evaluating student performance.

In some of the chapters, we provide general criteria for evaluating helping skills. You might also wish to develop a standard form or checklist for observers. For instance, you could include the dimensions suggested by Barkham (1988):

- Type of behavior (primary empathy, open question, etc.)
- Skillfulness of the genetic counselor (timeliness, plausibility, relevance, appropriateness, discrepant from patient's viewpoint, etc.)
- Interpersonal manner (empathic, respectful, distant, mechanical, etc.)

Observers can check off any categories the counselor demonstrates, and/or rate the degree of effectiveness (e.g., poor, adequate, good, excellent).

In our course, we stress that behavioral feedback is more important than checks on a rating form. Students learn by hearing specific examples of what they did (e.g., "When you said the patient might be a little nervous about talking to you, she seemed to relax"). They also learn by receiving specific suggestions as to how they might improve (e.g., "Try asking one question at a time so the patient doesn't get too overwhelmed").

1.3.3 Development or Deficiency?

Research has demonstrated that systematic training can improve helping skills. For example, individuals can be taught to formulate more concise primary empathy responses. *Timing* and *choosing* of responses, however, are more advanced skills that will develop gradually as students gain supervised counseling experience (Bernard and Goodyear 2013; McCarthy Veach and LeRoy 2009). It also appears to be the case that the *rich will get richer*. In other words, students who have adequate levels of cognitive development and who possess enough self-awareness and interpersonal sensitivity to choose appropriate responses in different situations will tend to become more effective helpers. One challenge you will face is evaluating whether poor performance is due to developmental issues (e.g., lack of experience, naivete) or to deficiencies that may or may not be teachable [e.g., poor communication skills, immaturity, lack of self-awareness, lack of intellectual reasoning (Veilleux et al. 2012)].

Criteria for helping to make this determination include four identified by Lamb et al. (1987):

- The problem behavior is pervasive.
- The student does not acknowledge, understand, or try to do anything about the behavior when it is identified.
- The problem behavior does not improve with training, feedback, or other remediation efforts.
- The student and her or his problematic behavior require a disproportionate amount of instructor time.

We would add a fifth criterion:

- The student responds defensively to critical feedback by denying or projecting (e.g., "It's your fault I haven't done better"); defending the behavior as a difference in *learning style*, *interpersonal style*, or *cultural difference* when this is not the case; pleading or bargaining; challenging the validity of the helping skills approach; and/or avoiding further feedback.

1.3.4 Student Resistance

It is natural for students to feel varying amounts of anxiety and resistance when learning and using genetic counseling skills. Resistance "... may stem from decreased confidence, fear of causing harm or a lack of clarity of psycho-social goals" (Shugar 2017, p. 215). They may be resistant to different aspects of helping skills training for one or more additional reasons, including:

- They are afraid of the unknown.
- They are worried they are not/will not be good genetic counselors.
- They do not see the relevance of a particular topic, activity, etc.
- They don't want to look foolish or incompetent in front of others.
- They are used to being *A* students who, in many courses, could memorize material and receive a perfect grade. Helping skills training is distinct because there is always something the counselor could have done differently.
- Your instructions/expectations are not clear and/or are inconsistent.

Furthermore, when students go through basic helping skills training without having ever done genetic counseling, they may tend to (a) think genetic counseling is easier to do than it is; (b) discount some of the feedback they receive because it's not from a patient or clinical supervisor; and (c) discredit some aspects of the helping skills model, theory, and skills. For instance, they may be dogmatic about how they think genetic counseling should be done; this is common for novices who need some certainty in order to deal with their anxiety about being beginners.

1.3.5 Strategies for Addressing Student Resistance

There are several things you can try to work through student resistance:

- Ask yourself whether the resistance is justified (e.g., you did not provide clear instructions; the relevance of a particular activity is questionable; etc.).
- Create situations where you gradually increase the difficulty/threat level of what you ask students to do so they can *ease into* these activities and be more successful in doing them.
- Provide a rationale for each topic and activity. If you are challenged (e.g., "Why are we doing this anyway? It seems like a waste of time!"), ask the group, "Why *do*

you think we're doing this? What's the point?" Usually someone will come up with a compelling rationale.

- Point out the resistance and talk about how it's natural to feel a little embarrassed or hesitant when trying out new things.
- Self-disclose about your own discomfort with certain helping skills and talk about some of the mistakes you've made as a genetic counselor, especially recent ones. This will help students realize genetic counseling is not easy and that everyone at any point in their professional development has something to learn.
- If feasible, have volunteers come in to serve as patients for the students during role-plays. Outsiders can provide influential feedback about what worked and what didn't during the role-play. Also, it usually is more difficult to discount a volunteer's feedback as opposed to a classmate's comments.
- Talk with students about the difference between helping skills training and their other courses with respect to performance and evaluation. Brainstorm with them ways to manage the stress and anxiety of being evaluated on their interpersonal skills and sensitivity (see Appendix 5 for guidelines on giving and receiving feedback).
- At times, you may be the only one who has a realistic or valid perception of what happened during a role-play or other activity and how well or poorly a student did during the activity. You will need to be tactful (especially when the rest of the group says a student did a wonderful job). You could try saying, "Here's another way to consider doing it…" or "Let's talk about the plusses and minuses of how you responded when the patient said…."

1.4 Skills Integration

The basic skills are introduced one chapter at a time, and therefore students may have difficulty seeing how they all fit together. You need to help them understand how to integrate the skills into a model of helping. We recommend four activities to help students make connections across the basic skills and broader concepts. The first activity, Student-Generated Discussion Questions Activity (Appendix 6), asks students to periodically develop questions based on the readings, classroom activities, and their own personal reflections about genetic counseling and then discuss one or more questions in small groups. This activity is intended to give student opportunities to critically reflect upon clinical issues that are important to them. In our experience, these questions change as the semester progresses, so we advise students against writing all of their questions in advance. We retain everyone's discussion questions and attempt to address them at various times throughout the semester.

The second activity, Genetic Counseling Interview Analysis (Appendix 7), involves a paper which can be assigned later in the course after students have been introduced to most of the basic helping skills. This paper is based on students watching a live, 50-min simulated genetic counseling session between a genetic counselor and "patient" from outside the course. The activity and resulting paper provide students with an opportunity to consolidate their learning and allow the instructor to assess student depth of understanding of basic skills and concepts. We've found that students become more *caught up* in a live interview, rather than viewing a video. They also benefit from sitting quietly and intently observing the genetic counseling interaction. A live demonstration allows for an optional activity—asking the genetic counselor and/or patient to remain at the conclusion of the session and inviting students to pose questions to them about the interaction.

The third activity, Integration of Skills: Stimulus Questions (see Appendix 8), involves a list of questions that stimulate students to consolidate their learning in the course; we use this exercise during the last class session. The fourth activity, Personal Reflection about Genetic Counseling Paper (Appendix 9), requires students to articulate in writing their perspective regarding genetic counseling. This paper, which comprises our final course assignment, asks students to consolidate their self-reflection about activities completed earlier in the course and allows them to assess their professional strengths and growth areas specific to clinical practice.

1.5 Closing Comments

Teaching and supervising genetic counseling students are skills that will improve with practice and experience. At their best, training and supervision are continuous learning processes for both teachers/supervisors and their students. Learning is enhanced through a variety of activities and exercises, a willingness to take risks, continual reflection upon one's experiences, and consideration and incorporation of feedback into one's practice. Keep in mind that helping is as much an art as it is a science, and every genetic counselor has a highly personalized style of helping. Encourage students to talk with their clinical supervisors about why different genetic counselors in different settings approach genetic counseling differently. Reflection upon these *differences* will assist students in developing their own individual styles.

Appendix 1.1: Basic Counseling Skills

Attending	
Physical attending	Counselor nonverbal behavior
Psychological attending	Counselor attention to patient nonverbal behavior
Empathy and Confrontation	
Primary empathy (content)	Reflection of surface content of patient's experience
Primary empathy (affect)	Reflection of patient's surface feelings
Advanced empathy	Reflection of patient's underlying experience
Confrontation	Challenge to patient's perceptions, beliefs, viewpoint

Questions	
Open questions	Cannot be answered easily with one or two words
Closed questions	Can be answered easily with one or two words
Self-reference	
Self-disclosure	Counselor revelation of information about her/himself
Self-involvement	Counselor "here-and-now" expression of feelings about/reactions to the patient
Additional skills	
Advice	Suggest something the patient should/should not do
Information giving	Provide data about something
Influence	Counselor states her/his opinion

Appendix 1.2: Genetic Counseling Role-Play Scenarios

You are to develop six patient roles for use during role-play exercises. Limit each to no more than half of one page. Use the following ten categories to create *six*, word-processed scenarios. *Use a separate page* for each role-play. *Note*: You should assume the counselor has already given genetic information to the patient. Focus the scenario instead on patient reactions, decisions, questions, etc. (b) Patients can be individuals or couples. (c) *Two scenarios* should involve giving patients "bad news" (positive or abnormal test results).

1. Counseling *setting*: Genetic counseling.
2. Patient *demographics*: Gender, age.
3. Describe the *situation*: What is the presenting concern? Why is the patient seeing you?
4. What are the patient's *surface feelings*?
5. What are the patient's *hidden feelings*?
6. What is the patient *thinking*?
7. What is the patient *doing*? What behaviors are involved in the presenting concern?
8. How is the patient *coping*? What strategies (positive and negative) has the patient tried to address her/his concern, with what success? What resources, including people, has the patient drawn upon?
9. Describe the *trigger event*: What precipitating factor(s) led to seeking counseling at this time? What does this patient want from the counselor?
10. Briefly *describe genetic condition*: two to three lines so classmates have a working notion of the condition.

Role-Play Scenario Example

Counseling setting: Genetic counseling agency.
Demographics: 35-year-old female lawyer, first pregnancy 10 weeks gestation.
Situation: Advanced maternal age, sister had baby with trisomy 18.
Surface feelings: Fear.
Hidden feelings: Worry, confusion, unclear about what she would do if the child had a trisomy.
Thoughts: Concerned about termination and general decision-making.
Behaviors: Diving into details and fidgeting.
Coping strategies/resources: Seeks knowledge, avoids talking about her situation with others.
Trigger event: Sister informed her of risk.
Description of genetic condition: Advanced maternal age is…. Trisomy 18 is….

Objective This assignment provides practice in perspective-taking, thereby promoting empathy.

Appendix 1.3: Guidelines for Student Role-Plays

A significant amount of class time will be spent doing role-plays. Despite their artificial nature, role-plays have been shown to be effective in increasing students' skills (e.g., Duys and Hedstrom 2000).

A 1.3.1 Role-Play #1: Triad/Quad Groups

Format

Role-playing will typically be done in a triad or quad consisting of three or four students. When feasible, one co-instructor will sit in on the triad/quad group. Students will take turns acting as counselor, patient, and observer. Role-play groups will be rearranged frequently so that you get the opportunity to work with different people.

Students sometimes will work with the same "patient" over two class sessions, which allows them to spend more time using basic skills and to gain a deeper conceptualization of the patient issues and genetic counseling process. The second role-play could be an extension of the first genetic counseling session, a "do-over" of the first genetic counseling session, or a second genetic counseling session (e.g., genetic test results discussion).

Length

Early in the course, role-plays will be brief—5–10 min. They will be longer as the course progresses and new skills are introduced.

Roles

1. Counselors will be asked to demonstrate the skills covered up to that point in the course.
2. Patients will be expected to convincingly present the patient's concerns. Their presentation should involve a certain amount of complexity, and their behavior should be realistic but not be so difficult that the genetic counselor is unable to practice the skills being covered. Examples of *inappropriate* patient behaviors are patient is too quiet or too talkative, mentally ill, and highly resistant.
3. Observers will be expected to watch the role-play and provide the counselor with feedback about the behaviors she/he used well (positive feedback) and about the behaviors which could be improved (corrective feedback). It is strongly recommended that observers make a written record of the role-play so that feedback is specific and chronological. One method is to divide a piece of paper into three columns:

Genetic counselor (co)	Patient (Pt)	Observer (Obs)

In the genetic counselor and patient columns, write down key phrases or sentences. In the observer column, note any comments you might have about the role-play.

Give your forms to the genetic counselor at the conclusion of feedback.

A 1.3.2 Role-Play #2: Interactive Training Model (ITM)[1]

Format and Roles

This is a whole classroom role-play model to help develop counseling skills, self-awareness, and working conceptualization skills. Class members take turns playing one of the following roles: Counselor, patient, counselor advisors, patient advocate, and audience. The audience will act as observers, and they will complete feedback forms if a written form is used in the course. They will give these forms to the counselor

The various roles involve the following:

- *Patient*—Gives realistic portrayal of details in scenario
- *Patient advocate*—Occasionally gives voice to patient's inner dialogue by verbalizing thoughts, feelings, and needs the patient does not share directly and the counselor is not addressing. This role should be played by the instructor for all or most role-plays when the students are novices
- *Counselor*—Treats commentary from patient advocate as if she/he were listening to an intercom in the grocery store, taking it in, but carrying on in the role-play

[1] From: Paladino et al. (2011).

- *Counselor advisors*—Support the counselor. They remain silent until asked by counselor to comment. They speak at an audible level. Usually two students act assume this role for each role-play
- *Audience*—Act as observers, taking notes regarding skills and processes used

Processing of each ITM role-play is done by the instructor in the following order, using some of the following questions

Counselor

- What was something you said/did that you thought went well?
- What would you like to have done differently?
- If the role-play continued, what focus would you like to take?
- Identify a time when you could have used the counselor advisors but did not

Patient

- What did you like about the counselor's approach?
- What would you have liked to hear from the counselor?

Counselor Advisors (Typically Two Students)

- What did you like about the counselor's intervention?
- If you were the counselor, what would you have added to the session?

Patient Advocate (As Stated Above, Typically This Role Is Enacted by the Instructor as It Requires a Fair Amount of Expertise)

- Discuss your perspective of the session with a focus on counselor strengths, opportunities
- If necessary, reframe counselor and counselor advisor responses
- Discuss what you might have added to the session if you were the counselor

Audience

- What did you like about the counselor's approach?
- What questions do you have for the patient and the counselor?
- If you were the counselor, what would you have added to the session?

Instructor Note

- This role-playing model can be a bit complicated to explain and implement. We suggest you read the article by Paladino et al. (2011) and then do a practice run in which the counselor and patient discuss an innocuous topic
- One of the most common misunderstandings in using this model is the patient thinking the patient advocate's comments are meant to shape her or his behavior. Patient advocate comments are intended to guide the *counselor's behavior*. You may have to remind students about this when initially using this model

A 1.3.3 Additional Guidelines for Processing Role-Plays

Two Important Criteria

- Being sure feedback is balanced (positive and corrective)
- Being sure feedback is precise (focused on specific actions/dialogue)

Instructor Feedback

- Discuss positive and less positive aspects, with attention to the basic skill of the day, but also all skills covered in the course up to this point.
- If necessary, reframe observers' feedback.
- If you were the counselor, what would you have added/done differently?

Working Conceptualization

- Ask students (except for the patient) for their hypotheses about what is going on with the patient.
- Add you own hypotheses and ideas of additional avenues to explore if there were more time/further sessions.
- Ask patient to read description of hidden feelings, thoughts, and what she/he wanted from the counselor (see Appendix 2 for patient role-play scenario components).

Appendix 1.4: Addressing Typical Student Concerns About Role-Plays

Student Concern: "Should I use any real material when I'm the patient?"

Response: There is no definitive answer to this question. Real material has the benefit of being closer to an actual genetic counseling situation, and you don't have to struggle making up information. On the other hand, you risk being caught off guard, revealing more than you intended, and/or you might feel frustrated when the role-play is cut short and feedback emphasizes the counselor's behaviors. Hypothetical material has the benefit of being less emotionally charged, and it allows for a greater variety of situations and patient types.

Student Concern: "Is it normal to feel anxious during role-plays?"

Response: Yes! But you will find that your anxiety decreases as you become more accustomed to doing role-plays. It may also help to remind yourself that there is no perfect genetic counseling session and no terminal skill level. Counselors at all levels of experience can benefit from practice and feedback.

Student Concern: How is a role-play supposed to be done?

Response: Here are some ground rules for role-plays.

1. When you are in the patient role, think through the role before you begin, so you can respond to the counselor as naturally as possible (e.g., What thoughts, feelings, and behaviors might this patient have?).
2. When in the genetic counselor role, think about whether there are certain skills or behaviors you would like the members of your group to watch for, and tell them what those skills/behaviors are before you begin the role-play.
3. Realize that you will receive a great deal of feedback from many different individuals during this course. The feedback will vary in its validity and importance. Listen for "themes" across different observers and role-plays. Repetitious feedback is generally a good indicator of your counseling strengths and growth areas.
4. Do not discuss the role-plays outside of your triad/quad or class. Whether hypothetical or real, patients and counselors deserve confidentiality.

Appendix 1.5: Giving and Receiving Feedback

Feedback is a way of helping another person to consider changing his or her behavior. It involves communicating your impressions, feelings, and observations about another person's behavior in order to be helpful to the person.

A 1.5.1 Types of Feedback

There are four types of feedback:

- Positive
- Corrective
- Performance
- Personal

	Positive	Corrective
Performance	*Reinforcement to continue behavior* Emphasizes sharing a perception or thought Example: I thought your summary was well-organized	*Reinforcement to modify behavior* Emphasizes sharing a perception or thought Example: I think your questions were too lengthy
Personal	*Reinforcement to continue a behavior* Emphasizes sharing feelings Example: When you listened to my concerns as the patient about being at risk, I really appreciated it	*Reinforcement to modify a behavior* Emphasizes sharing feelings Example: When you asked me why I felt the way I did about having genetic testing, I felt uncomfortable.

A 1.5.2 Giving Effective Feedback[2]

Effective feedback is:

- Requested by the receiver, if possible.
- Given as promptly as possible after the observed behavior.
- Concise; it does not contain unnecessary detail or information.
- Focused on the person's observable behavior, not the person's character. For instance, "You didn't look at the patient when you talked to her," not, "You were strange and distant."
- Given in a personal and non-threatening manner, avoiding moral or value judgments. For example, "When you look away when you talk to the patient, I get the impression you're disconnected," not, "Nobody likes people who look away when they talk."
- Concerned only with behavior the person can modify. For instance, counselors cannot change their gender in order to connect better with a patient.
- Focused on the person's strengths as well as limitations.
- Discussed by both giver and receiver until they can see each other's perspective.
- Definite, not given and then "taken back."

A 1.5.3 Receiving Feedback Effectively

When an individual receives feedback, the following behaviors can maximize its effectiveness:

[2] Adapted from: Danish et al. (1980).

- Clarify feedback. Let the person giving you feedback know you heard what she/he said. If you do not understand, ask for clarification.
- Share your reaction. When receiving feedback, you will have both a cognitive and an emotional reaction. Try to be aware of both and decide which aspects you want to share with the feedback giver.
- Accept positive feedback. If feedback is positive (especially when it is information you already know), you may tend to gloss over it quickly. Perhaps you are embarrassed, do not believe positive feedback, feel bored with the same old comments, etc. Try to remember that awareness of your strengths as well as your weaknesses is important in building strong skills. Try to think of new ways to creatively adapt your strengths in different situations.
- Accept corrective feedback. If feedback is corrective (especially when it's information that is new to you), you may tend to have a negative response. You may deny it, discredit the source, feel threatened or embarrassed, etc. Try to remember that corrective feedback is not a global criticism of you as a person (or as a genetic counselor!). Try to identify strategies for correction. You may want to ask for specific suggestions.
- Test validity of feedback. If the feedback does not fit well with your self-perceptions, pursue it further. You can ask for clarification. You can ask others if their perceptions are the same. While everyone's perspective is valid in his or her own frame of reference, it is not necessarily the absolute "truth." Usually you will discover the essential and useful element of feedback if you persist in attempting to understand it.
- Exercise personal responsibility. As you develop as a genetic counselor, you will become more aware of your own strengths and limitations. It is important for you to take responsibility for you own growth early in your development. One way to do this is to ask for feedback about specific behaviors and issues you know are problematic for you. It can be helpful to ask for this feedback before you are observed. Then observers can focus on these areas as well as other aspects of your counseling skills.
- Avoid feedback overload. At times, you may feel swamped with ideas, and at those times it's OK to let people know you've had enough for one session. You can always schedule another time to finish receiving feedback. Remember that feedback is for your own growth. If it is coming in too fast to assimilate, it will not help you develop your skills.

Feedback Exercise

This is an exercise that can be used with students early in a course or in a clinical supervision relationship.

- First, ask students to think of a time in their life when they received feedback that was particularly helpful and then to think about what made this feedback so helpful. Next, ask them to think about a time they received feedback that was not helpful and to reflect upon what made the feedback unhelpful. Then ask students to share what made their feedback situations helpful and unhelpful, and list these on the board. Add to the list any characteristics they may have overlooked.

- Next, using the definition of feedback presented at the beginning of this appendix, ask students to generate examples of the four types of feedback.
- Finally, ask students to find a partner and discuss this question: "What can you do to help yourself feel safe enough to receive all types of feedback?" Then open a discussion with the whole group about strategies to make feedback easier to give and receive in this course or clinical rotation.

Estimated time: 45 min.

Appendix 1.6: Student-Generated Discussion Questions Activity

Inform students they will meet several times during the course for a facilitated discussion. Tell them they will remain with the same group of students for each of these discussions. They are required to develop questions (one per discussion), as follows:

a. Develop *one question* based on readings, classroom activities, your own personal reflections about genetic counseling, etc. Your question can address broad topics/issues or be more specific in nature.
b. Give your written question to the instructor on the day of each discussion. Write your name on your question so you receive proper credit for it.

The instructor randomly selects one or two questions from those received and leads the group in a 15–20-min discussion. Authors of selected questions are *not* identified by the instructor.

Instructor Note

- The questions tend to change as the semester progresses, so advise students against writing all of their questions at one time.
- We suggest you retain everyone's discussion questions and attempt to address them at various times throughout the semester.
- Students seem to have the most appreciation for this activity when the discussion includes generation of concrete ideas for how to best address the issues reflected in the discussion questions.
- If there are multiple small discussion groups, you can lead a whole class discussion asking each small group to summarize their comments for one question, adding your own elaborations and clarifications.

Objective This activity provides opportunities for students to critically reflect upon important counseling issues, including those that are important to them.

Appendix 1.7: Genetic Counseling Interview Analysis

The instructor (or "guest counselor") models an entire genetic counseling session with a volunteer "patient" who is not a class member, while the students observe. The session is video recorded so students can review it later when preparing the written assignment. Students should be instructed to refer to Appendix 1 for a list of basic skills to guide them when observing the session.

Estimated time: 60 min.

Process

At the end of the session, students break into small groups to discuss what they observed.

Estimated time: 30 min.

A 1.7.1 Written Assignment

Based on the counseling session you observed, prepare a 6–7-page, word-processed, double-spaced paper describing the following:

A 1.7.2 Background Information

Demographics: A demographic description of the patient (e.g., age, gender, ethnicity, general appearance, socioeconomic status, manner of presentation, and motivation for participating in genetic counseling).

Patient Presenting Concerns/Session Expectations: How did the patient describe her/his concerns? Why is she/he seeking genetic counseling?

Medical and Family History: Summarize the patient's history and provide a risk assessment, if appropriate.

Working Conceptualization: How would *you* describe the patient's concerns? What is your working conceptualization/hypotheses about this patient's major (a) medical, (b) genetic, and (c) psychosocial issues? Give evidence to support your conceptualization.

A 1.7.3 Counseling Process

a. *Evaluate* the counseling relationship the genetic counselor formed. What did the counselor *do* to establish such a relationship? [*Hint*: Using the types of skills presented in this course, *name each skill used by the genetic counselor*, and *describe the general effect(s)* of each skill on this patient. Include brief quotations from the session to illustrate each skill.]
b. What *goals* did the counselor seem to have *for this session*?
c. What could the counselor have *done differently*?

A 1.7.4 Notable Genetic Counselor Skills

a. Identify two specific counselor behaviors (something the counselor said or did) that you would be likely to use in your genetic counseling sessions.
b. For each of the two genetic counselor behaviors identified, explain when in a genetic counseling session you might use the behavior and why.
c. How would you modify each behavior, if at all, to use it in your genetic counseling?

Objective This assignment is similar to a case debriefing, a common activity in genetic counseling clinical supervision. It also allows the instructor to assess student understanding of basic skills and concepts covered in the course.

Appendix 1.8: Integration of Skills—Stimulus Questions Activity

Pairs of students take turns answering each of the following questions, or they can select any questions they wish to answer in the order they wish to answer them.

1. How would you describe your current level of confidence in your counseling skills?
2. What have you learned about yourself as a genetic counselor in training?
3. What do you think is the most important skill?
4. Are there things you are still confused about?
5. What is the hardest skill we've talked about?
6. What is one of the most helpful things you've learned in this course?
7. How has this course affected your communication style?
8. What else do you feel you need to learn?
9. What makes genetic counseling so difficult?
10. What differences do you see between genetic counseling and listening to a friend?
11. What could make you feel "burned out" as a counselor?
12. What is one thing you expected to learn, but did not? One thing you did not expect to learn, but did?
13. How have your ideas changed about genetic counseling?
14. How helpful is genetic counseling? Why?

Estimated time: 20–75 min.

Instructor Note

- Processing in the large group is optional.
- A variation of this exercise is to write each question on a separate sheet of paper. Students randomly draw questions and respond to them.

Appendix 1.9: Personal Reflection About Genetic Counseling Paper

Prepare a 5–6-page, double-spaced paper in which you present your perspective on genetic counseling. You should incorporate readings, classroom activities, and personal experiences. Include in your reflection a discussion of the following areas:

1. What is genetic counseling? What makes it so challenging? What role does diversity (culture) play in genetic counseling relationships?
2. In this course, we discussed the importance of identifying client concerns as the client states them as well identifying them via the counselor's working conceptualization. Why is a working conceptualization important?
3. Which of the skills that we have covered in this class is easiest for you? Which skill is the most difficult? What makes it so difficult for you?
4. *Describe a counseling interaction from a *clinical rotation* in which you used a skill from this course that worked well. What did you do? Why/how was it effective?
5. Describe one piece of *positive feedback* you received in this course and one piece of *corrective feedback* you received in this course that were particularly illuminating for you.
6. How have your *beliefs* about genetic counseling changed since the beginning of this course?

Objective This assignment builds upon self-reflective activities from earlier in the course. It also provides students an opportunity to consolidate their learning and "take stock" of their professional development to date.

Instructor Note
- *If students have not yet begun a clinical rotation, you can ask them to describe a role-play interaction from the course.

References

Barkham M. Empathy in counselling and psychotherapy: present status and future directions. Couns Psychol Q. 1988;1:407–28.

Bennett-Levy J. Self and self-reflection in the therapeutic relationship: a conceptual map and practice strategies for the training, supervision and self-supervision of interpersonal skills. New York: Routledge/Taylor & Francis Group; 2007.

Bernard JM, Goodyear RK. Fundamentals of clinical supervision. 5th ed. Boston: Pearson Merrill Counseling Series; 2013.

Callanan N, Redlinger-Grosse K. Time flies: an examination of genetic counselor professional development: introduction to special issue on genetic counselor development. J Genet Couns. 2016;25:611–6.

Danish SJ, D'Augelli AR, Hauer AL. Helping skills: a basic training program. New York: Human Sciences Press; 1980.

Davis BB, Wood L, Wilson R. ABC's of teaching with excellence: a Berkeley compendium of suggestions for teaching with excellence. Berkeley: Office of Educational Development, University of California; 1983.

Duys DK, Hedstrom SM. Basic counselor skills training and counselor cognitive complexity. Couns Educ Superv. 2000;40:8–18.

Flash P, Tzenis C, Waller A. Helpfulness of feedback given you about your performance. In: Using student evaluations to increase classroom effectiveness. Minneapolis, MN: Faculty and Teaching Assistant Enrichment Program, University of Minnesota; 1995. p. 58–61.

Johnson DW, Johnson RT, Smith KA. Active learning: cooperation in the college classroom. Edina, MN: Interaction; 1991.

Joireman J, Parrott L, Hammersla J. Empathy and the self-absorption paradox: support for the distinction between self-rumination and self-reflection. Self Identity. 2002;1:56–65.

Lamb DH, Presser NR, Pfost KS, Baum MC, Jackso VR, Jarvis PA. Confronting professional impairment during the internship: identification, due process, and remediation. Prof Psychol Res Pr. 1987;18:597–603.

Lowe M, Rappolt S, Jaglal S, MacDonals G. The role of reflection in implementing learning from continuing education into practice. J Contin Educ Heal Prof. 2007;27:143–8.

McCarthy Veach P, LeRoy B. Student supervision: strategies for providing direction, guidance, and support. In: Uhlmann WR, Schuette JL, Yashar B, editors. A guide to genetic counseling. 2nd ed. New York: Wiley; 2009. p. 401–34.

Miranda C, Veach PM, Martyr MA, LeRoy BS. Portrait of the master genetic counselor clinician: a qualitative investigation of expertise in genetic counseling. J Genet Couns. 2016;25:767–85.

Paladino DA, Barrio Minton CA, Kern CW. Interactive training model: enhancing beginning counseling student development. Couns Educ Superv. 2011;50:189–206.

Parikh SB, Janson C, Singleton T. Video journaling as a method of reflective practice. Couns Educ Superv. 2012;51:33–49.

Ridley CR, Lingle DW. Cultural empathy in multicultural counseling. In: Pedersen PB, Draguns JG, Lonner WJ, Trimble JE, editors. Counseling across cultures. 4th ed. Thousand Oaks, CA: Sage; 1996. p. 21–46.

Ridley CR, Mollen D. Training in counseling psychology: an introduction to the major contribution. Couns Psychol. 2011;39:793–9.

Ridley CR, Mollen D, Kelly SM. Beyond microskills: toward a model of counseling competence. Couns Psychol. 2011;39:825–64.

Shugar A. Teaching genetic counseling skills: incorporating a genetic counseling adaptation continuum model to address psychosocial complexity. J Genet Couns. 2017;26:215–23.

Silverman E. Ongoing self-reflection. Am J Speech Lang Pathol. 2008;17:92.

Smith KA, Sheppard SD, Johnson DW, Johnson RT. Pedagogies of engagement: classroom-based practices. J Eng Educ. 2013;94:87–101.

Veilleux JC, January AM, Vanderveen JW, Felice Reddy L, Klonoff EA. Differentiating amongst characteristics associated with problems of professional competence: perceptions of graduate student peers. Train. Educ. Prof. Psychol. 2012;6:113–21.

Wells DM, Veach PM, Martyr MA, LeRoy BS. Development, experience, and expression of meaning in genetic counselors' lives: an exploratory analysis. J Genet Couns. 2016;25:799–817.

Zahm KW, Veach PM, Martyr MA, LeRoy BS. From novice to seasoned practitioner: a qualitative investigation of genetic counselor professional development. J Genet Couns. 2016;25:818–34.

Chapter 2
Overview of Genetic Counseling: History of the Profession and the Reciprocal-Engagement Model of Practice

Learning Objectives

1. Appreciate major aspects of the history of the genetic counseling profession.
2. Recognize the tenets, goals, and values comprising the Reciprocal-Engagement Model (REM) of practice for genetic counselors.
3. Describe some genetic counseling strategies and behaviors for meeting REM goals.

2.1 History of Genetic Counseling

Genetic counseling as a recognized, independent medical profession remains relatively young. Nevertheless, people have used genetic information for quite a long time throughout history to make medical and reproductive decisions. For instance, the Talmud advises against circumcising brothers of bleeders, and in most cultures throughout history, incest is forbidden. Historically, people made associations by observing patterns of disease in families, even though they did not understand why these diseases happened (Walker 2009; Weil 2000). Although there were, and still are, many nonscientific beliefs about the causes of disease, information from such observations was sometimes used to prevent the same problems in future children.

During the turn of the twentieth century to the mid-1900s, genetic counseling became the purview of public health and took on the mission of social reform. Heredity was credited as the cause of not only medical conditions but also of many social problems such as poverty, crime, and mental illness. The field of eugenics had dawned, and it was quite a public social movement (Sorenson 1993). In an early publication, Sorenson (1976) describes this movement as a mission: "It was Arcadian to the extent that many within the movement looked to the past as an ideal and they were attempting to reconstruct an assumed lost purity of the American race, or to recapture the simplicity of an earlier form of social existence.

P. McCarthy Veach et al., *Facilitating the Genetic Counseling Process*,
https://doi.org/10.1007/978-3-319-74799-6_2

The movement was also Utopian in that it looked to the future as an opportunity to improve men and society, through selective breeding, immigration, and social planning. In both its Arcadian dreams and Utopian fantasies, it looked to genetics as the method" (p. 474).

The general public as well as psychologists, medical professionals, and politicians were eager to use this new science of genetics to improve the human race, believing this goal would benefit everyone. In the early 1900s, many states in the USA had laws mandating the sterilization of the mentally defective. Informed consent was not involved, and over 60,000 people were sterilized involuntarily (Stern 2009). "Inferior" ethnic groups were not allowed to immigrate, and by the 1930s these ideas were well accepted not only in the USA but also in many other countries as well. In Germany, these ideas became the horrible excuse for killing many people considered to be inferior. This part of the history of genetics in medicine and public health is important to remember because it may still color the public perception of the profession of genetic counseling. Although less so today, many people may be reluctant to seek genetic counseling, fearing they will be told not to have a child because of their "bad" family history.

Additionally, the potential for genetic discrimination often remains a perceived risk, affecting patient decisions about testing and genetic counseling. Maio et al. (2013) studied awareness and perceptions of the Canadian public about genetic counseling and among other results, found that, "a sizable proportion of participants also felt that a purpose of genetic counseling was to prevent inheritable disease and abnormalities, advising couples regarding whether to have children, and helping couples [have] children with desirable characteristics" (p. 768). Riesgraf et al. (2015) studied the public's perceptions and attitudes about genetic counseling in a rural midwestern area and found that "Respondents generally seemed to understand how genetic counseling is performed and delivered. For example, a majority agreed genetic counseling is confidential and genetic counselors provide emotional support and receive special training…A majority also agreed seeing a genetic counselor would not lead to loss of insurance or a job, and genetic counseling would not be used to help expecting parents choose the gender or eye color of a future child. These findings differ from previous studies on genetic testing which showed genetic discrimination and eugenics were substantial concerns among members of the general public in Finland and the UK…While these data may reflect a difference between the perceptions of genetic counseling versus genetic testing, they may also reflect a changing climate in the years since the earlier research was conducted or cultural differences" (p. 575).

In 1947, Dr. Sheldon C. Reed coined the term *genetic counseling*. He delineated the three requirements of genetic counseling: (1) knowledge of human genetics; (2) respect for sensitivities, attitudes, and reactions of clients; and (3) teach and provide genetic information to the full extent known (Reed 1955). This era of genetics marks a significant turn where the scientific community took ownership of the practice of genetic counseling and adopted the belief that individuals should make decisions for themselves about their genetic risk. In commenting about the Preface of the first edition of the very first book published on the practice of genetic counseling, *Counseling in Medical Genetics*, Reed (1980) writes, "The first edition was written as an introduction for physicians to the new subject of counseling in medical genetics. It was my hope that it would have a wide distribution, and it did. Thousands of physicians enjoyed the comic bits in it, hopefully some learned a little genetics, and all were introduced to genetic counseling" (Preface).

In 1975, the American Society of Human Genetics (ASHG) published a definition of genetic counseling (ASHG 1975). The most important aspects of the definition include the acknowledgment that genetic counseling is a communication process and patient autonomy is the guiding principle of that process. In the third edition of his book, Reed acknowledges the formal definition of genetic counseling from the ASHG but defines it for himself as "a kind of social work which is often medical but not always so" (Reed 1980, p. 9). These definitions form the framework for contemporary genetic counseling practice. The underlying principles and values are important in that they distance the field from eugenics and, at the same time, strive to empower the patient. Patient autonomy is valued over any other factor.

Over time, although the definition of genetic counseling has evolved, patient autonomy and patient empowerment remain central. In 2006, the National Society of Genetic Counselors assembled a task force to update the definition and adopted the following, which remains the definition today:

> "Genetic counseling is the process of helping people understand and adapt to the medical, psychological and familial implications of genetic contributions to disease. This process integrates the following:
>
> - Interpretation of family and medical histories to assess the chance of disease occurrence or recurrence
> - Education about inheritance, testing, management, prevention, resources and research
> - Counseling to promote informed choices and adaptation to the risk or condition" (Resta et al. 2006, p. 77).

In 1980 Dr. Seymour Kessler described the major change in emphasis in genetic counseling as a *paradigm shift*. He was talking about a shift that originally emphasized a eugenics framework, to a preventive medicine framework, and then to a psychosocial medicine approach that emphasized patient self-determination and the genetic counselor's role as a patient advocate, grief counselor, researcher, and health-care professional providing supportive care, education, resources, and referrals (Kessler 1980). This shift positioned the practice of genetic counseling to be a unique, multifaceted health-care service.

As heredity clinics sprang up at major medical centers in the USA, genetics was well on its way to becoming an established medical service. In the third edition of his book, Reed (1980) also talks about a potential demand for genetic counseling that will exceed the supply of genetic counselors. He was referring mostly to physicians and Ph.D. geneticists at that time. The practice of genetic counseling as it exists today was just beginning to develop, but his prediction proved to be right on target.

In 1969, at Sarah Lawrence College in New York, the first graduate program designed to educate health-care professionals specifically to provide the service of genetic counseling enrolled its first class of students. The curriculum evolved over the first few years to incorporate the study of the psychosocial dimensions of genetic counseling with the medical aspects of genetic disease (Marks 1993). The profession was destined to be a hybrid, drawing skills from both the medical and the counseling professions. This graduate program, and others that soon followed, educates students to be unique health-care professionals who help their patients cope with both the medical and the psychosocial aspects of genetic risk and disease. Genetic counselors saw their responsibilities as not only involving the provision of genetic risk information but also working with families to help them understand their condition and their options for dealing with the condition, facilitating decision-making, and providing psychosocial supportive services (Eunpu 1997).

In 2017, there were more than 4000 practicing genetic counselors in North America, with growth in the profession evidenced by the addition of about 350 new professionals each year. Moreover, there were 41 graduate genetic counseling programs established in North America and several others in the planning stages. International growth in the genetic counseling profession was also evident, with long-standing programs in the UK, Australia, and South Africa and more recent programs in Armenia, Cuba, France, Italy, Israel, Japan, Korea, the Netherlands, Norway, the Philippines, Portugal, Saudi Arabia, Spain, and Taiwan (TAGC 2017).

According to The National Society of Genetic Counselors (NSGC 2017), the scope of practice for genetic counselors includes the following:

> **"Genetic Counselor Scope of Practice:**
>
> a) obtain and evaluate individual, family, and medical histories to determine genetic risk for genetic/medical conditions and diseases in a patient, his/her offspring, and other family members;
> b) discuss the features, natural history, means of diagnosis, genetic and environmental factors, and management of risk for genetic/medical conditions and diseases;
> c) identify and coordinate genetic laboratory tests and other diagnostic studies as appropriate for the genetic assessment;
> d) integrate genetic laboratory test results and other diagnostic studies with personal and family medical history to assess and communicate risk factors for genetic/medical conditions and diseases;
> e) explain the clinical implications of genetic laboratory tests and other diagnostic studies and their results;
> f) evaluate the client's or family's responses to the condition or risk of recurrence and provide client-centered counseling and anticipatory guidance;
> g) identify and utilize community resources that provide medical, educational, financial, and psychosocial support and advocacy; and
> h) provide written documentation of medical, genetic, and counseling information for families and health care professionals" (n.d.).

Today's genetic counselors help thousands of patients each year either through direct care or indirectly through their work in education, research, and commercial arenas. They work in a wide variety of settings and possess a multiplicity of skills from basic science to counseling, teaching, research, management, education, and more. Genetic counselors have taken, and will continue to take, the profession in new and different directions. Nevertheless, the patient/genetic counselor relationship is central, and strong communication and counseling skills will always serve as the basic framework for genetic counseling.

2.2 The Reciprocal-Engagement Model of Genetic Counseling Practice

> "Genetic counseling is directly concerned with human behavior. Thus it must be based on a knowledgeable understanding of psychodynamics and of the principles of interpersonal functioning. Also needed is an understanding of the psychological meanings of the issues with which genetic counseling is involved, namely the issues of health-illness, procreation, parenthood, as well as the complex processes by which the goals of genetic counseling are achieved" (Kessler 1979, p. 21).

Although written in 1979, Kessler's appraisal of the factors that are critical to genetic counseling hold true today. As the profession has progressed and practice has matured, it became clear that genetic counseling is a specific practice with a definite and unique guiding model that is not best defined by borrowing aspects from other professions. Defining the model of practice for genetic counseling was a goal that many have grappled with for quite some time.

2.2.1 What Are the Components of a Model of Practice?

A model of practice is *not* the same thing as a scope of practice (which defines what activities are involved in a service) nor is it a model of service delivery (which describes how a population accesses services). A model of practice defines the tenets, goals, strategies, and behaviors that guide the practice (McCarthy Veach et al. 2007). It embodies the underlying values of the practice, and it clarifies "the complex processes by which the goals of genetic counseling are achieved" (Kessler 1979, p. 21). A model of practice directly addresses these questions: "(a) What is the theoretical framework for the practice? (b) What are the goals of practice? (c) How do we know when we have met those goals? (d) How do we evaluate the service? (e) How do we improve services? and (f) How do we teach the practice?" (McCarthy Veach et al. 2007, p. 714). A model of practice is critical in that it provides the framework for teaching the skills necessary for practice, and a model is the basis for generating the methods used to evaluate the service. Without a model, it is difficult to teach others how to practice, and it is impossible to measure the impact of the service and improve the practice.

In 2005, McCarthy Veach et al. convened a consensus conference bringing together leaders in the profession and educators representing most genetic counseling graduate programs in North America with the goal of defining the elements of the genetic counseling model of practice. Educators and leaders in the profession were able to describe five primary genetic counseling tenets. In addition, some foremost goals, strategies, and behaviors that comprise genetic counseling practice were identified. From this consensus process, the Reciprocal-Engagement Model (REM) of genetic counseling practice was generated.

The five tenets of genetic counseling practice include (McCarthy Veach et al. 2007):

- *Genetic information is key*: This is the first tenet because it recognizes the primary reason patients seek or are referred for genetic counseling. This tenet reflects the conviction that information is critical to understanding and coping with a condition and for informed decision-making. It assumes that "being informed is better than being uninformed" (p. 719).
- *Relationship is integral to genetic counseling*: This tenet refers to the critical nature of the patient/genetic counselor relationship and the role this relationship plays in furthering the patient's ability to understand genetic information and use that information to her or his benefit. This relationship is central to genetic counseling.
- *Patient autonomy must be supported*: This tenet reinforces the long-standing value in genetic counseling that patients best understand their situations and are in the best position to make personal decisions about how to use their genetic information. This tenet reflects the belief that patients must be supported in their ability to self-direct.
- *Patients are resilient*: This tenet acknowledges that most people have the capacity to learn and to cope with their situation when provided with the appropriate psychological support and relevant information.
- *Patient emotions make a difference (also referred to as patient emotions matter)*: This tenet recognizes the important role emotions play in the genetic counseling process. Emotions are a critical part of dealing with a genetic condition; they are a significant factor (both positive and negative) in understanding information and making decisions, and they affect relationships and coping ability.

McCarthy Veach et al. (2007) proposed 17 goals for genetic counseling sessions corresponding to the five tenets. These goals, along with examples of genetic counselor strategies and behaviors, are presented in Table 2.1.

The REM is a model that demonstrates how the *patient/genetic counselor relationship* is central to the genetic counseling process. Through this relationship, information is communicated in a way that supports the autonomy of the patient, takes patient emotions into account, and supports the natural resilience of the patient. "The term *reciprocity* reflects that each element of the model is complementary and *completes* the other, while *engagement* refers to counselor and patient mutual participation in genetic counseling. As shown in Fig. 2.1, the model is represented visually with a triangle that embodies the five tenets articulated by conference participants: *Education* primarily represents the tenet of genetic information. *Individual Attributes* reflects the tenets of patient autonomy, resiliency, and emotions. *Relationship* embodies the tenet of counselor patient relationship" (McCarthy Veach et al. 2007, pp. 724–725).

The REM is specific to genetic counseling practice. It is grounded in the underlying values of the profession and was developed by examining the components of practice. As mentioned earlier, the central foundation of the model is the patient/genetic counselor relationship. Through this relationship, information critical to the

Table 2.1 Reciprocal-Engagement Model (REM) of genetic counseling practice—preliminary strategies and behaviors corresponding to REM tenets and goals

Goal[a]	Strategy[a]	Behavior[a]	Additional strategies[b]
Tenet: Genetic information is key[a]			
Patient is informed	Assess patient educational level Assess patient decision-making style	Open and closed questions to gather history and to determine what patient understands Open and closed questions	Information giving Use psychosocial counseling skills/strategies Establish working alliance
Counselor knows what information to impart	Assess medical literacy Listen for inaccuracy	Ask questions Open and closed questions to determine patient understanding; repeat or rephrase information	Information giving Use psychosocial counseling skills/strategies Assessment
Counselor presents genetic information	Two-way communication Use visual aids	Explain materials; use language patient can understand	Information giving Assessment Use psychosocial counseling skills/strategies
Patient gains new perspectives	Assess patient understanding	Open and closed questions to learn what the information means to the patient	Assessment Use psychosocial counseling skills/strategies Information giving
Tenet: Relationship is integral to genetic counseling[a]			
Counselor and patient establish a bond	Active listening	Sit quietly; reflect patient thoughts and feelings; summarize patient statements; rephrase; use similar body language	Establish working alliance Use psychosocial counseling skills/strategies Information giving
Good counselor-patient communication	–	–	Information giving Use psychosocial counseling skills/strategies Establish working alliance
Counselor characteristics positively influence process	Behave ethically Recognize impact on session Maintain objectivity Maintain boundaries Self-care Peer supervision	Self-disclose; request feedback; provide feedback	Use psychosocial counseling skills/strategies Information giving Establish working alliance Practice self-awareness Provide pre-and post-GC session care

(continued)

Table 2.1 (continued)

Goal[a]	Strategy[a]	Behavior[a]	Additional strategies[b]
Tenet: Patient autonomy must be supported[a]			
Establish working contract	Assess patient expectations Provide informed consent Establish realistic agenda	Ask questions Describe process State goals	Establish GC goals and expectations Information giving Establish working alliance
Integrate familial and cultural context into counseling relationship and decisions	Recognize multiple strategies Maintain counseling flexibility	–	Use psychosocial counseling skills/strategies Information giving Establish working alliance
Patient feels empowered and more in control	Discuss what patient wants to discuss Create safe environment Respect patient decision/viewpoint Enable informed decisions	–	Information giving Use psychosocial counseling skills/strategies Provide care before and after GC session Establish working alliance
Facilitate collaborate decisions	Ask about options	Reflect patient thoughts and feelings re: options	Use psychosocial counseling skills/strategies Assessment Information giving
Tenet: Patients are resilient[a]			
Recognize patient strengths	Identify patient strengths Make connections Anticipatory guidance Instill hope	Ask questions about patient coping skills	Assessment Use psychosocial skills/strategies Information giving
Adaptation	Assimilation Accommodation	–	Information giving Assessment Use psychosocial counseling skills/strategies
Empowerment	Create safe environment Maintain/enhance patient self-esteem Identify possible outcomes	–	Information giving Use psychosocial counseling skills/strategies Provide care before and after GC session Establish working alliance
Tenet: Patient emotions make a difference[a]			
Counselor and patient know patient concerns	Recognize ethical dilemmas in patient's life Anticipate patient needs	–	Use psychosocial skills/strategies Information giving Assessment

Table 2.1 (continued)

Goal[a]	Strategy[a]	Behavior[a]	Additional strategies[b]
Patient family dynamics are understood by counselor and patient	–	–	Use psychosocial counseling skills/strategies Information giving Assessment
Patient self-esteem is maintained or increased	Define patient support network Identify resources Convey empathy	–	Use psychosocial counseling skills/strategies Provide resources Empower patient

GC genetic counseling

[a]REM tenets, goals, preliminary strategies and behaviors from McCarthy Veach et al. (2007, pp. 720–721)

[b]Most prevalent strategy domain for each REM goal from research by Redlinger-Grosse et al. (2017, pp. 1378–1379)

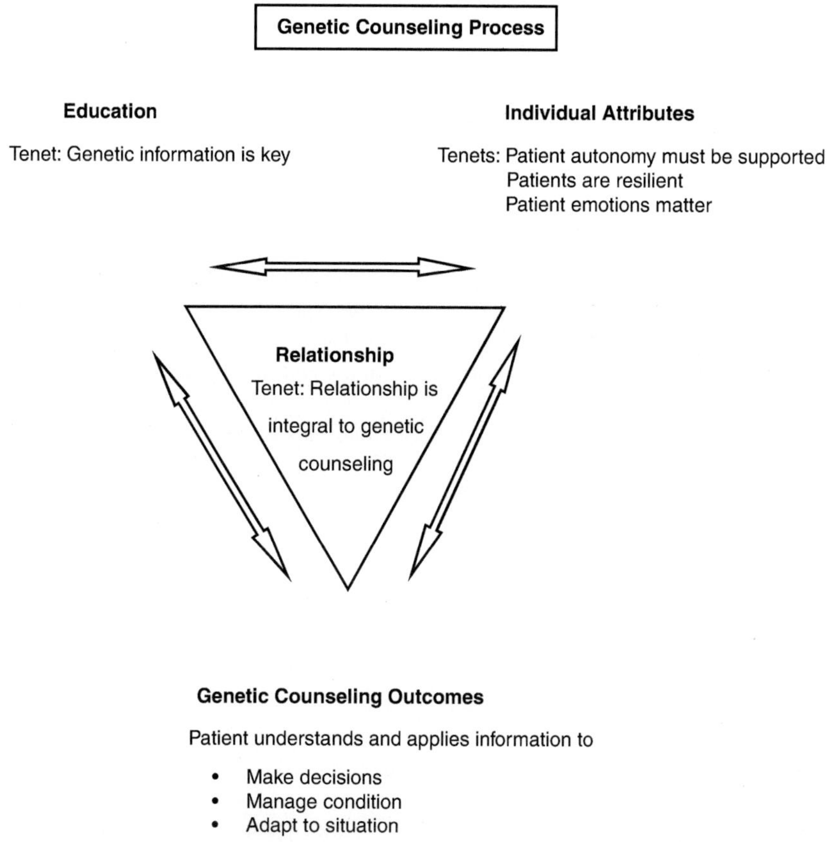

Fig. 2.1 Reciprocal-Engagement Model (REM) of genetic counseling practice. *Note*. Each element interacts with every other element. None stand alone or work isolation. Reprinted with permission of the Journal of Genetic Counseling

patient's situation is conveyed, patient autonomy is supported, patient emotions are addressed, and the patient is better able to cope. The process of genetic counseling is channeled through this relationship. The REM clarifies that basic helping skills described in this book are the tools necessary to forming this critical relationship, without which genetic counseling goals cannot be achieved.

2.2.2 Research on the REM Goals and Outcomes

Hartmann et al. (2015) surveyed practicing genetic counselors and asked them to rate each of the 17 REM goals in terms of their importance to their practice and how often they were able to achieve the goal. All 17 REM goals were rated on average as somewhat to very important. The analysis identified four factors that accounted for variance in importance ratings. The authors noted that the five REM tenets could apply to more than one factor. The 17 REM goals with corresponding factors are shown in Table 2.2. The four factors are as follows:

- *Understanding and Appreciation*: This factor includes six goals emphasizing counselor and patient awareness of how patients' situations and characteristics may influence their decision-making or feelings about a diagnosis or risk. Many of the goals in this factor correspond to REM tenets *Patients are resilient* and *Patient emotions make a difference*.
- *Support and Guidance*: This factor includes six goals emphasizing development of a supportive genetic counselor/patient relationship. The goals imply that the counselor works with patients in ways that allow patients to feel involved, autonomous, and efficacious. These goals correspond to REM tenets *Patient autonomy must be supported*, *Patients are resilient*, and *Relationship is integral to genetic counseling*.
- *Facilitative Decision-Making*: This factor includes three goals with some of the highest importance ratings. These goals focus on informed, collaborative decisions, and they correspond to REM tenets *Patient autonomy must be supported* and *Information is key*.
- *Patient-Centered Education*: This factor includes two goals involving counselor presentation of genetic information in a way that patients can understand and having good communication. These goals correspond to REM tenets *Genetic information is key* and *Relationship is integral to genetic counseling*.

Building on the work of Hartmann et al. (2015), other researchers (Redlinger-Grosse et al. 2016) have explored the relationships between REM goals and measurable genetic counseling outcomes. Starting with a REM goal, it is possible to identify the desired outcome, which in turn can be measured. For example, for the REM goal "patient is informed," which falls within Factor 3 (facilitative decision-making), Redlinger-Grosse et al. (2016) identified six possible measurable outcomes: (1) change in communication regarding genetic information within the patient's family; (2) change in patient's ability to ask appropriate questions regarding

Table 2.2 Reciprocal-Engagement Model (REM) goals and corresponding factors

REM goal	Factor
The counselor knows what information to impart to each patient	Facilitative decision-making
Counselor presents genetic information in a way that the patient can understand	Patient-centered education
Counselor helps the patient to feel informed	Facilitative decision-making
Counselor helps the patient to gain new perspectives	Support and guidance
Counselor and patient establish a bond	Support and guidance
Good counselor-patient communication occurs	Patient-centered education
Counselor's characteristics positively influence the process of relationship-building and communication between counselor and patient	Support and guidance
Counselor establishes a working contract with a patient	Understanding and appreciation
Counselor integrates the patient's familial and cultural context into the counseling relationship and decision-making	Understanding and appreciation
Counselor helps the patient to feel in control	Support and guidance
Counselor facilitates collaborative decisions with the patient	Facilitative decision-making
Counselor recognizes patient strengths	Support and guidance
Counselor helps patient to adapt to his or her situation	Support and guidance
Counselor facilitates the patient's feelings of empowerment	Understanding and appreciation
Counselor works with patient to recognize concerns that are triggering the patient's emotions	Understanding and appreciation
Counselor and patient reach an understanding of patient's family dynamics and their effects on the patient's situation	Understanding and appreciation
Counselor promotes maintenance of or increase in patient self-esteem	Understanding and appreciation

Adapted from Hartmann et al. (2015)

their medical care; (3) change in patient's ability to engage in the genetic counseling process; (4) change in patient's genetic knowledge; (5) patient is empowered; and (6) patient receives short-term counseling. These studies demonstrate the dynamic interaction of the tenets and goals of the model and their relationship to desired outcomes and, thus, reflect the complex nature of genetic counseling.

2.3 Carl Rogers' Person-Centered Counseling

Prior to the development of the REM, the profession looked to Carl Rogers' theory of Person-Centered Counseling as the basis for the genetic counseling approach to patient care. A closer look at Rogers' Person-Centered Counseling provides some context for two of the basic tenets of the REM—Patient autonomy must be supported and Patients are resilient—that serve as underlying values of the profession. The basic philosophy fundamental to Rogers' theory involves a positive view of humans and a trust in the self for greater inner directedness. Rogers believed that people possess the capacity to become self-aware, to self-direct, and to actualize into whole, fully functioning individuals (Rogers 1992). The aim of therapy in Rogers' view is to help clients in their personal growth process so they are better able to cope with the difficulties they are facing now as well as those that occur in the future (Corey 1996).

Rogers' basic assumptions about human nature and psychosocial development have been described as follows (Hjelle and Ziegler 1984):

- People are inherently free to *self-actualize*. They are able to overcome conditions of worth (other's expectations) to make the choices that help them develop into the persons that they become.
- People are basically rational beings—planful, thoughtful, etc. Irrational behaviors stem from being out of touch with one's true inner nature.
- The human self is global, all-inclusive, and whole, not compartmentalized. Therefore, one must try to understand a person in her or his entirety.
- People have the innate potential to self-actualize, but this potential can be compromised by environmental events. Nevertheless, individuals can rise above such events.
- A person's essence is her or his self-concept or self-perception. The private world of experience shapes the self-concept.
- The actualizing tendency is purposeful and oriented toward the future. People grow from, rather than react to, external experience.
- The actualizing tendency moves an individual toward growth, self-realization, and personality enhancement.
- The actualizing tendency itself leads to constant growth and unfolding potential.
- No one can fully understand another's private world.

These assumptions form the foundation of Person-Centered Counseling. For instance, Rogers theorized that the attitudes of the counselor and the quality of the counselor-client relationship determine the outcome of the counseling process. It is important to note that the major focus is on the counselor's way of thinking. Rogers believed that when the counselor is able to convey key elements, a positive outcome would follow. He described three key counselor attitudes that he referred to as *facilitative conditions*:

- *Unconditional positive regard*: a positive view of clients, the belief that clients are coping to the best of their ability, a total respect for who they are as individuals, acceptance of client strengths and weaknesses, a belief that clients have the capacity for self-direction, and a focus on the present moment and experience.
- *Empathy*: strives to understand the client's reality, to get into the world of the client, and to see things from the client's perspective.

- *Counselor genuineness*: the counselor establishes an open relationship with the client, is open to his or her own emotional reactions to the client, and establishes a safe setting where clients are free to self-actualize.

Upon examination of Rogers' theory, one can see how the basic foundations of this approach are a good fit with the REM of genetic counseling practice. Both Person-Centered Counseling and the REM empower the patient, value the patient's belief system, and strive to understand the patient's experiences.

2.4 Person-Oriented Versus Content-Oriented Genetic Counseling

We only need to look at the work of Seymour Kessler to better understand two other tenets of the REM: Relationship is integral to genetic counseling and Patient emotions make a difference. No one individual has examined the complex psychological dimensions of genetic counseling in more detail than has Kessler. His work in this area reaches back to the time when genetic counseling was first establishing itself as a health-care service in major medical settings. Kessler was tireless in his efforts to examine the psychological issues associated with the provision of this service and to teach genetic counselors about the skills they need to enhance their practice as the profession has advanced over the years.

In 1979, Kessler discusses the emergence of a more psychologically or person-oriented genetic counseling in contrast to the previous content-oriented genetic counseling. He states that the person orientation "...starts with the premise that genetic counseling deals with human behaviors, important ones at that; health and illness, procreation, parenthood, and sometimes life and death. It views the problems posed by a genetic disorder as being intimately related to the overall situation of the persons, their ways of solving problems, making decisions and adapting to life crises. Whereas the content oriented approach emphasizes facts, the person oriented approach places the focus on the various meanings that facts have for the counselees as well as on the intrapsychic and interpersonal consequences of these meanings" [p. 19].

In the *content orientation*:

- The counselor believes that objective facts and figures are the basis on which decisions are made and actions proceed.
- The counselor gives high priority to providing information.
- The counselor functions as authority, educator, and advisor.
- The approach fosters emotional distancing on the part of the counselor.

In the *person orientation*:

- The counselor believes decisions and actions are based on the subjective understanding and varied meanings of the facts and figures.

- The counselor helps patients understand and integrate their experiences.
- The counselor functions as facilitator, guide, and model.
- The approach fosters counselor involvement with the patient's emotional issues.

2.5 The Teaching Versus Counseling Approach to Genetic Counseling

Kessler (1997) later describes two basic approaches to genetic counseling: teaching and counseling. Although he names these models, they are, in fact, approaches to genetic counseling patient care. These approaches dovetail well with the descriptions of the two basic orientations of the genetic counselor (content orientation and person orientation) that Kessler described 18 years earlier.

2.5.1 The Teaching Model of Genetic Counseling

- The major outcome goal is educated patients.
- A premise is that patients come to genetic counseling for information.
- An assumption is that informed patients are able to make autonomous decisions.
- Cognitive and rational processes form the foundation of the approach; psychological aspects are minimized.
- The counseling process involves providing all-inclusive, accurate information in an impartial manner; the counselor does not become involved.
- Teaching is the only means to meet the end goal: an educated patient.
- The counselor-patient relationship is based on counselor authority.

2.5.2 The Counseling Model of Genetic Counseling

- The major outcome goals are to understand the patient, advance the patient's sense of self-competence, help the patient gain a sense of control, alleviate some psychological stress, provide support, and help the patient with problem solving.
- A premise is that patients come to genetic counseling for complicated reasons such as needing information, wishing for validation, wanting support, and looking for a way to reduce their anxiety.
- Human behavior and psychological aspects of genetic counseling are complex.
- The counseling process is multifaceted, involving the psychological assessment of patient strengths, limitations, needs, values, and decision-making styles; a range of counseling skills are needed for a positive outcome; counseling must be specific to the patient and flexible; and the counselor must attend to his or her inner self.
- Education is only one means that is used to meet the end goals described above.
- The counselor-patient relationship is mutual.

In comparing the models, Kessler (1997) states, "The net psychological impact of this strategy [the teaching model] is to enrich the authority, status, and ego of the professional at the expense of the client. The purpose of any counseling strategy is to reverse this process and leave the client psychologically enriched even if it is at the expense of the professional" (p. 291). Maturation into the profession requires students to grow away from being the content-oriented counselor utilizing the teaching model into the psychologically oriented counselor who makes use of the counseling model. "Counselors strive to perfect their ability to understand clients, give them a sense of being understood, and help them feel more hopeful, more valued, and more capable of dealing with their life problems. Because genetic counselors work with people filled with uncertainty, fear of the future, anguish, and a sense of personal failure, they have unusual opportunities to accomplish these tasks" (Kessler 1999, p. 341).

2.6 Closing Comments

Genetic counseling is a unique medically based health-care practice. Genetic counselors help patients and their families navigate a wide variety of situations. In one session, a patient is told her baby has a disorder that will limit his or her ability to experience life fully, and in another session, parents are given a long-awaited diagnosis for their child that helps them finally understand what happened. In still another session, a young woman is relieved to learn she has not inherited a gene that would have increased her risk for cancer, and therefore her children are free of that increased risk as well. Regardless of a patient's circumstances, the process of genetic counseling is dynamic and complex. The REM provides a theoretical framework and defines the tenets of genetic counseling that apply to all areas of clinical practice. The empirically derived REM goals are identifiable and measurable. Understanding the model allows us to teach, assess, and improve practice over time. When we look at the history of genetic counseling, clearly, the core underlying values have remained constant and are evident in the five tenets of the Reciprocal-Engagement Model of genetic counseling practice.

2.7 Class Activity

Activity: Identifying Goals, Strategies, and Behaviors in Genetic Counseling (Dyads)

Students select a partner. They can either select one of their own cases or use one of the following situations:

- Case #1: A 40-year-old woman who is 16 weeks into her first pregnancy comes to clinic in follow up to an abnormal ultrasound. She had the ultrasound because her doctor thought the baby was small for gestational age. Her doctor suspects a chromosomal anomaly.

- Case #2: A couple brings their 2-year-old son to clinic. He is delayed in many of his milestones, and he is small and has some dysmorphic features. The geneticist suspects a syndrome and has ordered genetic testing.
- Case #3: A 49-year-old man comes to clinic in response to a referral from his primary care doctor. His father, paternal grandmother, and now recently a brother have all had pancreatic cancer. His father and grandmother died of the disease at about 45 years of age. His brother was just diagnosed at 42.

Students are asked to describe five goals for their session. The goals can either be those identified in the REM (see Table 2.1), or they can be other goals identified by the students. For each goal, they should identify one strategy and corresponding behavior that would support that goal. Lastly, students are asked to describe at least one desirable and measurable outcome for the session.

Example
For Case #1, one possible goal, strategy, behavior, and outcome could look like the following:

Goal	Patient understands the meaning of the ultrasound finding
Strategy	Assess patient knowledge of situation
Behavior	Ask patient to relate what she was told by her doctor
Outcome	Patient asked relevant questions about management options

Estimated time: 20–30 min.

Process
Students share their responses with the class, and the class provides feedback to each dyad.
Estimated time: 30 min.

Instructor Note
- An additional activity would be to ask students to seek out measures that would indicate the goals have been met. Some examples include measures of patient satisfaction, quality of life, decisional regret, etc.
- Another activity would be to have each dyad role-play the situation for 15 min while the class identifies the goals, strategies, and behaviors demonstrated in the role-play.

References

American Society of Human Genetics. Genetic counseling. Am J Hum Genet. 1975;27:240–2.
Corey G. Theory and practice of counseling and psychotherapy. 5th ed. Pacific Grove, CA: Brooks/Cole; 1996.
Eunpu DL. Systemically based psychotherapeutic techniques in genetic counseling. J Genet Couns. 1997;6:1–20.

Hartmann JE, McCarthy Veach P, MacFarlane IM, LeRoy BS. Genetic counselor perceptions of genetic counseling session goals: a validation study of the Reciprocal-Engagement Model. J Genet Couns. 2015;24:225–37.
Hjelle DJ, Ziegler LA. Personality theories. 2nd ed. New York: McGraw-Hill; 1984.
Kessler S. Genetic counseling: psychological dimensions. New York: Academic Press; 1979.
Kessler S. The psychological paradigm shift in genetic counseling. Soc Biol. 1980;27:167–85.
Kessler S. Psychological aspects of genetic counseling: IX. Teaching and counseling. J Genet Couns. 1997;6:287–95.
Kessler S. Psychological aspects of genetic counseling: XIII. Empathy and decency. J Genet Couns. 1999;8:333–44.
Maio M, Carrion P, Yaremco E, Austin JC. Awareness of genetic counseling and perceptions of its purpose: a survey of the Canadian public. J Genet Couns. 2013;22:762–70.
Marks JH. The training of genetic counselors: origins of a psychosocial model. In: Bartels DM, LeRoy BS, Caplan A, editors. Prescribing our future: ethical challenges in genetic counseling. New York: Aldine de Gruyter; 1993. p. 15–24.
McCarthy Veach P, Bartels DM, LeRoy BS. Coming full circle: a Reciprocal-Engagement Model of genetic counseling practice. J Genet Couns. 2007;16:713–28.
National Society of Genetic Counselors Web. Scope of practice. https://www.nsgc.org/p/cm/ld/fid=18#scope. Accessed Nov 2017.
Redlinger-Grosse K, Veach PM, Cohen S, LeRoy BS, MacFarlane IM, Zierhut H. Defining our clinical practice: the identification of genetic counseling outcomes utilizing the Reciprocal Engagement Model. J Genet Couns. 2016;25:239–57.
Redlinger-Grosse K, Veach PM, LeRoy BS, Zierhut H. Elaboration of the Reciprocal-Engagement Model of genetic counseling practice: a qualitative investigation of goals and strategies. J Genet Couns. 2017;26:1372–87.
Reed SC. Counseling in medical genetics. Philadelphia, PA: WB Sanders; 1955.
Reed SC. Counseling in medical genetics. 3rd ed. New York: Alan R. Liss; 1980.
Resta R, Biesecker BB, Bennett RL, Blum S, Hahn SE, Strecker MN, et al. A new definition of genetic counseling: National Society of Genetic Counselors' task force report. J Genet Couns. 2006;15:77–83.
Riesgraf RJ, McCarthy Veach P, MacFarlane IM, LeRoy BS. Perceptions and attitudes about genetic counseling among residents of a midwestern rural area. J Genet Couns. 2015;24:565–79.
Rogers CR. The necessary and sufficient conditions of therapeutic personality change. J Consult Clin Psychol. 1992;60:827–32.
Sorenson JR. From social movements to clinical medicine: the role of law and the medical profession in regulating applied human genetics. In: Mulinsky A, editor. Genetics and the law. New York: Plenum Press; 1976. p. 467–85.
Sorenson JR. Genetic counseling: values that have mattered. In: Bartels DM, BS LR, Caplan A, editors. Prescribing our future: ethical challenges in genetic counseling. New York: Aldine de Gruyter; 1993. p. 3–14.
Stern AM. A quiet revolution: the birth of the genetic counselor at Sarah Lawrence College, 1969. J Genet Couns. 2009;18:1–11.
Transnational Alliance for Genetic Counseling (TAGC). Education programs. http://tagc.med.sc.edu/education.asp. Accessed 29 Nov 2017.
Walker AP. The practice of genetic counseling. In: Uhlmann WR, Schuette JL, Yashar B, editors. A guide to genetic counseling. 2nd ed. New York: Wiley; 2009. p. 1–36.
Weil J. Psychosocial genetic counseling. New York: Oxford University Press; 2000.

Chapter 3
Listening to Patients: Attending Skills

Learning Objectives
1. Define attending skills and describe their functions in genetic counseling.
2. Distinguish between physical and psychological attending.
3. Recognize some ways in which attending skills are tailored to individual and cultural patient characteristics, practice specialties, and service delivery modalities.
4. Develop attending skills through self-reflection, practice, and feedback.

3.1 Definition of Attending Skills

Attending skills consist of the genetic counselor's observations of patient verbal and nonverbal behaviors as one way to understand what patients are experiencing and displaying effective nonverbal behaviors to patients during genetic counseling sessions. These two broad domains of attending skills are known, respectively, as "psychological attending" and "physical attending" (Egan 1994).

3.1.1 Psychological Attending

Psychological attending is an important skill set for recognizing genetic counseling patients' unspoken feelings, intentions, and experiences. Psychological attending occurs when you sense experiences, to the extent possible, through the patient's eyes rather than through your own. You intuit emotions, attitudes, and intentions patients have or might have had by being *in tune* with their verbal and nonverbal communications. Patients' nonverbal behaviors may be particularly informative, as many individuals, for example, will not directly state what they are feeling and thinking. Thus, psychological attending relies heavily upon noticing and interpreting messages from patients' nonverbal behaviors.

P. McCarthy Veach et al., *Facilitating the Genetic Counseling Process*,
https://doi.org/10.1007/978-3-319-74799-6_3

A number of authors note that nonverbal behaviors serve important interpersonal functions which include demonstrating how individuals feel, as well as providing clues about their internal physiological state and their intentions (Patterson 2003; Philippot et al. 2003). Hall et al. (2008) note, "In daily life, we are constantly processing and evaluating cues that are conveyed by others through the face, body, and voice or embodied in their appearance, and we can do so with surprising accuracy based on fairly small amounts of information…" (p. 238). When psychologically attending to patients, it is important that you attempt to discern the possible reasons for their actions. For example, a patient may smile as you explain she is at high risk for a lethal genetic condition. Clearly, she is not happy about this news. Smiling may be her way of expressing cooperation and politeness.

Psychological attending not only provides a window into another person's inner processes, it also conveys your interest and concern (interpersonal sensitivity) and contributes to genetic counseling outcomes. In health-care settings, research evidence indicates greater physician interpersonal sensitivity is related to higher patient satisfaction (e.g., Mast 2007; Roter et al. 2006).

3.1.2 Physical Attending

Physical attending skills involve nonverbal ways in which you use your body to communicate with patients. They can be more powerful than verbal communication, because nonverbal communication is constant (Egan 1994); much of the meaning of a message may be perceived from nonverbal behaviors. Furthermore, feelings and thoughts have a way of working themselves into our nonverbals (e.g., looking down at notes when you feel discomfort, flipping through your notes or the electronic medical record while the patient is speaking because you disagree with her or his decision, looking at your watch when you are impatient about the pace with which the patient is coming to a decision, etc.).

Roter et al. (2006) assert that in medical visits, "the emotional context of care is especially related to nonverbal communication and that emotion-related communication skills, including sending and receiving nonverbal messages and emotional self-awareness are critical elements of high quality care" (p. S28). They point out that physicians and patients both show emotions, sometimes even when they attempt to hide them, and both parties form judgments about each other's feelings that affect the processes of care. In genetic counseling, for instance, some patients may be fearful or uncertain about what is going to happen. They may also believe you are withholding information or will tell them what to do. They will attempt to *read* your nonverbals for any signs of dishonesty, discomfort, disapproval, or judgment.

Good physical attending can alleviate patient apprehension, build rapport, and facilitate a strong working relationship (e.g., Leach 2005; Philippot et al. 2003). For example, Solomon et al. (2012) interviewed Xhosa-speaking mothers/caregivers of boys with hemophilia in South Africa. Their data collection methods included an interpreter who they described as "…empathetic and friendly and established an easy and good relationship with the participants. She established rapport through positive verbal and nonverbal encouragement. Good eye contact, smiling and open body language ensured that the participant felt comfortable with the process and sufficiently relaxed to 'talk back'" (p. 729). These behaviors are consistent with recommendations in the literature on physical attending behaviors.

3.1.3 Why and How Psychological and Physical Attending Skills Matter

Tickle-Degnen and Gavett (2003) postulate a three-phase model of relationship development: (1) rapport building, (2) development of working alliance, and (3) ongoing working relationship. Three nonverbal components promote relationship processes and outcomes corresponding to these phases, namely, attentiveness, positivity-negativity, and coordination (p. 76): Attentiveness is the degree to which two individuals (e.g., a genetic counselor and patient) focus their attention on each other (through eye contact, body position, etc.). Positivity-negativity is the degree to which they respond in ways that convey cooperation and a "readiness to do no harm" (e.g., smiling, moving closer), versus in ways suggesting dislike or hostility and a "readiness to hurt the other person, at least emotionally" (e.g., frowning, looking angry). Coordination is the extent to which their behaviors mimic each other (e.g., similar arm and leg positions, voice tone). Later in this chapter, we use the terms "synchrony" and "synchronicity" to refer to the coordination nonverbal component.

Applied to genetic counseling, this three-phase model emphasizes the importance of nonverbal behavior throughout the relationship in order to make a connection, establish agreed-upon genetic counseling goals, exchange relevant information, and work toward goal accomplishment. When counseling patients, you should strive to use good physical attending skills, psychologically attend to patients' behaviors and their possible meanings (attentiveness and positivity), and try to be aware of the extent to which your behaviors match those of the patient. Matching of behaviors (coordination) should occur only when *appropriate*, however (e.g., you would want to speak softly with a crying patient but avoid raising your voice when a patient speaks loudly in frustration).

Attentiveness, eye contact, and open posture are important practitioner behaviors for improving trust, communication, and rapport (Leach 2005), and they are positively related to other clinician skills and qualities. Studies of psychotherapy demonstrate that increased therapist eye contact is related to better rapport, respect, empathy, and genuineness (Darrow and Johnson 2009); increased therapist facial expressions of a positive nature (happiness, interest, concern) have been associated with greater rapport (Sharpley et al. 2005); nodding and gesturing resulted in more favorable ratings of therapists (Darrow and Johnson 2009); and good eye contact in combination with forward leaning by the therapist enhanced ratings of empathy, the working alliance, and treatment credibility (Dowell and Berman 2013). Henry et al. (2012) found that greater clinician warmth and listening were related to higher patient satisfaction. Philippot et al. (2003) similarly report that clients who perceive their psychotherapists as in tune with them feel positively about their therapists and the relationship.

Some authors theorize that the positive effects of attending skills are due to "perceived responsiveness" (Dowell and Berman 2013; Lemay et al. 2007; Murray et al. 2006; Reis et al. 2000) or the extent to which an individual believes the other person "understands, values, and supports key aspects of the self" (Dowell and Berman 2013, p. 159). We believe perceived responsiveness is an essential aspect of effective genetic counseling, and therefore *all* genetic counseling practice relies upon a solid base of attending behaviors. Effective psychological and physical attending can convey your involvement and understanding; build rapport; encourage patients to self-disclose; increase patient perceptions that you are expert (competent and professional), socially attractive (warm, likeable), and trustworthy; and build a foundation from which you may understand and assist patients in their decision-making.

Good attending, however, can be difficult to achieve for any number of reasons. A genetic counselor may find it difficult to focus on a patient if she/he is aware of other pressing clinical responsibilities or time constraints. A genetic counselor's pager may be vibrating, the patient may be late for another scheduled appointment or procedure, other health-care team members may interrupt the session, etc. Sometimes, factors inherent to the session, such as the presence of small children and patients who are experiencing physical symptoms (e.g., nausea in a pregnant woman), may make it difficult for both the genetic counselor and the patient to focus their attention. In some cases, student or novice genetic counselors may have difficulty fully attending to a patient if they are anxious about their own performance.

3.2 Effective Genetic Counselor Psychological Attending Skills

Effective psychological attending consists of three major activities: observing and responding to patient nonverbal behaviors, understanding patient body and facial movements, and noticing subtle cues. We suggest the following strategies as general guidelines:

3.2.1 Observing and Responding to Patient Nonverbal Behaviors

- Pay attention to patient nonverbals and think about their possible meaning (e.g., if the patient is gripping the arms of the chair, it may indicate that she/he is anxious).
- Notice incongruences between patient nonverbal and verbal behaviors (e.g., saying "yes" while shaking one's head "no"). In general, you should *go with* the

nonverbal behavior when there are incongruences. Nonverbal behaviors are more spontaneous and less under a person's conscious control, and therefore they may be more indicative of patients' psychological/emotional state than are their verbal behaviors.

- Consider pointing out nonverbals to the patient (e.g., "You say you're fine with this decision, yet you look tearful").
- Comment on nonverbals when a patient is silent (e.g., "You are very quiet right now. I wonder what you're thinking?" [or, depending on the context, "…what you're feeling?"])
- Look for patterns of behavior that *together* suggest the patient is feeling or thinking a certain way. *Beware of over-interpreting a single nonverbal behavior* (e.g., sighing by itself might indicate any number of feelings from impatience, fatigue, regret, and hopelessness. Sighing in combination with eye rolling and crossed arms is a stronger clue that the patient feels frustrated or misunderstood).
- Observe the following patient characteristics as these may give you clues about a patient's traits and/or emotional state, attitudes about genetic counseling, and motivations: activity level (agitated or lethargic), speaking slowly or quickly, manner of dress (sloppy or careful, appropriate to the situation or haphazard), movements (easy or difficult, fluid or staccato), state of health, tension behaviors (swallowing, nervous laughter, excessive throat-clearing), voice (firm or shaky, loud or soft), and patient projection of self (mature and in control or childlike, submissive or aggressive) (Fine and Glasser 1996). Of course, it's important to always consider the extent to which patient behaviors reflect symptoms of a genetic condition. For example, a patient being seen in neurology may be exhibiting symptoms of a neurodegenerative disease.

3.2.2 Understanding Patient Cues

- Attend to the face because it is a very rich source of nonverbal communication (Batty and Taylor 2003). As much as 55% of a person's feeling messages come through the face (Egan 1994). Over 1000 facial expressions have been identified, and many of these expressions appear to have similar meanings to people from all countries and cultures (Ekman and Friesen 2003). Moreover, facial expressions can provide clues about cognitive processes such as attention (based on where a person is gazing) as well as how they are evaluating events that are triggering their emotions (Sander et al. 2007, p. 470).
- Facial muscles can be controlled in all areas but the eyes (Hill 2014), thus revealing more of one's true self. Watch a patient's eyes for signs of fear and anger; frightened or anxious people will have dilated pupils, and angry people will have constricted pupils. Additionally, anger, distress, and fear can be communicated in the temples (the pulse will quicken), in the carotids (blood visibly pulses to the head), in the upper and lower jaw muscles (clench together), and in the nostrils (dilate and constrict).

- Look for leg and foot movements and physiological reactions. Leg and foot movements are most subject to nonverbal leakage because we move them more automatically, without conscious thought (Ekman and Friesen 2003). Very controlled individuals often show emotions in their hands and feet (e.g., gripping their hands together, tapping their foot) or in physiological behaviors such as blushing, sweating, breathing (e.g., shallowly or rapidly), and blinking.
- Notice frozen expressions (avoidance of showing emotion, poker face), masking (replacing a felt emotion with another *more appropriate* one), minimizing expressions (to make a feeling seem milder), and exaggerating an expression (e.g., nodding the head vigorously and saying "uh-huh" when confused by the information you present).
- Nonverbal expression may be dependent upon age, gender, and/or culture (e.g., older patients' facial expressions may be more difficult to read as they have a diminished blushing response, and wrinkling may mask subtle reactions; women may be more likely than men to cry; and some cultures discourage public displays of emotion). Furthermore, although research suggests recognition of emotions is a universal ability, accuracy may vary as a function of cultural background and exposure (Elfenbein and Ambady 2002). Specifically, facial recognition generally is higher when both parties are from the same "national, ethnic, or regional group" (Elfenbein and Ambady 2002, p. 203), although accuracy can be improved when one has greater exposure to the cultural group. Additionally, research suggests members of a majority group show less accurate judgements of minority group members' facial expressions, while minority group members are more accurate in their judgments of majority group members' expressions (Elfenbein and Ambady 2002).
- Listen for incomplete sentences. Patients may trail off or shift to another sentence/topic because what they are saying is emotionally charged. Ask patients to finish incomplete sentences.
- Watch for sudden shifts in behavior in any direction (moving from open posture to closed posture, speaking more rapidly to more slowly, breathing more deeply to more shallowly, etc.). For example, a patient may have a sudden shift in behavior depending on the content of the session (presentation of risk information, introduction of abortion as an option, etc.).

3.3 Effective Counselor Physical Attending Behaviors

There are five major domains of physical attending: face and eyes, body, voice, distracting behaviors, and touch.

Face and Eyes

Effective attending with the face and eyes generally involves the use of occasional head nods, smiling at appropriate times, and looking at the patient without staring. Be careful, however, about nodding your head at times when patients are saying something that is inaccurate and/or disparaging, for instance, if a patient says "I'm sure this is my fault. If I'd only been more careful earlier in the pregnancy, my baby would be ok." In this case you may intend to communicate that you understand what the patient said, but the patient might interpret your head nod as agreeing it is in fact her fault.

Body

Effective use of your body refers to maintaining relaxed but alert posture, using occasional hand and arm gestures for emphasis, keeping your legs and feet still (no leg or foot jiggling), positioning yourself so you face the patient as directly as possible and sitting with an open stance (uncrossed arms and legs), and sitting at a distance that is comfortable for the patient. If you work behind a desk, position the patient chairs to one side and move your chair to that end of the desk in order to minimize the desk as a physical barrier.

Voice

Effective vocal attending includes speaking at an adequate volume, maintaining an appropriate pace or speed, using inflections, using words the patient can understand (be careful about "talking down" to patients, which usually happens if you use simple words in combination with a "singsong voice" and exaggeratedly slow pace), and using a tone that matches the content and tenor of the conversation.

Distracting Behaviors (Behaviors to Avoid)

We are all prone to engage in distracting behaviors when we feel anxious, preoccupied, and/or otherwise are not fully engaged with a patient. Distracting behaviors include habitual, informal word choices (e.g., "you guys" which, although quite common in US vernacular, is very unprofessional in a genetic counseling setting); excessive use of filler words (you know, right, ok, it's like…, um, etc.); shuffling through notes and/or focusing on a computer rather than looking at the patient; playing with something like a pen, jewelry, or paper clip; twisting your fingers or hair or clenching your hands together; jiggling your foot; and chewing gum (also very unprofessional).

Touching Patients

Touch can be beneficial if it leads to an improved relationship but harmful if the patient views it negatively. In the context of genetic counseling, as with other medical interactions, lightly touching a patient after giving bad news may be a normal, compassionate human response. Touch, however, can raise a number of social and cultural issues and therefore is a controversial behavior: "The only thing that is commonly agreed in this controversy is that touch can have different meanings for different people" (Dewane 2006, p. 546).

We suggest you be aware that touching patients might be misinterpreted. People vary in their comfort with being touched by strangers. Abuse survivors may be particularly sensitive to touch they did not invite/initiate. Some patients may feel they are being patronized or put in a submissive position when you place a hand on their shoulder or arm. There are also wide cultural variations in who may touch and how they may do so. Touch can be particularly risky if you initiate it. Some patients will initiate touch (reach out to shake your hand, extend their arms and/or ask for a hug); children generally are more likely than adults to communicate through touch, and some patients with intellectual disabilities such as Down syndrome may use touch to express connection.

Please note that shaking hands, while generally appropriate in Western cultures, may be regarded as offensive in some cultural groups (e.g., some individuals from Middle Eastern cultures will only shake hands with a person who is of the same gender). One strategy is to wait to see if your patient offers her or his hand first.

Finally, there are ways to connect with patients without touching them. You can convey your sentiments by moving your chair closer, leaning forward, putting down your visual aids, softening your voice tone and volume, and slowing your pace. When patients convey that they are pleased or relieved with news, you can express your happiness and support with a hearty "great news" or "I'm happy for you."

Other Considerations

- *Formality*: People vary in their comfort with informal approaches. We find it's best to begin by being more formal with every patient unless and until their behavior invites less formality. Ask how they would like to be addressed (Mr., Mrs., Ms., Dr.). Avoid initiating physical contact such as a handshake unless they extend their hand first. Tell them how they may address you.
- *Courtesy*: All cultures have politeness norms. Early in a session if you wish to ask a question, begin by seeking the patient's permission, "Could you please tell me…" or "I'd like to ask about____, if that is ok with you." Give an explanation for why you are addressing certain topics and/or asking certain questions. If you take notes, explain what you are doing and why. Be sure to always turn off your pager and phone or put them on mute. Excuse yourself if you are called away, and apologize to the patient for the inconvenience when you return.
- *Interpersonal dynamics*: When other people accompany the patient (whether partner, family members, friends), watch for nonverbal indicators of who the decision-maker may be. Who speaks first? Does the patient look at the other person before responding to you? How hesitant is the patient in her/his speech? What is the interaction among all parties? In many cases, it may be appropriate to provide family genetic counseling. The fact that your patient brought other people to the session may signify a preference for having those individuals

involved in the discussion and or decision-making. Keep in mind, however, that this might not always be the case. By attending to nonverbal communication, you should be able to ascertain when it is appropriate to either request or offer to meet individually with the primary patient.

3.3.1 Setting the Stage for Good Attending

Now that you've reviewed a rather lengthy list of recommended physical attending behaviors, you may be thinking you must use every one of them. Please keep in mind two important points. First, no one is able to control any nonverbal behavior for more than a few minutes at a time. Eventually, we all go back to our natural responses. Second, not all of these behaviors will feel "natural/right" for you. Don't try to force behaviors that simply do not work. Do try, however, to offset behaviors on the "generally not recommended" list with other, recommended ones. For instance, if you are a "leg crosser," don't try to eliminate it completely. When you do cross your legs, try to keep your other behaviors more open (uncrossed arms, facing patients, giving eye contact). The most important thing to communicate to patients is that you genuinely care about them.

Finally, we suggest you arrange your physical environment whenever possible to maximize good attending. Select a chair that does not swivel or rock, one that has arms so you can rest your hands on them rather than clenching them in your lap, and one that fits your body so you can rest your feet on the floor. Select your clothing to avoid jewelry you would be tempted to play with when counseling; wear high-necked clothing if you have an extreme blushing response on your neck; and rearrange furniture when possible to reduce physical barriers between you and the patients.

3.4 Additional Suggestions for Attending Effectively

In order to build rapport and convey your interest and understanding to the patient, we recommend the following:

- *Be congruent.* Your body should parallel your verbal message. When your words and nonverbal behaviors are discrepant, the patient will tend to believe your nonverbals. For example, if you say, "I can respect your decision to terminate the pregnancy" while you are frowning and clenching your hands together, the patient will probably decide you disapprove of the decision.
- *Get in sync.* Your communication will be more effective if your demeanor is in harmony with your patient's. Synchronicity may increase empathy, promote a common understanding, and/or lead to similarity of views (Ramseyer and Tschacher 2011). Ramseyer and Tschacher (2011) studied nonverbal synchrony (also known as coordination of movement [Tickle-Degnen and Gavett 2003; and

what we term *synchronicity*]) between patients and therapists. Higher levels of synchrony were associated with more positive therapy processes and outcomes, including clients rating the relationship as higher in quality and reporting an increase in their self-efficacy.

So, for instance, if your patient is very sad and speaking in a slow, barely audible manner, you will have synchronicity if you also slow the pace of your speech and speak more quietly. Or, if a patient is crying, you would not want to smile; instead your nonverbals should convey caring. If you are *tuned in* to your patient's emotions, synchronicity will happen *automatically*, with little or no conscious effort on your part. Be careful, however, not to carry this *mirroring* too far. For instance, if a patient is very anxious, talking rapidly and loudly, you would only foster further anxiety if you were to respond in a similar fashion.

- *Relax physically*. You will be more open to hearing patients if your body is relaxed and you are breathing regularly and deeply. Try to take a few minutes before a genetic counseling session to calm yourself and focus your attention.
- *Do an internal process check*. Genetic counselors sometimes become aware that they are moving too quickly through a session or skipping over important content in response to patient verbal or nonverbal cues. For example, they may respond by talking faster or louder when a patient is nodding vigorously or saying "yes, yes" to content the counselors are providing. Watching for these behaviors may offer insight into how the patient is feeling and how you are responding (synchronicity) and allow you to "regroup," that is, sit back, take a deep breath, slow your pace, and relax your body.
- *Use eye contact*. Eye contact helps you focus on the patient and indicates you are listening. It's generally a good idea to look at your patient even if she/he is not looking at you and is instead staring at the floor or looking at the wall. Eventually most patients will venture a glance at you, and when they do, it's important that they can see you are looking at them. One disclaimer, mentioned later in this chapter, is to decrease your eye contact if it appears to be making a patient uncomfortable.
- *Convey sensitivity*. Your nonverbals should communicate concern, alertness, and vigilance.

3.5 Challenges in Attending

In our experience, challenges in attending are more likely to occur when a genetic counselor generally has either too much or too little involvement or has an intensity that is too low or too high. Moderation is key to effective attending. Consider the following challenges:

- *Enthusiasm*—In this situation, a genetic counselor displays too much enthusiasm and energy, to the point of practically violating the patient's personal space; talking loudly, quickly, and too cheerfully; nodding excessively (think of a

bobblehead doll); and saying "uh-huh" after every patient utterance. At best, these behaviors can be tiring and, at worst, seem intrusive and patronizing.
- *Anxiety*—A genetic counselor who is feeling overly anxious may avoid eye contact, fiddle with a pen or paper, or exhibit one or more distracting mannerisms that suggest self-protection.
- *Detachment*—Sometimes, a genetic counselor may seem to be too much of a *blank screen*, for instance, using a piercing stare; taking a cold, *clinical* stance (facial expression does not change); displaying little or no emotion; and sitting completely still with no hand or arm gestures. The counselor comes across as analyzing and/or judging the patient.
- *Overly Concerned*—In this case a genetic counselor displays too much concern through sad facial expressions, deep sighs, and furrowed brow. These behaviors suggest the genetic counselor feels the patients' problems almost more than the patient does. Patients may even say, "Don't be so worried! I'll be ok."
- *Low-Key Involvement*—When a genetic counselor is *too* laid-back during a session, slouching in the chair, yawning, and dressed unprofessionally (e.g., blue jeans, low-cut top, short and/or tight clothes), this can be misperceived as a lack of concern about the patient.

These attending challenges can arise for any genetic counselor at any time. They are usually prompted by certain aspects of the genetic counseling situation or by events in one's personal life. Therefore, it is important to recognize the types of patient characteristics, genetic conditions, and/or personal life events that may provoke these challenges for you.

3.5.1 Silence or the "Space Between"

Silence is a critical part of psychological and physical attending, and yet it is one of the more challenging skills to cultivate. The difficulty is due in part to common misperceptions such as the following: silence is the "absence" of skills ("If I'm silent, then I'm not doing anything"); silence will make patients (or my supervisor) think I don't know what to say or do; silence is a waste of the limited time I have to engage with patients ("Why be silent when I can always tell patients more of the ever growing biomedical information?"); and silent patients are simply waiting for my next question or directive. These perceptions probably make you feel anxious, and usually they are untrue. We maintain that when you make an effort to challenge your misperceptions, you will become less afraid of silence and will be able to use it with greater intentionality. We suggest you work on gaining comfort with silence and think of it as "part of the interaction rather than the absence of the interaction" (Sharpley et al. 2005, p. 158). As you become less afraid of silence and more able to fully attend to the patient "in the moment," you will find silence occurs naturally and appropriately. We also suggest you try to discern the meaning of silences that you initiate and those that are patient-initiated, as "no two silences are the same."

In the psychotherapy literature, Lane et al. (2002) assert that silence must be done skillfully in order to convey "safety, understanding, and containment (p. 1091). When done unskillfully, they note it can imply 'distance, disinterest, and disengagement' and thus damage trust" (p. 1091). Two studies of therapist views of silence found their reasons to use silence included to facilitate reflection, encourage responsibility, facilitate expression of feelings, and convey empathy (Hill et al. 2003; Ladany et al. 2004) and also to give therapists some time to think of what they want to say (Ladany et al. 2004). Sharpley et al. (2005) studied the relationship between silence and rapport in initial therapy sessions and found significantly higher amounts of silence during portions of the sessions rated as "very high rapport." Moreover, silences initiated by therapists and terminated by clients were more likely to contribute to rapport than were silences which were both initiated and terminated by the therapist.

Levitt (2002) asked clients to discuss pauses in video-recorded therapy sessions and found three sorts of productive pauses: emotional pauses, in which clients moved more deeply into their specific feelings; expressive pauses, in which clients were searching for words to express their ideas and/or name their feelings; and reflective pauses, in which clients were questioning, gaining further awareness of an issue, and/or connecting ideas and gaining insight/realization.

3.5.2 Patient Characteristics that Pose Attending Challenges

Limited Communication Ability

Providing genetic counseling to patients with limited communication ability is challenging. Sometimes limited communication is due to psychophysiological reasons. For instance, Kring and Stuart (2008) describe individuals with major depressive mood disorder as having dampened facial, vocal, and gestural expressive behaviors. They tend to exhibit less eye contact and have a flat, dull, and slow tempo when speaking. This is not to be confused with cultural differences [cf. Kim et al. (2003) about Asian-American culturally endorsed behavior] or with thinking the behavior reflects motivation or intent as opposed to an underlying physiological state (Patterson 2003).

Smith et al. (2014) described a genetic counseling case in which the patient's disease progression posed communication challenges. The patient had sporadic ALS and maternal history of HD. The authors noted that, "Assessment of our patient's nonverbal communication was also limited given his disease progression, which significantly limited his physical movements…Therefore, alternative approaches had to be used in order to establish a working relationship with the patient and understand his needs and desires. Our approach was to limit the information conveyed to what was most necessary to communicate and to utilize yes/no questioning to facilitate our patient's involvement. Additional counseling time was also provided to accommodate the patient's limitations" (p. 730).

Patient Anger

Schema et al. (2015) interviewed genetic counselors about patient anger directed at them. Their participants noted that patient expressions of anger range from "yelling or screaming" to more subtle, indirect nonverbal behaviors "such as acting uninterested in the information shared" (p. 723). One of the counselors described typical indirect expressions as "'walking in, arms folded, short answers to questions, not smiling, and tense tone'" (p. 723). Baty (2010) similarly describes nonverbal expressions of patient anger as disengagement during a genetic counseling session, characterized by not listening closely and/or not thinking critically about information the counselor presents. Additional nonverbal clues of possible anger include failure to complete requested paperwork before coming to the session, arriving late, and responding minimally to genetic counselor statements (Smith and Antley 1979). Good psychological attending skills will allow you to recognize these clues and consider whether they indicate patient anger.

Couple Interactions

Schoeffel et al. (2018) interviewed genetic counselors about their experiences with couple conflict in prenatal sessions. Every counselor noted the couples' nonverbal behaviors provided clues that they were in conflict. These clues variously included turned or leaning away from each other, crossed arms, lack of participation, physical/facial reaction to what partner is saying, sighs of exasperation, looking away, rolling their eyes at partner, glaring/scowling, tone of voice, sitting apart in the waiting room, leaving the room, energy/tension in the room, fidgeting, not talking to partner, and not touching partner when in a difficult situation.

Lafans et al. (2003) interviewed prenatal genetic counselors about their experiences of paternal involvement during prenatal sessions. They identified a number of nonverbal behaviors suggesting:

1. *Appropriate paternal involvement*: appears to be attentive and gives eye contact to the counselor, sits close to partner, touches her and/or holds her hand, leans forward to observe visual aids, faces the counselor, and nods at the counselor (pp. 222–223).
2. *Paternal under-involvement*, that is, "disengaged, distracted, uncooperative, and/or defensive" (p. 235): looks away/stares into space, appears passive/disinterested/yawns, engages in other activities (reads magazine/newspaper, uses cell phone/computer), slumps/slouches/leans back in chair, and falls asleep during the session.
3. *Paternal over-involvement*, that is, "exhibiting behaviors that control the content and flow of sessions, ignore their partner's needs or feelings, and/or promote their own agenda" (p. 235): one of these behaviors could be considered nonverbal, namely, interrupts the genetic counselor.

3.5.3 *Genetic Counseling Modalities*

The format for genetic counseling may pose attending challenges. Goodenberger et al. (2015) note that a majority of a laboratory genetic counselor's communication takes place by telephone and often involves brief interactions with health-care providers or patients. They stress that the way in which lab genetic counselors present themselves "…is especially important because the [recipient of the communication] has only verbal cues to react to as opposed to the nonverbal cues present in a face-to-face encounter" (p. 8). Moreover, counseling over the phone precludes physically attending to the sorts of patient body language available in face-to-face interactions and does not allow the genetic counselor to mirror that body language. They further note restrictions on the use of visual aids to inform and educate. They recommend a laboratory genetic counselor adapt to these limitations by "increasing his or her sensitivity to vocal cues, such as listening carefully for key words or phrases that can be used to assess understanding or needs... For example, he or she may try to counter a client's hurried pace if it is felt that more time is needed for adequate understanding. The specific words a genetic counselor chooses when describing technologies and discussing test results over the phone become very important because of the inability to use visual aids and nonverbal cues" (p. 15). These recommendations are also useful if you work as a clinical genetic counselor as you often engage with patients by phone (e.g., to call out test results, answer patient questions that arise outside of the session).

Telehealth, such as telephone counseling, also limits the available nonverbal cues (Peshkin et al. 2016; Zilliacus et al. 2010). Research demonstrates that key differences between telephone genetic counseling and face-to-face counseling involve ways in which counselors go about "establishing rapport through verbal and nonverbal interactions…recognizing factors affecting the counseling interaction... assessing client/family emotions, support, etc.…and educating clients about basic genetic concepts [e.g., in the absence of visual aids]" (Burgess et al. 2016, p. 112).

Participants in the Burgess et al. (2016) study "…pointed to the inability to read the patient's body language and assess nonverbal cues as factors that adversely impacted their ability to build rapport, assess understanding, and make psychosocial assessments" (p. 116). Several of their participants described modifying their genetic counseling approach in the absence of nonverbals. For example, "At the beginning of the conversation I usually explain to the patient that since we are not in the same room I cannot read their non-verbal cues and need them to speak up if they have questions or get confused. I am almost never this blunt during in-person discussions"; "…counseling when not in person requires much more verbal checking in to ensure and confirm understanding"; and "Evaluating a client's risk perception and response and modifying counseling requires closer attention to verbal cues in telephone counseling since facial expressions and body language cannot be assessed" (p. 118). One participant mentioned an approach for addressing patients' psychosocial needs: "I have actually said to people 'I know this is an emotional topic, and since I can't see you, I may miss a sign that the information is upsetting to you. This can be helpful information to me, so that we can address your concerns, so please feel free to stop me and tell me if something is upsetting to you'" (p. 121). Many participants suggested "…tailoring training in psychosocial assessment skills to include asking more direct questions and identifying different nonverbal patient cues (like inflection, pauses or sighing) to determine a patient's emotional status" (p. 124).

Video telehealth may also require modifications with respect to nonverbal attending. Some of the genetics practitioners in Zilliacus et al.'s (2009) study described focusing the camera on facial expressions in order to promote rapport. For example, "I focus in fairly sharply on me so that they can see the expression on my face and I'm trying to see the expression on theirs and so I feel as though there's a reasonable contact and communication link with them" (p. 602).

3.6 Cultural Considerations in Attending

As with any clinical encounter, cultural differences are important to consider in genetic counseling. It's impossible, however, to be an expert on issues relevant to genetic counseling for every cultural group. Even when you have cultural knowledge, cultural sensitivity, and cultural skills for certain populations, a constant interplay of individual characteristics and prior life events interacts with culture to make every patient unique. As Steinberg Warren (2011) notes, cultural competence is a complex mixture of "…the client, the counselor, the multiple cultures to which they each belong, the verbal and *nonverbal interactions between the two* [emphasis ours], their respective family, educational and social backgrounds, their respective past and current living and working environments, the communities in which they live, the health care system in which they meet, and, of course, the genetic and family history, diagnosis, testing, and/or decisions that bring the two individuals together in a genetic counseling setting" (p. 545).

Nonetheless, learning about communication preferences in different cultures can be helpful. It can also be helpful to develop an appreciation of how culture affects health beliefs and practices. That said, as Lewis (2010), referencing Gelman (2004), states, "Culture is dynamic, so the contents of a single culture can change over time and location. Members of a culture add new ideas, values and behaviors and become disenchanted with prior beliefs and behaviors, thus transforming culture over time. People are also members of multiple social groups, many of which generate a coherent set of beliefs and expectations. Within a technologically sophisticated, multicultural society, it is clear that (1) individual decisions about cultural values, (2) exposure to and membership in multiple cultures, and (3) rapid change in the contents of culture itself make it difficult to invest in a static model of culture. To base our understanding of others solely or largely on our perceptions of their ethnocultural profile (e.g., Latinos are Roman Catholics and thus do not wish to consider pregnancy termination) without further investigation ignores the diversity in individuals as well as in their ethnic and racial groups" (p. 205).

You should adapt your attending style to your patient's style as much as possible rather than expecting patients to adapt to yours. When you are uncertain about the effects of your attending behaviors, ask your patient what feels comfortable or uncomfortable, and observe the impact of your nonverbals. For instance, if you are sitting close and your patient seems uncomfortable, try moving your chair back a bit and see if that helps. Also keep in mind that you should vary your attending behaviors based on both a patient's immediate needs and his or her cultural background. As mentioned earlier in this chapter, you might pull your chair closer to a patient who is crying. You would slow the rate of your speech and become less animated with an extremely anxious patient. You would be careful about touching patients whose backgrounds prohibit physical contact with nonfamilial members of the opposite sex (e.g., members of some Muslim sects). Some couples who seek counseling will prefer that you communicate with the husband who then translates to his wife; for instance, in some Asian and Middle Eastern couples, the husband may prefer that you communicate through him rather than speaking directly to his wife (Lafans et al. 2003).

Some studies offer helpful insights about the role that culture might play in attending behaviors and communication in genetic counseling. The results of these studies suggest variability in patients' verbal and nonverbal communication. Some relevant examples are summarized below.

3.6.1 Verbalizations/Language

Ishii et al. (2003) noted that there are cultural differences in attention to certain nonverbals. Specifically, they asserted that "Americans primarily attend to verbal content [while] Asians pay closer attention to vocal tone…" (p. 39). In their study they found American participants had an easier time ignoring vocal tone than verbal content, while the reverse was true for Japanese participants. They also found that Tagalog-English bilingual participants in the Philippines were biased toward attending to vocal tone regardless of the language spoken.

Cura (2015) discusses cultural meanings of nonverbal communication among Filipinos. He asserts that "Filipino culture is characterized as less verbal, and nonverbal cues usually provide meaningful signals during communication" (p. 221). Patient silence may represent unwillingness to disagree with other family members about a decision and wish to preserve family harmony. The author suggests health-care providers attend to patient body language, such as bowing one's head, lack of verbal response (silence), blankly staring, or a lack of eye contact as cues they are reluctant to express their views and/or are experiencing uncertainty. Cura also notes Filipino patients may wish to rely upon health-care providers' expertise. They may seek their recommendations and adhere to them in "the midst of uncertainty and unfamiliarity with the genetic condition… [even when] they are actually unsure of [their] answers/decisions" (p. 219).

Kim et al. (2003) report findings from the literature that Asian-Americans "…in general tend to value emotional self-control and tend not to openly display their feelings, even if the feelings are positive… [They are] often taught to limit their emotional expressiveness even with family members…because traditional Asian cultural values consider the ability to control emotions as a sign of strength. In contrast, European Americans tend to believe that individuals should openly and directly express their affection for each other" (p. 205). Thus, some Asian-American patients may present in a calm manner, smiling less frequently, sitting more still with fewer shifts in posture, being less vocal, and so forth. You should be aware they may be experiencing a range of emotions internally (e.g., distress, confusion, shame). One strategy for assessing their internal reaction is to normalize it and invite direct expression. For example, "Sometimes when patients hear this information they feel frightened. I wonder what you're thinking right now"; or "Sometimes when patients hear this information they feel confused. Could you please tell me about any confusions you are having?"

3.6.2 Nonverbal Communication

Individuals who are deaf "tend to be highly attuned to messages delivered through facial expressions and body language when communicating with others. As Corker (1996) pointed out, 90% of communication occurs in a nonverbal way, and these unspoken conversations are vital to establishing and maintaining a therapeutic relationship with a client" (Williams and Abeles 2004, p. 644).

Sagaser et al. (2016) explored prenatal genetic counselors' strategies for assessing patients' religious/spirituality beliefs. Several of their participants noted the utility of psychological attending, in particular, looking for "nonverbal or contextual clues" (p. 930) including patient clothing that implies ministry, jewelry suggesting a religious affiliation (e.g., crosses, other religious images), and bringing a prayer book to the session. The researchers concluded that genetic counselors could easily use this type of psychological attending to assess the importance of religion/spirituality to their patients and suggested they make mention of these sorts of clues as "a helpful starting point for initiating discussion of spiritual matters in pregnancy decision-making" (p. 930).

3.7 Closing Comments

Although attending is the lynchpin to effective genetic counseling, it is not always an easy process. Attending is complicated by the fact that you must simultaneously focus on the patient and yourself. We would like to close with two caveats:

- *Attending to Your Patients.* Remember that universally valid statements about effective physical and psychological attending and the meaning of nonverbals are impossible because of the many individual and cultural differences in patients and their situations. Psychological attending will help you discern how patients prefer to discuss their experiences, and you can adjust your responses accordingly. When unsure, ask your patient about the general meaning of a behavior in her or his culture.

- *Attending to Yourself.* Initially you may find that focusing on behaviors, which you typically do *automatically*, will make you extremely self-conscious. You may feel somewhat awkward and mechanical as you practice attending (and other) skills. Self-awareness, however, is an important first step toward developing your genetic counseling skills. Over time and with practice, you will learn to relax and therefore be able to focus less on yourself and more on your patients.

3.8 Class Activities

Activity 1: Attending Behaviors (Think-Pair-Share Dyads)

Students respond individually in writing to four questions and then discuss their responses with a partner:

1. What is attending?
2. As a genetic counselor, what attending behaviors do you think are helpful?
3. What attending behaviors are not so helpful?
4. Is there a cultural group that might have an attending style different from your own?

Next, pairs of students discuss their written responses.
Estimated time: 20 min.

Process
The instructor lists the four questions in four columns on the blackboard or on newsprint. Students then share their responses to each of the questions and the instructor summarizes them under the appropriate column. Then the instructor verbally summarizes major themes and presents any ideas which did not emerge from the dyads.
Estimated time: 15 min.

Activity 2: Attending (Group Discussion)

The instructor shows photographs of people and asks students to speculate about how the people are feeling. The pictures should represent a range of emotions. Also, to make it more challenging and to move into primary empathy, include pictures in which the person(s) has incongruous facial expressions (e.g., an athlete who looks as if she/he is in pain after winning a sporting event).
Estimated time: 20 min.

Activity 3: Psychological Attending Role Play

The instructor engages in a 10–15-min, video-recorded role-play with a volunteer from outside of the class. The volunteer leaves, and then the students recall everything they can about the "patient's" demographic characteristics (gender, ethnicity, eye and hair color, height, weight, dress, etc.) and nonverbal behaviors. Then the instructor plays back the videotaped session and students compare it to their recalled responses. Usually the students will have overlooked or forgotten some characteristics or behaviors. This leads into a discussion of how difficult it is to fully attend to all aspects of another person.

Estimated time: 30–35 min.

Activity 4: Psychological Attending (Genetic Counseling Video)

The instructor shows students a segment of a video-recorded genetic counseling session (either an actual or a simulated session) with the volume turned-off. In a large group, the students identify what they think the counselor and patient are talking about and what feelings each person is experiencing. Next, the instructor replays the segment with the volume on. The students compare their description of the *volume-off* segment with the *volume-on* segment.

Estimated time: 30 min.

Instructor Note

- The instructor could also ask students to identify counselor and patient nonverbal behaviors that are in sync (synchronicity) and those that are discordant. If students desire additional practice, they could try this same exercise at home with television programs or videos.

Activity 5a: Psychological Attending Role-Play (Dyads)

Dyads discuss any topic (e.g., how it feels to be taking a course on counseling skills, how it feels to be in school this year, etc.) with their eyes closed. One person is the speaker (patient) and one person is the listener (counselor). They engage in a dialogue for 5 min. The student who is the listener (counselor) should try to *sense* the patient's experience from what she/he says and how she/he says it.

Estimated time: 5 min.

Process

In the large group, dyads respond to these questions: How did it feel to converse with your eyes closed? What cues did you respond to? What was hard? Easy? How much do you rely on visual cues? What strategies did you use to establish rapport? To understand the "patient"? How well do you think these strategies would translate to telephone counseling or another sort of telehealth?

Estimated time: 10 min.

Activity 5b: Psychological Attending Role-Play (Dyads)

The same dyads take turns being the counselor and the patient for two, 10-min role-plays, using the same discussion topic as in the previous exercise. The counselor watches for a significant patient nonverbal (e.g., change in breathing, shift in eye contact, voice tone). The counselor should not focus on small nonverbals that are out of context with spoken words. After the counselor has observed one significant nonverbal, she/he should focus by asking the patient whether the patient is aware of what is happening to his/her breathing, eye contact, voice tone, etc. The counselor *should not interpret* or assign meaning to the patient's behavior. The counselor should merely notice where the focus takes the patient.

Estimated time: 20 min.

Process

After both role-plays are completed, students discuss the following questions: What kinds of nonverbals did you focus on? What happened when you pointed them out? Both the counselor and the patient should comment on the latter question.

Estimated time: 10 min.

Activity 6: Physical Attending Role-Play (Dyads)

Dyads engage in 10-min role-plays, taking turns as counselor and patient. The instructor gives the patient the following instructions (the counselors should not see these instructions).

Role-play 1: The patient *violates* the counselor's personal space (sits too close, leans in too far, touches the counselor).

Role-play 2: The patient acts uncomfortable with the counselor's eye contact. Whenever the counselor looks at the patient, the patient should turn away, fidget, stammer, etc.

Estimated time: 20 min.

Process

After both role-plays are completed, students discuss the following questions: How did the counselor feel? What did the counselor in each role-play think was going on? Was the counselor in Role-play #2 aware of the patient's discomfort with eye contact? What did the counselor do with this awareness?

Estimated time: 10–20 min.

Activity 7a: Low-Level Attending Skills Model

Instructor and a volunteer genetic counseling patient engage in a role-play in which the counselor demonstrates poor physical and psychological attending behaviors (see section on Challenges in Attending for some examples of poor attending). Students observe and take notes of examples of poor attending.

Estimated time: 5 min.

Process

Students share their examples of poor attending. Then they discuss the impact of the counselor's poor attending skills on the patient. The patient can offer her or his impressions of the counselor's behaviors after the other students have commented.

Estimated time: 10 min.

Activity 7b: High-Level Attending Skills Model

Instructor and the same volunteer repeat the same role-play, only this time the counselor displays good attending skills. Students take notes of examples of good attending behaviors.

Estimated time: 5 min.

Process

Students share their examples of good attending. Then they discuss the impact of the counselor's attending behaviors on the patient. They also contrast this role-play to the low-level role-play.

Estimated time: 10 min.

Instructor Note

- After each role-play, students could work together in Think-Pair-Share dyads to identify examples of attending behaviors and their impact on the patient before sharing as a whole class.

Activity 8: Attending Skills Role-Play (Triad)

Three students practice physical attending skills in 5-min role-plays taking turns as counselor, patient, and observer. Allow 10 min of feedback after each role-play. Students should focus on using good physical attending behaviors. They can refer to the section on Effective Counselor Physical Attending Behaviors for examples of good skills.

Estimated time: 45 min.

Process

In the large group, discuss the following: How was it to do this exercise? What are you learning about attending in general? About yourself?

Estimated time: 20 min.

Instructor Note

- Some individuals have very powerful nonverbals (e.g., a strong, loud voice, piercing gaze, etc.). If this is the case for any of the students, the instructor should give them feedback about how they might *tone down* intense nonverbals.

3.9 Written Exercises

Exercise 1[1]

Briefly describe *two* possible meanings for each of the following patient nonverbal behaviors:

Patient nonverbal behavior	Possible meanings

- Patient stares at the floor
- Patient grimaces at the term "defect"
- Patient jiggles her foot repeatedly
- Patient sighs deeply and says nothing
- Patient has drops of sweat on his forehead
- Patient grips her partner's hand
- Patient leans away from the counselor
- Patient stumbles over his words
- Patient frowns
- Patient draws in a deep breath

Exercise 2

Respond in writing to the following questions:

- What physical attending behaviors are most difficult for you to use?
- What physical attending behaviors are the easiest for you to use?
- What are your most powerful nonverbal behaviors (i.e., what do other people notice the most about the way you attend)?
- What strategies might you use to offset or lessen the intensity of your powerful nonverbal behaviors with patients who are uncomfortable with them?
- What distracting nonverbal behaviors do you engage in when you feel nervous? Bored? Distracted?

Instructor Note
- Students could write responses to the five questions as part of a journal or a case logbook.

[1] Adapted from: Cormier and Cormier (1991).

References

Batty M, Taylor MJ. Early processing of the six basic facial emotional expressions. Cogn Brain Res. 2003;17:613–20.
Baty BJ. Facing patient anger. In: LeRoy BS, McCarthy Veach P, Bartels DM, editors. Genetic counseling practice. Hoboken: Wiley-Blackwell; 2010. p. 125–54.
Burgess KR, Carmany EP, Trepanier AM. A comparison of telephone genetic counseling and in-person genetic counseling from the genetic counselor's perspective. J Genet Couns. 2016;25:112–26.
Corker M. Deaf transitions: images and origins of deaf families, deaf communities, and deaf identities. London: Jessica Kingsley; 1996.
Cormier WH, Cormier LS. Interviewing strategies for helpers (3. Baskı). Pacific Grove, CA: Brooks; 1991.
Cura JD. Respecting autonomous decision making among Filipinos: a re-emphasis in genetic counseling. J Genet Couns. 2015;24:213–24.
Darrow AA, Johnson C. Preservice music teachers' and therapists' nonverbal behaviors and their relationship to perceived rapport. Int J Music Educ. 2009;27:269–80.
Dewane CJ. Use of self: a primer revisited. Clin Soc Work J. 2006;34:543–58.
Dowell NM, Berman JS. Therapist nonverbal behavior and perceptions of empathy, alliance, and treatment credibility. J Psychother Integr. 2013;23:158–65.
Egan G. The skilled helper. Pacific Grove/Monterey, CA: Brooks/Cole; 1994.
Ekman P, Friesen WV. Unmasking the face: a guide to recognizing emotions from facial clues. Los Altos, CA: Malor Books/Ishk; 2003.
Elfenbein HA, Ambady N. On the universality and cultural specificity of emotion recognition: a meta-analysis. Psychol Bull. 2002;128:203–35.
Fine SF, Glasser PH. The first helping interview. Thousand Oaks, CA: Sage; 1996.
Gelman CR. Empirically-based principles for culturally competent practice with Latinos. J Ethn Cult Divers Soc Work. 2004;13:83–108.
Goodenberger ML, Thomas BC, Wain KE. The utilization of counseling skills by the laboratory genetic counselor. J Genet Couns. 2015;24:6–17.
Hall JA, Bernieri FJ, Carney DR. Nonverbal behavior and interpersonal sensitivity. In: Harrigan JA, Rosenthal R, Scherer KR, editors. The new handbook of methods in nonverbal behavior research (Series in Affective Science) (reprint ed.). New York: Oxford University Press; 2008. p. 237–82.
Henry SG, Fuhrel-Forbis A, Rogers MA, Eggly S. Association between nonverbal communication during clinical interactions and outcomes: a systematic review and meta-analysis. Patient Educ Couns. 2012;86:297–315.
Hill CE. Helping skills: facilitating exploration, insight, and action. 4th ed. Washington, DC: American Psychological Association; 2014.
Hill CE, Thompson BJ, Ladany N. Therapist use of silence in therapy: a survey. J Clin Psychol. 2003;59:513–24.
Ishii K, Reyes JA, Kitayama S. Spontaneous attention to word content versus emotional tone: differences among three cultures. Psychol Sci. 2003;14:39–46.
Kim BS, Liang CT, Li LC. Counselor ethnicity, counselor nonverbal behavior, and session outcome with Asian American clients: initial findings. J Couns Dev. 2003;81:202–7.
Kring AM, Stuart BK. Nonverbal behavior and psychopathology. In: Harrigan JA, Rosenthal R, Scherer KR, editors. The new handbook of methods in nonverbal behavior research (Series in Affective Science) (reprint ed.). New York: Oxford University Press; 2008. p. 313–34.
Ladany N, Hill CE, Thompson BJ, O'Brien KM. Therapist perspectives on using silence in therapy: a qualitative study. Couns Psychother Res. 2004;4:80–9.
Lafans RS, Veach PM, LeRoy BS. Genetic counselors' experiences with paternal involvement in prenatal genetic counseling sessions: an exploratory investigation. J Genet Couns. 2003;12:219–42.

Lane RC, Koetting MG, Bishop J. Silence as communication in psychodynamic psychotherapy. Clin Psychol Rev. 2002;22:1091–104.
Leach MJ. Rapport: a key to treatment success. Complement Ther Clin Pract. 2005;11:262–5.
Lemay EP Jr, Clark MS, Feeney BC. Projection of responsiveness to needs and the construction of satisfying communal relationships. J Pers Soc Psychol. 2007;92:834–53.
Levitt HM. The unsaid in the psychotherapy narrative: voicing the unvoiced. Couns Psychol Q. 2002;15:333–50.
Lewis L. Honoring diversity: cultural competence in genetic counseling. In: LeRoy BS, McCarthy Veach P, Bartels DM, editors. Genetic counseling practice. Hoboken: Wiley-Blackwell; 2010. p. 201–34.
Mast MS. On the importance of nonverbal communication in the physician–patient interaction. Patient Educ Couns. 2007;67:315–8.
Murray SL, Holmes JG, Collins NL. Optimizing assurance: the risk regulation system in relationships. Psychol Bull. 2006;132:641–66.
Patterson ML. Commentary: evolution and nonverbal behavior: functions and mediating processes. J Nonverbal Behav. 2003;27:201–7.
Peshkin BN, Kelly S, Nusbaum RH, Similuk M, DeMarco TA, Hooker GW, et al. Patient perceptions of telephone vs. in-person BRCA1/BRCA2 genetic counseling. J Genet Couns. 2016;25:472–82.
Philippot P, Feldman RS, Coats EJ. The role of nonverbal behavior in clinical settings. In: Philippot P, Feldman RS, Coats EJ, editors. Nonverbal behavior in clinical settings. New York: Oxford University Press; 2003. p. 3–13.
Ramseyer F, Tschacher W. Nonverbal synchrony in psychotherapy: coordinated body movement reflects relationship quality and outcome. J Consult Clin Psychol. 2011;79:284–95.
Reis HT, Collins WA, Berscheid E. The relationship context of human behavior and development. Psychol Bull. 2000;126:844–72.
Roter DL, Frankel RM, Hall JA, Sluyter D. The expression of emotion through nonverbal behavior in medical visits. J Gen Intern Med. 2006;21(S1):S28–34.
Sagaser KG, Hashmi SS, Carter RD, Lemons J, Mendez-Figueroa H, Nassef S, et al. Spiritual exploration in the prenatal genetic counseling session. J Genet Couns. 2016;25:923–35.
Sander D, Grandjean D, Kaiser S, Wehrle T, Scherer KR. Interaction effects of perceived gaze direction and dynamic facial expression: evidence for appraisal theories of emotion. Eur J Cogn Psychol. 2007;19:470–80.
Schema L, McLaughlin M, Veach PM, LeRoy BS. Clearing the air: a qualitative investigation of genetic counselors' experiences of counselor-focused patient anger. J Genet Couns. 2015;24:717–31.
Schoeffel K, McCarthy Veach P, Rubin K, LeRoy BS. Managing couple conflict during prenatal counseling sessions: an investigation of genetic counselor experiences and perceptions. J Genet Couns. 2018. https://doi.org/10.1007/s10897-018-0252-6.
Sharpley CF, Munro DM, Elly MJ. Silence and rapport during initial interviews. Couns Psychol Q. 2005;18:149–59.
Smith AL, Teener JW, Callaghan BC, Harrington J, Uhlmann WR. Amyotrophic lateral sclerosis in a patient with a family history of Huntington disease: genetic counseling challenges. J Genet Couns. 2014;23:725–33.
Smith RW, Antley RM. Anger: a significant obstacle to informed decision making in genetic counseling. Birth Defects: Orig Articles Series. 1979;15:257–60.
Solomon G, Greenberg J, Futter M, Vivian L, Penn C. Understanding of genetic inheritance among Xhosa-speaking caretakers of children with hemophilia. J Genet Couns. 2012;21:726–40.
Steinberg Warren NS. Introduction to the special issue: toward diversity and cultural competence in genetic counseling. J Genet Couns. 2011;20:543–6.
Tickle-Degnen L, Gavett E. Changes in nonverbal behavior during the development of therapeutic relationship. In: Philippot P, Feldman RS, Coats EJ, editors. Nonverbal behavior in clinical settings. New York: Oxford University Press; 2003. p. 75–110.

Williams CR, Abeles N. Issues and implications of deaf culture in therapy. Prof Psychol Res Pr. 2004;35:643–8.

Zilliacus E, Meiser B, Lobb E, Barlow-Stewart K, Tucker K. A balancing act—telehealth cancer genetics and practitioners' experiences of a triadic consultation. J Genet Couns. 2009;18:598–605.

Zilliacus EM, Meiser B, Lobb EA, Kirk J, Warwick L, Tucker K. Women's experience of telehealth cancer genetic counseling. J Genet Couns. 2010;19:463–72.

Chapter 4
Listening to Patients: Primary Empathy Skills

Learning Objectives

1. Define primary empathy and its functions in genetic counseling.
2. Distinguish between different types of primary empathy responses.
3. Develop primary empathy skills through self-reflection, practice, and feedback.

4.1 Definition of Empathy

Empathy is the *vicarious experiencing* of another person's feelings and situation and an ability to *communicate* one's understanding of another's feelings and experience. Empathy involves the capacity to put yourself in another person's place to understand from her or his frame of reference (Bellet and Maloney 1991). When you are engaged empathically, you enter into patients' worlds to feel *with* them rather than *for* them and to think *with* them rather than *for* or *about* them (Chung and Bemak 2002). Empathy forms the very basis of all human interactions (Duan and Hill 1996), it is an essential condition within Carl Rogers' person-centered approach to counseling, and it is a hallmark of the Reciprocal-Engagement Model (REM) of genetic counseling practice (McCarthy Veach et al. 2007).

The psychological literature contains varied definitions of empathy. Most authors emphasize two major dimensions: empathic emotions (having an affective reaction that is *in tune* with the patient's experience) and intellectual empathy (engaging in role-taking or perspective-taking) (Bellet and Maloney 1991; Duan and Hill 1996; Gladstein 1983). In medical literature "clinical empathy" is a commonly used term, and it refers to both a skill and a process (VandenLangenberg 2012). In genetic counseling, "Empathic communication includes timing and selection of biomedical information that is relevant to the patient's situations and provision of this information in ways that the patient can understand. Empathic communication also indi-

P. McCarthy Veach et al., *Facilitating the Genetic Counseling Process*,
https://doi.org/10.1007/978-3-319-74799-6_4

cates the counselor understands how the patient is feeling about this information" (VandenLangenberg 2012, p. 130).

Most authors (e.g., Barrett-Lennard 1981; Duan and Hill 1996; Gladstein 1983) agree that empathy is a multistage, interpersonal process that contains at least three elements:

- Can I sense what you experience?
- Can I communicate this sense to you?
- Can you perceive this communication as my understanding you/your experience?

This third element depends to a great extent on the characteristics of the recipient of the empathy response (Barrett-Lennard 1981).

4.1.1 Types of Empathy

There are two major types of empathy responses, primary empathy and advanced empathy:

Primary empathy communicates initial understanding of what a patient is experiencing. Primary empathy is particularly important for rapport building and problem exploration. In genetic counseling, you use your own words to concisely convey an understanding of surface, fairly explicit patient experiences.

Example Pt (tearfully says): "I don't want anything to be wrong with my baby."

Co: "It's upsetting to think that something could be wrong."
Pt: "This is so much information! I'm so confused about what I should do. I don't think I can make this decision."
Co: "You're feeling overwhelmed by the amount of information."

Advanced empathy communicates an understanding of underlying, implicit aspects of patient experience. This type of empathy is useful for dynamic understanding (assessing the patient's deeper, less obvious feelings and experiences). Your responses are *additive* in that they go beyond surface patient expressions.

Example A patient is focusing on her fear of having a genetic test because she dislikes having her blood drawn. You believe there is more to her reaction and say, "In addition to being fearful of having your blood drawn, maybe you're also scared about what the test results might reveal?"

This chapter is about primary empathy. We consider advanced empathy in greater detail in Chap. 8.

4.2 Importance and Functions of Primary Empathy

Psychotherapy research consistently demonstrates that therapist empathy is positively related to therapy processes and outcomes (Elliott et al. 2011; Norcross and Wampold 2011). Specifically, empathy enhances the working alliance (therapeutic relationship), and a strong working alliance leads to desired therapy outcomes (Elliott et al. 2011; Norcross and Wampold 2011). Rubin (2002) notes that empathy "…is essential because it fosters a safe, trusting environment and opens up the possibility of deeper levels of understanding and compassion between patient and therapist" (p. 31). Empathy also builds a "deep emotional connection" between the patient and therapist (Rubin 2002, p. 33). Within medicine, clinical empathy plays a key role in the quality of care received as it allows clinicians "…to fulfill key medical tasks more accurately, thereby achieving enhanced patient health outcomes" (Neumann et al. 2009, p. 339). Gladstein (2012) speculates that empathy is essential in part because it encompasses multiple strategies such as actively attending, interpretation, working in a mutual relationship with patients, and placing patient needs first.

Stone (1994) asserts that "In counseling relationships we earn the right to say certain things or use certain interventions. Most troubled individuals do not take helpers seriously unless they respect them. Respect is not a gift that comes automatically with one's vocation; it is earned primarily through skillfully establishing relationships with counselees" (p. 36). Empathy is a critical component of establishing a relationship characterized by mutual respect.

A growing body of literature demonstrates that genetic counselors regard empathy as central to genetic counseling (e.g., Abrams and Kessler 2002; Kao 2010; McCarthy Veach et al. 2002a, b; McCarthy Veach and LeRoy 2012; Miranda et al. 2016; Runyon et al. 2010; Wells et al. 2016; Zahm et al. 2016). Similar to psychological and medical health fields, within genetic counseling empathy is viewed as critical to serving patients (Kao 2010; McCarthy Veach et al. 2007). For instance, in Runyon et al.'s (2010) survey of practicing genetic counselors, one counselor expressed, "I have learned that I can be an important source of support to others in devastating emotional states, just by providing a calm and compassionate 'presence'" (p. 377).

Duric et al. (2003) analyzed empathic expression in 111 cancer genetic counseling sessions and found patients who received more empathic responses to initial cues about their feelings were more likely to give more feeling cues over the course of the session. Moreover, patients who received more empathy responses showed a greater decrease in depression post-session than did patients who received fewer empathy responses. Importantly, the researchers noted "Patients who may be in most need of psychological support are not likely to emotionally disclose more than nondistressed patients during sessions. Therefore, the responsibility should rest with the clinician for actively eliciting emotional needs" (p. 261). These findings suggest that when you initiate discussion of patients' emotions and respond to their affective cues, patients may more fully express their feelings.

Pieterse et al. (2005) administered pre- and post-genetic counseling surveys to cancer genetic counseling patients regarding their needs and preferences, their perceptions of the counseling they received, and genetic counseling outcomes. They found that 20% of the patients who rated as important "receiving explanations about (emotional) aspects of counseling and about their own risk of cancer" (p. 31) were not satisfied with the extent to which these needs were addressed during counseling. Moreover, they found "addressing counselees' major needs results in higher perceptions of control and, to some extent, in lower levels of anxiety" (p. 33). These findings suggest the importance of empathy during genetic counseling sessions in order to assess patient needs, particularly with respect to emotional factors.

In a critical review of studies of communication during genetic counseling sessions and counseling outcomes, Meiser et al. (2008) found higher levels of genetic counselor empathic responses and lower levels of verbal dominance (ratio of counselor to patient talk) were key factors associated with more positive patient outcomes. The authors concluded that empathy is an important part of genetic counseling.

Tluczek et al. (2006) interviewed parents whose infants had abnormal cystic fibrosis newborn screening results about their genetic counseling preferences at the time of their infant's sweat test. Some parents expressed a preference for emotional support which included the counselor or nurse showing empathy about their distress. Parents' comments about practitioner empathy included that the practitioner conveying warmth and genuine concern was calming; and they variously described empathic practitioners as "personable, kind, compassionate, caring, [and] friendly" (p. 286).

Selkirk et al. (2009) surveyed parents of children affected with autism and solicited their advice for genetic counselors. Their advice included listening to them with empathy and nonjudgmentalness; understanding and acknowledging their views, feelings, and experiences; and taking their concerns seriously. These researchers recommended that genetic counselors work with geneticists to address the psychosocial effects of determining a genetic diagnosis. They noted, "…frustration and anger may be common. Some of the parents in the present study advised genetic counselors to acknowledge their anger over professionals ignoring their concerns and over difficulty receiving a diagnosis for their child…Moreover, some parents described feelings of guilt. Genetic counselors should initiate discussion of such challenges and resulting feelings, rather than waiting for parents to articulate these emotions" (p. 517).

Kao (2010) investigated how and why genetic counselors use empathy in genetic counseling sessions. She asked participants to write empathy responses to a series of patient scenarios and to explain their responses. Her participants primarily used empathy to express their understanding of a patient's situation, provide support, and help a patient cope with her/his emotional reactions. Kao hypothesized that empathy creates a supportive and understanding relationship which allows patients to hear medical information and proceed with the decision-making process. These findings and conclusions support a basic component of the Reciprocal-Engagement Model (REM) (McCarthy Veach et al. 2007), namely, the genetic counselor-patient relationship and the role of empathy in promoting that relationship and facilitating genetic counseling outcomes.

Primary empathy serves several functions, including:

- *Encouraging* the patient to continue talking
- Providing *clarification* for both the counselor and the patient
- Making the genetic counselor seem similar to the patient, thus increasing *social attractiveness* (the counselor is viewed as warm and likeable)
- Providing a *model* for the patient of how to be empathic

- Facilitating the establishment of *rapport* and trust
- Helping patients *feel understood* by the counselor
- Helping patients *manage their feelings*
- Facilitating patient *risk-taking*, discussion of unpleasant emotions, and reduction of nonproductive anger, overwhelming anxiety or other strong feelings (Greenberg and Pascual-Leone 2006; Hill 2014; Schema et al. 2015)

4.3 How Empathy Occurs: Origins and Mechanisms

Empathy is both innate and learned. Many theorists and researchers believe the essence of one's ability to sense another person's experience is present in infancy and develops during childhood and adolescence through the interaction of genetic and environmental factors (e.g., Gladstein 1983; Knafo et al. 2008). Have you ever noticed, for instance, in a nursery or daycare setting, when one infant becomes distressed and cries, other infants begin to cry as well? Some researchers think this behavior is evidence of the beginnings of empathy (Azar 1997). As children mature, they may be socialized through their interactions with parents and others to resonate with people's feelings and perspectives. Once a sufficient level of cognitive ability develops, the older child/adolescent is capable of communicating this understanding in a more sophisticated manner. Although the **ability** to understand another person's experience probably cannot be taught to adults, adults can, through appropriate learning activities, develop better skills for **communicating** their understanding to others (Gladstein 1983). They also can learn to focus their empathic ability.

Opportunities to expand empathy skills come from professional experiences (cf. Zahm et al. 2016). Runyon et al.'s (2010) sample of practicing genetic counselors noted they cultivated empathy by listening to patients and determining patients' needs. A number of their participants mentioned that interactions with patients taught them the importance of empathy and how to manage difficult patient feelings as well as their own emotions. Opportunities for developing empathy skills also come from personal life experiences (cf. Zahm et al. 2016). Genetic counselors' essays illustrate the influence of personal life events on their empathy in the clinical setting, including being the recipients themselves of genetic counseling services (Cohen 2002; Hatten 2002; Keilman 2002; Valverde 2002), having a pregnancy affected with multiple abnormalities (Anonymous 2008), having a child with a medical condition (Bellcross 2012), and being diagnosed with a serious medical condition (Glessner 2012). These authors describe how their experiences led to a qualitatively different perspective about their work, including deeper empathy (e.g., they are better able to anticipate patient questions and concerns). Importantly, however, these authors also describe a need to strike a balance between empathy and projecting their own experiences onto patients (see Chap. 12 countertransference).

Different theories describe the mechanisms of empathy. As mentioned earlier, empathy requires a "shift of perspective. It's not what I would experience *as me* in your shoes; empathy is what I experience *as you* in your shoes..." (Glanzer 2006, p. 135). Glanzer (2006) notes that "Empathy requires (1) an internal model of the other and (2) the capacity to experience from the perspective of this internal model of the other" (p. 125). Eisenberg and Eggum's (2009) theory of empathy proposes three processes: "(a) emotional stimulation – mirroring of the other's experience, (b) perspective taking – understanding the client, and (c) emotion regulation – soothing interpersonal distress" (as described in Imel et al. 2014; p. 146). Consistent with this model, Imel et al. (2014) studied vocal synchrony (imitation) and its relationship to empathy in 89 psychotherapy dyads. They found vocal synchrony was strongly associated with ratings of therapist empathy, and they recommended therapists pay attention to both clients' words and also "track the extent to which they are in tune with clients' vocal tone" (p. 151). Their findings demonstrate the interrelatedness of physical and psychological attending in the experience and expression of empathy.

4.4 Effectively Communicating Empathic Understanding

Rather than having no idea what patients are feeling and thinking, you will probably find that your bigger challenge is how to express your understanding to them. The good news is that as long as you have some sense of what patients might be experiencing, you can always learn ways to convey your empathy. First and foremost, you need to tune into what you are hearing and observing. The following suggestions will help you do that.

- Imagine yourself in your patient's place and ask yourself what you might think and feel in their situation. This is called *perspective-taking*.
- Try to differentiate between what patients are feeling regarding the genetic counseling *experience* as opposed to their feelings about the *problem at hand.*
- Mentally relate your patient's experience to a *similar life experience* of your own.
- Pay attention to *patient verbalizations*. Listen to what your patient is saying and how she/he is saying it.
- Attend to *patient nonverbals.* As discussed in Chap. 3 (attending skills), nonverbals provide powerful clues to patient emotions.
- Become aware of *your own nonverbal reactions* as you listen to a patient. Is your stomach tightening? Do you find yourself close to tears? Are you sighing?
- *Gain experience*. As you see more patients, you will recognize that certain experiences and emotions frequently coincide with particular genetic conditions and patient situations. For example, prenatal genetic counselors anticipate that most women with abnormal screening test results will be fearful about the possibility of an abnormality. Genetic counselors could anticipate that a couple who has lost one child to a familial cardiomyopathy may be very ambivalent about having another pregnancy.

- Read the genetic counseling *literature*. You can gain an intellectual understanding of what it might be like to be a genetic counseling patient by reading about different genetic conditions, family challenges, and patient experiences with genetic counseling and decision-making.
- Read books or articles written by patients and their family members to learn more about their firsthand experiences with genetic conditions or risks. There are movies that address these themes as well.
- Draw upon your *intuition.* Play a hunch. If you suspect your patient is feeling or thinking something, tentatively suggest it.
- *Become comfortable with your patient.* If you feel threatened or defensive, you will have difficulty experiencing and expressing empathy (Barrett-Lennard 1981).
- *Focus on your patient rather than on yourself.* With practice and experience you will gradually become less self-conscious and more patient-focused. If you find yourself becoming overly self-conscious, try taking a couple of deep breaths, and relax in your chair. You will be *in the flow* when you are no longer thinking, "How do I sound? What am I going to say next? What do I do if my patient cries?"
- *Acknowledge and set aside your biases.* It's virtually impossible to communicate authentic empathy when you feel judgmental.
- *Communicate acceptance.* Fine and Glasser (1996) wisely point out that "Feelings belong to the person who has them and are neither right nor wrong… Feelings are useful, even negative and painful feelings. They cannot and should not be argued or debated away" (p. 60). They further state that communicating acceptance means "...not debating, not arguing, never using the *b* word: but" (p. 60).
- *State your understanding of your patient's experience <u>concisely</u> and in your <u>own words</u>.* You should highlight the *essence* of what your patient has expressed, rather than giving a verbatim account. For example, the patient says, "I just found out that my sister's baby has this genetic condition. I can't believe that *my* baby is at risk. I'm afraid of what the prenatal tests are going to show. If only I'd known this before I became pregnant!" You might say: "It sounds like you're very worried about your baby." This response emphasizes what you believe to be the most salient aspect of her concerns.
- *State your empathy tentatively.* Tentative statements give the patient room to correct you if you are off-target. For example, "Is it possible that…?"; "Maybe you're feeling…?"; "Perhaps you feel…?"; and "So it seems you might be feeling...?"
- *Aim for the ballpark* rather than the *bulls-eye*. Although it's always gratifying when a patient responds to your statement by saying, "That's exactly it," it's sufficient if your words have approximately the same intensity and are close in meaning to your patient's. A *ballpark* goal reduces some of the pressure on you and frees you to focus on your patient.
- *Reflect content and affect.* Aim for responses that tap both the feeling (emotional empathy) and content (intellectual empathy) dimensions of your patient's experi-

ence (e.g., "It sounds like you're angry because your parents never told you about your risk for this condition").

- *Be thorough.* State all sides of your patient's message, including conflicting and contradictory parts. For some situations where your patient is mixed or conflicted, try saying something like, "You're torn between these two very different feelings."
- *Respond empathically and then STOP*! Patients will almost always respond. Beginning genetic counselors frequently make the mistake of giving a great empathic response and then immediately following it with a question, not allowing the patient an opportunity to respond.

4.5 Primary Empathy Responses

Primary empathy responses vary on a continuum from head nods, silence, and minimal encouragers to more complex responses that reflect the content and feeling of patients' experiences. Pedersen and Ivey (1993) identify six major types of primary empathy responses shown on the following continuum:

The primary empathy continuum					
<Simple			Complex>		
Minimal encourager	Paraphrase	Summary	Reflect content	Reflect feelings	Reflect content and feelings

Minimal Encouragers: Minimal encouragers prompt patients to continue talking, but do not interrupt the flow of the session. They may include occasional head nods, hand gestures, brief comments such as "uh-huh" and "mm-hm," repeating a few key words, and even silence. A minimal encourager response is "…the simplest of the listening skills – but it is also one of the most powerful. Research indicates that effective and experienced counselors use this skill significantly more often than ineffective and inexperienced helpers" (Pedersen and Ivey 1993, p. 121).

Example Pt: "It's my first baby, and I'm afraid something's going to go wrong."

Co: "You're afraid?"

Paraphrasing: Paraphrases reflect back to patients the essence of what they said. In order to paraphrase, you use your own concise words, while including some of the patient's key phrases (Pedersen and Ivey 1993). Be careful, however, not to parrot the patient's statements—do not repeat verbatim.

Example Pt: "We want to adopt a child, but we're worried about how this genetic condition will affect the baby we've been offered."

Co: "You want to know what you'd be taking on if you adopted a child?"

Summarizing: Summarizations are somewhat longer than paraphrases, and they contain more information (Pedersen and Ivey 1993). When patients have disclosed a large amount of information, summarization is useful because it synthesizes disparate parts of their stories. Furthermore, "Many cultures [e.g., the Deaf culture (Williams and Abeles 2004)] use story-telling as a major vehicle in disseminating their culture" (Pedersen and Ivey 1993, p. 119). When working with a patient who uses a storytelling vehicle, you may be able to communicate your understanding with a summarization that ties together the major themes.

Example Pt: "I really want to be tested for this gene. My mom and her sister died of breast cancer, and my sister was diagnosed two months ago. I have two daughters myself. What will happen to them?"

Co: "What I'm hearing is, you're very scared. And with all of the cancer in your family, you're worried about getting it and passing it on."

Content Reflection (Content Responses): Content responses concisely emphasize the cognitive gist of a patient's experience. Content responses help patients explore their goals and values and gain deeper understanding of their experience. They also allow counselors to identify "...different or conflicting culturally learned perspectives without necessarily resolving them in favor of either viewpoint" (Pedersen and Ivey 1993, p. 156).

Example A deaf couple wants a non-hearing child. However, their desire may conflict with the values of the broader culture.

Pts: "We don't know how to raise a child to live in the hearing world. We're fully prepared to raise a deaf child. But you can't believe what people are saying about our decision!"
Co: "It seems like you're kind of caught between your Deaf culture and the judgments of others."

Feeling Reflection (Affective Responses): Affective responses concisely stress the emotional aspects of a patient's experience. They contain explicit labeling of a patient's feelings.

Example Pt: "I've tried to find out information about Trisomy 18, and nobody's telling me what I need to know!"

Co: "You sound frustrated and angry."

Content and Feeling Reflections: These responses concisely combine statements about patient feelings and the situations/factors contributing to these feelings. One strategy for making this kind of reflection is to say, "You feel ... because ...." (Egan 1994).

Example Pt: "I'm glad we went ahead with the prenatal testing. I can't wait to tell my husband the good news! We were so worried about our baby having muscular dystrophy."

Co: "You feel very relieved because the results are negative."

Note that paraphrase and summary responses will be similar to content responses if they contain no feeling words (other than feeling words the patient already stated); and they will be similar to affect responses if they contain feeling words a patient has not said. Paraphrase and summary responses tend to be lengthier and use more of the patient's words, however.

The following is an example of the different types of empathy responses to the same patient statement:

Patient Statement: "I'm so upset about this diagnosis. I feel like crying all the time. I can't eat. I can't sleep. I haven't been able to keep my mind on my work."

Minimal Encourager:	"[Head nod] Mm-hm."
Paraphrase:	"You've been so upset that you're having difficulty eating, sleeping, and working."
Summary:	"This diagnosis has really upset you. Not only do you feel like crying all the time, it's getting in the way of your daily activities like eating, sleeping, and working."
Content Response:	"This diagnosis seems to have turned your world upside down."
Affect Response:	"You seem very distressed."
Content + Affect:	"You seem very distressed by this diagnosis."

A number of genetic counseling studies illustrate the essential role of counselor empathy. For example, Runyon et al. (2010) surveyed genetic counselors about the most important learning they acquired about themselves in their practice as well as advice they would give to novice genetic counselors. A prevalent theme concerned cultivating empathy "...defined as listening, determining the patient's specific needs, and *being comfortable with silence* [emphasis ours]" (p. 380). Multiple respondents mentioned the importance of "being with patients" "...as opposed to either talking, demonstrating one's knowledge, or assuming one knows best what patients need or want" (p. 380).

Zanko and Abrams (2015) reported a genetic counseling case in which the patient was affected by both Wilson's disease and Huntington disease (HD). When they counseled the patient and his wife, they noted, "Tears repeatedly punctuated the discussion, requiring time for silence and reassurance" (p. 42).

Miranda et al. (2016) interviewed master genetic counselors in order to explore their personal and professional characteristics. One of their participants expressed the following perspective: "After you've done [genetic counseling] for a while, you get good at it, and you're not really afraid of silence in a session, and you're not really afraid if people start crying, or even if you cry yourself...It may not be as professional as you want...but it happens. It's OK. I think genetic counselors sometimes don't feel like sharing their personalities, being authentic. If you pull out your little diagrams and all you want to do is point to things, you're just hiding behind all that science. That's really not what it's all about" (p. 775).

4.6 The Importance of Attending to Patient Affect

Feelings are a universal human experience. Izard (1977) identified 10 universal emotions: interest, enjoyment, surprise, distress, anger, disgust, contempt, fear, shame, and guilt. These feelings can be broadly categorized by domain and by intensity:

- *Domain*—The type of emotion. Feelings are either pleasant (e.g., happy) or unpleasant (e.g., sad).
- *Intensity*—The degree or level of emotion. Feelings can range on a continuum from mild (e.g., irritated) to moderate (e.g., angry) to extreme (e.g., furious).

Although feelings may be experienced universally, the ways in which patients will express their emotions is very culture-specific. Also, the types of events and situations that trigger specific emotions have a strong cultural component.

Patient feelings are a critical part of the genetic counseling process (Kessler 1999). Some patients may use feeling words frequently, but not *hear* them. When reflected back to them, they may be able to hear their feelings and come to terms with them. Furthermore, patients often "...have mixed feelings and are not sure themselves about what they feel. This confusion can interfere with an interview unless the feelings are clarified" (Pedersen and Ivey 1993, p. 150).

Primary empathy allows you to recognize and label patient feelings. When you tentatively reflect patient feelings, you help to clarify them. However, be sure to observe patient reactions, as their responses may indicate the accuracy of your reflections. In order to recognize and label feelings accurately, Pedersen and Ivey (1993) suggest that you:

- Listen for feeling words.
- Watch for clues about feelings in patient nonverbals.
- Reflect feelings back to the patient in your own words.
- Use a basic sentence stem that reflects the way the patient talks (e.g., "It looks like…" for a visual patient, "It sounds like…" for an auditory patient, "It feels like…" for a tactile patient).
- State the situation in which the feelings occurred (e.g., "It looks like you feel… because….).
- Check for accuracy (e.g., "Am I correct in thinking you're scared to make this decision alone?").

4.7 Cultural Empathy

"Basic counseling skills such as attentive listening, empathy, and respect form the foundations of successful cross cultural communication. Genetic counselors should also explore the varied worldviews, beliefs and values of each client, as relevant to the situation at hand...By taking the culturally humble approach and learning from our clients, we avoid stereotyping and keep the focus on the client's specific needs" (Steinberg Warren n.d.). Steinberg Warren and Wilson (2013) note that as genetic counselors, "We use empathy in all genetic counseling sessions to understand the client's experiences, emotions, and perceptions of the world, and we determine how our client's behaviors and decisions are influenced" (p. 7).

Given growing attention to and awareness of cultural differences, some authors further refine the concept of empathy. Ridley (1995; Ridley and Lingle 1996) coined the term "cultural empathy" to describe empathy that is sensitive to patient culture in psychological counseling. Cultural empathy is based on three principles:

- Every patient should be understood from her or his unique frame of reference.
- Normative information (e.g., data about what people do on average, statistics about the *typical* person) does not always fit a particular patient, although it can be useful as background information.
- People are a dynamic blend of multiple roles and identities.

Cultural empathy occurs when counselors demonstrate and communicate "an understanding of the client's worldview and [acknowledge] the cultural differences between them" (Chung and Bemak 2002, p. 155). Cultural empathy involves two components—understanding and responsiveness:

Cultural empathic *understanding* entails:

(a) *Cultural self-other differentiation*—examining your own cultural identity and values and learning about the patient's cultural identity and values. Chung and Bemak (2002) note that "…one of the major cognitive tasks in achieving cultural empathy is for counselors to differentiate their cultural self and their strong cultural biases from those of their clients" (p. 157).
(b) *Perspective-taking*—developing an understanding of the patient's culture and using this understanding to see the patient in his/her cultural context.
(c) *Probing for insight*—collecting information about the patient's entire self-experience and asking clarifying questions. (Open-ended questions, discussed in Chap. 5, can be useful.)

Cultural empathic *responsiveness* entails:

(a) *Conveying interest*—in learning more about the patient's cultural values (e.g., "Tell me more about how this is viewed in your culture")
(b) *Expressing naïveté*—with respect to the patient's cultural experience (e.g., "What *is* it like for you as a member of this religious community?")
(c) *Verbally disclosing*—to the patient your understanding of the patient's self-experience (e.g., through paraphrasing, reflecting, summarizing)

Chung and Bemak (2002, pp. 157–158) recommend that counselors:

- Affirm their patient's cultural experience.
- Clarify language and other cultural communication modes.
- Express a desire to be helpful.
- Understand and accept the context of a patient's family and community.

- Incorporate the indigenous healing practices of the patient's culture when possible.
- Become knowledgeable about patients' historical and sociopolitical background and be sensitive to oppression, discrimination, and racism encountered by many.
- Be knowledgeable about acculturation issues for patients who have moved from one place to another.
- Facilitate empowerment for patients who feel under-advantaged and undervalued.

Ridley and Udipi (2002) provide several recommendations regarding cultural empathy, including asking patients whether your perceptions are correct, never pretending to understand, taking time to consider patients' comments and to formulate a response instead of responding immediately to what they said, respecting a patient's need for silence to digest what is being discussed, and engaging in self-reflection about one's own cultural assumptions and stereotypes. Specific to empathy, the authors recommend that "…counselors should not assume that clients of other cultures place the same importance on empathy as do members of the counselors' own cultures. Instead, they should try to determine their clients' attitudes towards empathy and how empathy is expressed in the clients' cultures" (p. 327).

Williams and Abeles (2004) provide an excellent example of cultural empathy in their article on counseling individuals from the Deaf community. They note that similar to other minorities, members of the Deaf community experience effects of oppression such as "a greater incidence of substance abuse, unemployment or underemployment, isolation/segregation from others, and distrust of members of the mainstream society (Glickman 1996). The fact that Deaf individuals do not communicate using the dominant language of the society may further isolate them from their parents and other family members (Harvey 1982)" (p. 643). They further note "More than 90% of Deaf children are born to hearing parents who have little or no previous experience with deafness and are not able to provide a language model for their children (Schirmer 2001). Without effective language interactions, Deaf individuals may have limited ability to express themselves with others and may also struggle to label their own experiences, thoughts, and feelings (Corker 1996; Pollard 1998)" (p. 643). The language barrier poses a major challenge. "Deaf clients may wait for the therapist to prompt conversation and may provide short, simple responses that lack richness and content (Hoyt et al. 1981; Pollard 1998)" (p. 644). The authors note the importance of self-awareness of how one feels about working with Deaf individuals, including the therapist's cultural assumptions and feelings of competence (or lack thereof) in counseling Deaf individuals.

Browner et al. (2003) interviewed pregnant Mexican-American women who screened positive for possible birth defects to explore the extent to which miscommunication with their genetic counselor affected their decision to pursue or decline amniocentesis. Among their results they found "clients who do not feel that their views have been listened to and respected, are less likely to listen to and respect the counselor's guidance" (p. 1945).

Barlow-Stewart et al. (2006) conducted a study illustrating the importance of cultural empathy. They studied Chinese-Australians' beliefs about inheritance and kinship and their implications for cancer genetic counseling and education regarding hereditary cancer. They found level of acculturation was not associated with an individual's beliefs (be they either Western or traditional concepts); members within families may hold differing beliefs; the family plays a role in decision-making; and a patrilineal concept of kinship, common in the Chinese-Australian community, can affect family history taking. The authors recommended gaining awareness of these factors, adopting a nonjudgmental attitude regarding cultural beliefs, and making efforts to avoid stereotyping individuals.

Charles et al. (2006) compared culturally tailored genetic counseling versus standard genetic counseling in a sample of African American women at risk for BRCA 1/2 mutations and found women who received the culturally tailored counseling reported greater satisfaction and a greater reduction in their worries than women who received the standard counseling. Specific to cultural empathy, the culturally tailored approach included questions that invited discussion of the women's cultural beliefs and values and how they apply to health-care decisions and coping with medical concerns. The questions addressed three aspects of worldviews common in the African American community—communalism, spirituality, and a flexible temporal worldview.

In sum, "Before counselors can respond in a culturally empathic manner, it is essential that they perceive each client as a unique individual with his or her own particular experiences" (Chung and Bemak 2002, p. 156). Cultural empathy requires you to *see the world* the way your patients see it, rather than imposing your own *take* on the situation. You must be able to step out of your own frame of reference to view a situation the way the patient views it and seek information about your patient's beliefs (Brown 1997).

4.8 Common Empathy Mistakes

Empathy mistakes tend to be due either to genetic counselors' covert processes (their beliefs, assumptions, attitudes, etc.) or to overt processes (their actual behaviors).

4.8.1 Mistakes Due to Covert Processes

- *Over-identifying*—When you over-identify, you *feel too much* with your patient. Empathy involves sensing "...the client's world as if it were your own, but without ever losing the 'as if' quality...[and sensing] the client's anger, fear, or confusion as if it were your own, yet without your own anger, fear, or confusion getting bound up in it" (Rogers 1992, p. 829). If you lose the *as if* quality, the result is not empathy but identification with the patient (Barrett-Lennard 1981) or what some authors (e.g., Kessler 1998) refer to as countertransference (we discuss countertransference in greater detail in Chap. 12). Feeling as angry or as sad as patients do about their situations usually is ineffective. You no longer understand your patient's experience, but rather you become caught up in your own feelings and perceptions. Another problem with counselor identification occurs when your emotional reaction to the patient is too intense, what Gladstein (1983) calls *empathic distress*. In this situation, you are likely to psychologically *move away* from the patient (e.g., avoiding a discussion of patient feelings, offering false reassurance that everything will be ok). An important aspect of empathy is the ability to maintain some boundaries between yourself and your patient's experience. You must be able to *step back* after sensing a patient's feelings, thus giving yourself some distance from the affect (Barrett-Lennard 1981; Rogers 1992). One way to understand and address over-identification is to discuss it with your clinical supervisor.

- *Making assumptions*—You should be careful about assuming your patients will feel exactly what you would feel, as this may not be the case. For example, suppose you have a baby with a cleft lip and palate and you quickly come to view this as a minor and treatable condition. Some of your patients may be devastated by the same condition in their child.
- *Being afraid of patient feelings*—During genetic counseling, patients may experience a range of emotions, some of which are frightening. Your fear of certain emotions may be due to mistaken beliefs. For instance, you (and your patients) may think that if certain feelings are identified (e.g., grief, anger), you will both be overwhelmed by them (Schema et al. 2015); or you might believe that only some feelings are acceptable (e.g., sadness), while others are not (e.g., anger, despair). In addition, you may mistakenly believe you must *fix* your patient's feelings, or if they are expressed, you won't know how to handle these emotions (Schema et al. 2015). It's important to remember there are no *right* or *wrong* feelings. People feel what they feel. Furthermore, when patients express emotions, they usually end up feeling more in control. Until patients can get out their sadness, anxiety, anger, etc., they will be less able to digest the information you provide and less capable of making decisions (Schema et al. 2015).
- *Thinking you can't understand if you have not had your patient's experience*—Although you may never have had a family member with a genetic condition, you do have experiences in your own life of loss, disappointment, grief, etc. Your own experience will help you empathize with patient feelings. Of course, you will not have a specific understanding of what it's like to be in every patient's situation (e.g., what it's like to live with a parent who has Huntington disease). In those cases, you might say, "Please tell me about what this is like for you so I can try to understand."
- *Thinking patients are different from non-patients*—They aren't. Patients have the same hopes, fears, anxieties, and beliefs as anyone. Although they might differ from most other people because they have come for assistance with a possible or known genetic condition, the empathic process is the same for genetic counseling patients as it is for all people. As we stated earlier, empathy is an essential ingredient in all human relationships (Duan and Hill 1996). Ask yourself, if you

were sitting with a friend who thought she/he might have a genetic condition, what would you say to empathize? Try using a similar response with your patients.

- *Assuming all patients will respond in the same way*—People may have very different reactions to similar events. One patient may be angry, another sad, and another disbelieving. Patients will also respond in unique ways to your interventions. Therefore, you cannot give a *cookbook response* and get positive results with every patient. There is no *answer key* in genetic counseling, because patients differ in subtle and not-so-subtle ways. For example, consider a prenatal patient who has four children and discovers her current pregnancy is affected with trisomy 18. How might her experience be similar to and different from a prenatal patient who has undergone several years of infertility treatment, has no children, and discovers her pregnancy is affected with trisomy 18? Or, consider the case of a couple who will be returning to their home country of China. They have one daughter, and their second baby is a boy with a fatal disease. In Chinese culture male children are valued highly. The hopes of many Chinese parents rest in having a son to support them in their old age and to carry on the family name. Consider how this couple's experience might be different if they were White and from the USA.
- *Assuming all patients desire the same type and amount of primary empathy*—Patients will vary in their preferences for counselor empathy (Duan and Hill 1996; Gladstein 1983; Ridley and Udipi 2002). Some patients, wanting a close relationship, will desire more affective empathy from you, while others, who wish for a more neutral emotional relationship, will prefer less affective empathy (Gladstein 1983). One clue about the type of relationship a patient wants is his or her reactions to your initial affective empathy statements. If patients do not elaborate and/or seem nonverbally *taken aback*, these may be indications they do not wish you to verbally express a lot of empathy. You should not take this personally or as a sign that something went wrong. Not every patient wants the same type of relationship, and not every patient will *share* no matter how many different ways you try to engage them emotionally.

4.8.2 Mistakes Due to Overt Processes

- *Not replying*—Failure to respond may suggest what your patient said is not worth a response or is not relevant to genetic counseling (Weil 2000). It's a matter of common decency to display some understanding of your patient (Kessler 1999).
- *Using clichés*—Although they often have an element of truth, clichés (e.g., "You can always try to have another baby," "Time heals all wounds," "New treatments are coming along all the time") may seem dismissive of the patient's experience, sound "canned" or trite, and/or suggest you don't want to make an effort to fully engage with them.
- *Offering false reassurance*—Some beginning counselors use a fair number of reassuring statements (e.g., "You seem like you are great parents," "The test results

will probably be negative," "You've really thought this through and can do it," "Most people find this easier to deal with as time passes"). Although well-intentioned and likely related to a belief that you are empowering patients, we caution you about using these types of statements. Unless you include a specific reason to support what you say, patients may feel your comment is gratuitous, and/or not believe you. Before offering reassurance, ask yourself, "Why am I doing this? Whose needs am I addressing? Am I trying to make the patient feel better?" We further caution that it is not always possible to make patients feel better.

- *Focusing too much on either content or affect*—Beginning counselors tend to emphasize content and overlook affect. In addition, Western cultures tend to stress intellect, often at the expense of feelings. To further complicate matters, patients might avoid expressing feelings because they are afraid of losing control and/or are not sure discussing feelings is appropriate in genetic counseling (McCarthy Veach et al. 1999). On the other hand, sometimes counselors emphasize patients' feelings at the expense of content. Too much attention to feelings can prevent you and your patient from moving to goal setting and decision-making. Ultimately, the issue is whether and how their feelings are either facilitating or impeding their ability to hear biomedical information and make decisions. Effective genetic counseling includes a balance of attention to content and affect.
- *Making a content response when you intended to reflect feelings*—If you wish to make an affective reflection, then be sure you identify a feeling. If your response begins "You feel *like*…" or "You feel *that*…," it is probably reflecting the patient's actions or thoughts and not feelings. Often, we think we are stating a feeling when we are actually stating a behavior (e.g., "You feel like you gave this condition to your child") or stating a thought (e.g., "You feel that it's your fault" [actually, you are saying the patient *believes* it is her/his fault]).
- *Prematurely using advanced empathy*—Even if your remark is *on-target*, it may be too threatening unless you have established an initial rapport with your patient, and your patient is ready to hear your interpretation.
- *Using empathy responses inappropriately*—Reflections can encourage patients to continue talking. So, when you are trying to change topics, want a patient to stop talking, or wish to end the session, you should generally avoid reflections.
- *Inaccurate labeling/distorting*—You make statements that are wrong or *miss the mark* with respect to either the feelings or content of your patient's experience (e.g., reflecting to a patient that she seems to have made a decision when she has stated that she can't decide or telling a furious patient that he seems a bit irritated).
- *Pretending to understand*—This is not genuine, and patients will pick up on your pretense.
- *Parroting*—Primary empathy is *not* simply repeating patients' words verbatim. You should communicate the core or essence of patient expressions and do so in your own words.
- *Being long-winded*—Long, rambling primary empathy statements confuse patients. Remember to keep your responses concise and to the point.

- *Jumping in too quickly*—You should avoid interrupting patients (unless their verbosity is hindering the accomplishment of session goals) or thinking you must respond immediately after they speak.
- *Using inappropriate language*—Jargon or words that are too complicated can distance patients. Try to match your patient's language level.
- *Forgetting to use silence*—Silence and a calm presence can be as empathic as anything you might say. Silence allows patients to become aware of their feelings, digest what has been discussed, and collect their thoughts (see Chap. 3 section on silence).
- *Not allowing enough time for patients to respond to your empathy statements*—Silence often seems much longer to a beginning counselor than it actually is. Try mentally counting to 10 or 15 before jumping in; by then, most patients will have responded to your statement. Of course, when patients cannot think of how to say what they want to express (watch for nonverbal indications of this), you can step in with a statement like "It's hard to put into words what you want to say" or "What do you think about what I just said?"
- *Taking sides*—Expressing a lot of empathy for one member of a couple or for certain family members and *forgetting* to do so with the other individuals is divisive and judgmental on your part.
- *Forgetting the cultural context*—As mentioned earlier, empathy can be conveyed quite differently in some populations. Clinicians must recognize the validity of cultural variation, in addition to overarching human commonalities and within group variation (Chung and Bemak 2002; Salzman 1995).

4.9 Typical Concerns About Primary Empathy

Beginning genetic counselors typically have a number of concerns about empathy. In the following sections, we address some common questions.

4.9.1 Why Is Empathy Sometimes Difficult?

Many patients will experience intense, unpleasant emotions. It is a natural human tendency to want to feel pleasant emotions and avoid unpleasant ones. So, patients may avoid expressing and/or acknowledging their unpleasant feelings. Similarly, we may avoid empathizing because we are afraid of feeling our patients' pain.

Reflecting feelings is challenging because "In our culture [U.S.] we learn to comfort people by encouraging them to run away from their feelings. We are taught to say, 'Don't cry, it'll be all right,' when it quite probably won't be all right and the person really needs to cry to release his emotional pain" (Geldard and Anderson 1989, p. 37). Although directly confronting feelings may be uncomfortable for your patients and for you, it is sometimes essential because "At crisis times in our lives the emotional pressure builds up until we are ready to explode. In this state, our thought processes are blocked and we are unable to cope. We feel out of control of ourselves. To regain control, we must first release some of the emotional pressure…" (Geldard and Anderson 1989, p. 39).

Your own background, abilities, and present situation will affect the ease with which you can empathize (cf. Miranda et al. 2016). Your empathy toward a patient is impacted by your "empathic capacity, past experience, motivation to empathize, and affective and cognitive state at the time of the session" (Duan and Hill 1996, p. 268).

Additional reasons (addressed earlier in this chapter) that empathy is difficult include:

- Worry that you won't be able to think of what to say/will lose your train of thought.
- Your own issues get in the way (over-identifying).
- You lack personal experience with a patient's concern and therefore think you're unable to understand.
- Fearing you will be overwhelmed by a patient's emotion.
- Fearing your patient will be overwhelmed.
- Believing you somehow "gave" patients their feelings because you named them.
- Thinking you are responsible for making their feelings stop, for fixing the reason(s) they feel as they do, etc.
- Feeling caught up in the threat—Their story could be your story (see countertransference in Chap. 12).
- Feeling helpless—that your empathy is not enough.
- Thinking you may never be able to stop worrying about/crying about/ruminating about a particular patient.

Strategies to help you engage empathically with patients include:

- Stay as physically relaxed as possible in sessions (deep breathing, relaxed body posture).
- Discuss difficult cases in detail with supervisors.
- Recognize empathy is always necessary and often it is enough.
- Take breaks from your work, when feasible, after a particularly intense case (even 1 day away can help) (Figley 2002).
- Do other professional activities in addition to direct clinical practice (e.g., teaching, public education, research).
- Maintain your physical health.

4.9.2 Is Empathy Different from Sympathy?

Empathy is not the same thing as sympathy (Clark 2010). Vincent (2005) differentiates sympathy and empathy. Sympathy involves "feeling *toward another*," while empathy involves "*insight* into the feelings of another" by "*projecting* your own personality into, fully comprehending and being *in-feeling* with another" (p. 15). Sympathy is *feeling for* a person, and it conveys a one-up/one-down relationship. Empathy is *feeling with*, and it conveys a more equal, collaborative relationship. Sympathy implies pity, while empathy implies trust: "I am saying to my client that he or she is strong enough to solve problems, that I will not condescend pityingly, and that our work together is not just hand holding" (Martin 2000 p. 9). Wispé (1986) asserts that sympathy is "…heightened awareness of another's plight as something to be alleviated, whereas empathy refers to the attempt of one self-aware [individual] to understand the subjective experiences of another" (p. 314).

Glanzer (2006) stresses that "an essential prerequisite to empathy is a sense of self…Empathy always involves differentiation of self and other. This is one reason it is so important for the counselor to know him- or herself" (p. 125). Relatedly, Neumann et al. (2009) note that "…when experiencing empathy, individuals are able to disentangle themselves from others, whereas individuals experiencing sympathy have difficulty maintaining a sense of whose feelings belong to whom" (p. 340). They say a prerequisite for empathy "is that an individual should not be overly preoccupied with himself and his own concerns, because, if the experience is to a greater extent focused on the individual himself, then the willingness to help the other person decreases" (p. 340). The authors further note research findings that fear, anxiety, and distress reduce one's ability to empathize.

In summary, empathy is not:

- Sorrow for a person, which is sympathy
- Concern/worry, which is anxiety
- Judgmental, which says you feel superior
- Critical, which is self-protection
- Reassurance, which is superficial

4.9.3 Is My Empathy Affected if I Have an Experience Like My Patient?

There can be both advantages and disadvantages to having a similar experience to your patient. It can be an *advantage* to have some firsthand experience of what it might be like to be this person. Also, you may gain credibility with a patient who is more likely to think you can really understand. It can be a *disadvantage* if you impose your experience on a patient, rather than listening to how it is for her or him. Additionally, the patient may not disclose as much information because she/he assumes you know it by virtue of having had a similar experience. As we said earlier, you can have empathy without having a similar experience. There is no need to feel inadequate or apologetic for not having had a similar experience. If a patient asks you whether you've had a similar experience, you might try responding matter-of-factly, "No, I haven't. I *have* worked with patients who have had similar situations, but I'd like to try to understand how it is for you" (of course, this response only works if you've actually had patients!). Or try saying, "No, I haven't, but I'd really like to understand what it's like for you. Would you please tell me about it?" (see Chap. 11 on self-reference).

4.9.4 *Won't My Patients Think I'm Just Parroting Their Words?*

No, as long as you use concise responses expressed in your own words. While your responses may seem forced or awkward to you, they allow patients to hear (sometimes for the first time) what they are experiencing and how they sound.

4.9.5 *What Can I Accomplish with Empathy Reflections?*

Sometimes students tell us they feel as if they aren't accomplishing anything if they "only repeat what the patient says." Their comments reflect a Western perspective that highly values problem-solving. What they don't realize is that empathy is a powerful component of effective problem-solving. It provides an initial understanding of the nature of patient concerns and helps patients gain insight about their attitudes, feelings, and real issues (Rubin 2002). Without accurate empathy, you may come up with a great solution. However, it may be a solution to the wrong problem (Egan 1994)!

Additionally, we agree with Kessler (1999) that "...the new genetics increasingly confronts professionals with issues that tend to place them into the role of counselors or therapists rather than educators. The fact that the information they provide is emotionally evocative and intimately connected to the survival of patients requires counselors to make a deeper exploration of the personal meaning patients give to the information" (p. 341). Empathy is an essential skill for this type of exploration.

4.9.6 *Is There Anything I Should Avoid Saying if I Want to Be Empathic?*

We recommend that you *never* say any of the following to your patients:

- "I know exactly how you feel." You don't. You can never get inside another person's skin and have the exact experience. This type of remark can be quite insulting to patients. Furthermore, if patients actually believe it, they may stop describing their experience because they assume you already know all about it.
- "You shouldn't feel that way." This statement is judgmental and may make patients think they are wrong to feel the way that they do. Furthermore, the reality is that the patient *does* feel that way.

- "Everybody feels (or would feel) that way." A remark like this can trivialize the patient's experience.
- "Nobody feels (or would feel) that way." This is another judgmental response suggesting patients are wrong to feel the way they do.
- "*Why* do you feel that way?" "Why" implies judgment and suggests the patient's feeling is not appropriate.

4.10 Closing Comments

Rogers (1992) said empathy and other essential therapist qualities are "qualities of experience, not intellectual information. If they are to be acquired, they must, in my opinion, be acquired through experiential training…" (p. 831). We agree with Rogers that your empathy will increase as you gain experience—lots of it! Moreover, experiences in your professional and personal lives will intertwine to build your empathy skills (Miranda et al. 2016; Wells et al. 2016; Zahm et al. 2016). As you see more genetic counseling patients, you will grow in your capacity to understand them. You may also be able to *speed-up* the process by experimenting, trying different approaches, and discussing the outcomes with your clinical supervisors. Very importantly, reflecting upon your experiences and their meaning for your work as a genetic counselor will help you deepen your empathic understanding and communication. You will increasingly appreciate the diverse responses of patients, recognize subtle differences in emotional responses due to individual and cultural circumstances, and counsel each patient according to his or her specific situation.

4.11 Class Activities

Activity 1: Primary Empathy (Think-Pair-Share Dyads)

Students respond individually in writing to three questions:

- What is empathy?
- Where does empathy come from?
- What functions does empathy serve in genetic counseling?

Next, pairs of students discuss their written responses.
Estimated time: 10–15 min.

Process
Dyads report on their discussion. Instructor summarizes major themes and presents any ideas which did not emerge from the dyads.
Estimated time: 10–15 min.

Instructor Note

- This activity could also be done in groups of three to four students.
- Instead of writing individually, students can think about their responses to the questions for a couple of minutes and then discuss with a partner.
- This activity could be assigned as a paper.

Activity 2a: Low-Level Empathy Skills Model

Instructor and a volunteer genetic counseling patient engage in a role-play in which the counselor demonstrates poor primary empathy (refer to common mistakes in primary empathy for ideas on how to model a low skill level). Students observe and take notes of examples of poor empathy.

Estimated time: 5 min.

Process

Students share their examples of poor empathy. Then they discuss with the instructor the impact of the counselor's poor empathy on the patient. The patient can offer her or his impressions of the counselor's behaviors after the other students have made their comments.

Estimated time: 10 min.

Activity 2b: High-Level Empathy Skills Model

Instructor and the same volunteer repeat the same role-play; only this time the counselor displays good primary empathy skills. Students take notes of examples of good empathy skills.

Estimated time: 5 min.

Process

Students share their examples of good empathy. Then they discuss with the instructor the impact of the counselor's empathy on the patient. As part of the discussion they contrast this role-play to the low-level role-play.

Estimated time: 10 min.

Instructor Note

- Students could work together in Think-Pair-Share dyads to identify empathy examples and their impact on the patient.
- Students can also comment upon attending skills, but the focus of the processing should be on primary empathy.

Activity 3: Cliché Brainstorming (Small Groups)

Small groups of students brainstorm clichés which might be said to genetic counseling patients (e.g., time heals all wounds). This exercise could also be done in dyads or individually. Students share their clichés with the large group and then discuss with the instructor why people use clichés and what impact they might have on genetic counseling patients.

Estimated time: 15–20 min.

Instructor Note

- In processing the large group discussion, ask students to think about positive reasons (e.g., to put a person at ease) and negative reasons (e.g., when you don't know what to say) people use clichés and also identify possible positive effects (might make the counselor seem more relatable) and negative effects (e.g., patient may feel devalued).
- A variation of this activity is to interview genetic counselors and ask them to describe the most offensive and outrageous things other people have said to their patients about their genetic situations.

Activity 4: Domain/Intensity of Feelings (Small Groups)

As stated in the chapter, in order to be effective, an empathic response needs to be accurate with respect to domain (positive or negative) and intensity (level of emotion). Students write a 4- or 5-sentence description of a concern they might have if they were a genetic counseling patient. They should not state any *feelings* about the concern in their description. Next the instructor asks for a student volunteer to read her/his sentences to the class *matter-of-factly* without conveying feelings either verbally or nonverbally. Students brainstorm possible feelings. As each feeling is identified, the instructor asks whether it is positive or negative and mild, moderate, or intense. The instructor list students' feeling words on a blackboard or newsprint. After the students have finished brainstorming, the instructor asks the volunteer to select the feelings that come closest to what she would feel as this genetic counseling patient.

For example, the situation involves a positive prenatal screening test. The student volunteer writes: "I just found out there might be something wrong with the baby. The pregnancy has been going along so well. This is not what I expected. What if it's something really awful? Maybe the test is wrong." The student reads these sentences in a monotone voice and perhaps sits with her back to the group in order to avoid giving any cues about her feelings. Next the group brainstorms possible emotions and where they think the emotions would be on the following chart:

	Positive feeling domain	Negative feeling domain
Mild intensity	Hopeful; doubtful	Uneasy
Moderate intensity		Surprised, anxious, worried, concerned, caught off guard, upset, frightened, afraid, alarmed
Strong intensity		Shocked, stunned, terrified, panicked

Finally, the student volunteer identifies which of the feelings are closest to what she is feeling.

Estimated time: 15 min.

Process

Students respond to the following questions:

- What was challenging about this activity?
- Were you able to choose the right domain? The right intensity?
- Can you see how easy it is to choose the wrong intensity?
- Do you think it's more ineffective to choose the wrong intensity or the wrong domain?

Estimated time: 15 min.

Instructor Note

- This activity can be repeated with several volunteers.

Activity 5: Primary Empathy Round Robin Exercise

Round 1

Students work in a circle with the instructor. The instructor goes first to demonstrate the activity. The instructor asks the student beside her/him, Student A, to say two or three sentences that a genetic counseling patient might say about her or his situation. Then the instructor uses *Concise Own Words*—summarizing the most important content *without* labeling feelings. Next Student A turns to Student B who says two or three sentences about a *different* patient situation, and Student A provides a Concise Own Words response to Student B's patient sentences. Continue this process around the circle until everyone has had the chance to be both counselor and a patient.

Round 2

For the next round, using the same patient situations/sentences, the counselor makes a *Content and Affective* response—the counselor should use the formula "You feel…because…."

Example Pt: "I'm glad we went ahead with the prenatal testing. I can't wait to tell my husband the good news! We were so worried about our baby having muscular dystrophy."

Round 1:
Co: The test gave you the news you wanted to hear. (Concise Own Words response—content without labeling feelings).

Round 2:
Co: "You feel very relieved because of this good news and you're excited to share it." (Content and Affective response).
Estimated time: 20–30 min.

Instructor Note
- For each round, the instructor should reinforce good responses. If a student's response is way off base or is too verbatim (mimicking) the patient's statement, ask the group, "Does anyone else have some other ideas about how to respond?

Activity 6: Primary Empathy Skills (Small Group Role-Play)

Form small groups (four to five students). In each small group, the instructor pretends to be a genetic counseling patient. The *patient* begins by talking about why she/he came for genetic counseling. Next, one of the small group members, Student A, counsels the patient for two or three interchanges in which Student A uses primary empathy responses. Then the next student, Student B, becomes the counselor and continues to counsel the patient for two or three responses. The process continues until each student has had the opportunity to be the counselor for this patient. Halfway through the process, the group should stop and discuss what they *know* about the patient so far, what else they may need to cover via primary empathy, etc. This discussion can also be done whenever a student gets *stuck* while in the counselor role.

Estimated time: 30–40 min.

Instructor Note
- This exercise helps students practice *conveying* empathy to patients. The discussion midway through the role-play helps them draw upon/strengthen their empathic *understanding*.

Activity 7: Triad Role-Play

Three students practice primary empathy and attending skills in 15 min role-plays taking turns as counselor, patient, and observer. They spend 10 min for feedback after each role-play. The observer should stop the counselor if the counselor appears to be *stuck*.

Criteria for Evaluating Counselor Primary Empathy

- Accuracy
- Aware of content
- Aware of feelings
- Well-timed
- Tentative
- Concise
- Primary, not advanced empathy

Estimated time: 75 min.

Process

In the large group, students discuss what they learned from the role-play, what questions they still have about primary empathy and attending skills, and what they think about the role of empathy skills in genetic counseling.

Estimated time: 10–15 min.

Activity 8: Cultural Empathy Presentations[1]

For this activity, each student will summarize a different selected chapter from Fisher (1996) about the particular cultural group *and* describe selected resources for providing culturally competent care for individuals in the identified population in a 20-min oral presentation.

Students should be given the following instructions:

1. Select a chapter from Fisher to summarize for your classmates.
2. Identify *additional references/resources* for providing culturally competent care for individuals from this population.
3. Prepare a 1–2-page handout summarizing major points of the chapter and the additional resources you identified. Include in your handout an annotated bibliography of the references and resources you used in preparing your presentation.

Estimated time: 20 min per presentation.

4.12 Written Exercises

Exercise 1

Identify two situations in your own life where you have experienced disappointment, loss, grief, etc.

- Describe the situation, what you were feeling, thinking, doing.
- How did you cope with the situation?
- What resources (including other people) did you turn to in order to seek assistance?

[1] Resource: Fisher (1996).

Instructor Note

- This exercise could be done as part of a journal, as a small reflection paper, or verbally with a dyad partner.
- Students should be encouraged to choose examples carefully so they do not inadvertently disclose more than they intended.

Exercise 2

Using the following list of feeling words, generate four or five synonyms for each:

Happy	Anxious	Embarrassed
Sad	Uncertain	Withdrawn
Angry	Responsible	Hopeless
Scared	Reluctant	Rejected
Confused	Torn	Uncomfortable

Example Interested: curious, engaged, involved, invested

Exercise 3

Using the following list of mild intensity feeling words, generate feelings that are at the moderate and strong intensity levels for each one.

Mild intensity	Moderate intensity	Strong intensity
Confused		
Sorry		
Nervous		
Dissatisfied		
Hesitant		
Uncomfortable		
Irritated		
Glad		

Example Mild = puzzled; moderate = surprised; strong = amazed.

Exercise 4

Use the following patient description to construct a dialogue between the genetic counselor and the patient in which the genetic counselor uses *only* primary empathy responses. Formulate eight patient statements and eight counselor statements. [*Hint*:

Avoid the same formula when creating counselor statements, e.g., do not begin every sentence "It sounds like…" and try to use a range of empathy statements (content, affect, content and affect). Read your empathy responses aloud to be sure they are concise and tentative and convey the patient's experience in your own words.]

Patient Description.
A professional couple, both about 25 years old, recently had their first baby. The baby was found to have PKU. The couple has just learned all about the diet and the risk of mental retardation.

Cl Response:
Co Response:

Cl Response:
Co Response:

Cl Response:
Co Response:

Etc.

Exercise 5: Primary Empathy Exercise[2]

I. Identification of Feelings

For each patient statement below, list three to four possible feelings the patient *could* be experiencing when saying the statement. Choose feelings that are close to the surface of what the patient is saying; do not move to advanced empathy (hidden feelings).

- If I'd known the baby would have hemophilia, I'd never have gotten pregnant in the first place.
- If my Huntington test is positive, then my life will be over.
- Why are you talking to me about an abortion? I've already told you that it's not an option!
- How can I even begin to tell my son that he has muscular dystrophy?
- I've already had three miscarriages; I'm not sure I can face another one.
- I don't know why I'm here. I just came because my doctor told me to.
- Can't you tell me anything for certain?
- You have no idea how hard it is to have another child with special needs!
- Since my mother died of breast cancer, my dad doesn't want me or any of my sisters to be tested.
- My sister refuses to give blood so I can figure out if I'm at risk.

[2] Adapted from Danish et al. (1980).

II. Making Content Responses

Construct one concise content response for each of the patient statements in Part I. Write each response as if you were actually speaking to the patient. Be sure that you have summarized the *content*.

III. Making Affect (Feeling-Oriented) Responses

Read each patient statement again. Then write down one affect response for each. When you complete each response, read the patient statement again. Does your response hit the *most important* feeling expressed? Does the response match the *intensity* of feeling expressed by the patient?

Example

Patient Statement:	I can't believe that I gave this disease to my child!
Genetic Counselor:	I. Guilty, remorseful, responsible, ashamed
	II. So, you feel like it's your fault?
	III. It sounds like you feel ashamed

[*Hint*: Read your content and affect responses aloud to be sure they are concise, tentative, and convey the patient's experience in your own words. Avoid using the same formula when creating statements (e.g., do not begin every sentence "It sounds like…" or "You feel…).]

Exercise 6: Primary Empathy Letter to Your Genetic Counselor[3]

Imagine that you and your partner have an appointment to see a genetic counselor because you (or your partner) had an abnormal ultrasound finding and subsequent testing confirms the diagnosis of Down syndrome in your baby (Slendokova 2005). Write a letter to the genetic counselor in which you describe your *thoughts* and *feelings*, what you *expect* about the genetic counseling appointment, and what you *want* from the counselor.

Instructor Note

- This exercise could be done as part of a journal, as a small reflection paper, or with a dyad partner.
- The exercise can be varied for any genetic counseling specialty and for any patient indication.

[3]Adapted from Slendokova (2005) and from research by Siemińska et al. (2002) involving an intervention to develop sensitivity to health-care patients.

- The letters generated by students could be used for genetic counseling role-plays. The "patient" could either act out the content from her/his own letter or from a classmate's letter.

Exercise 7: Role-Play

Engage in a 15-min role-play of a genetic counseling session with a classmate. The role-play can be based on a patient you saw in clinic or it can be a made-up patient situation. During the role-play, focus on primary empathy and attending skills. Audio record the role-play. Next transcribe the role-play and critique your work. Use the following method for transcribing the session:

Counselor	Patient	Self-critique	Instructor
Key phrases of dialogue	Key phrases	Comment on your own responses	Will provide feedback on your responses

Create a brief summary:

1. Briefly describe patient *demographics* (e.g., age, gender, ethnicity, socioeconomic status, relationship status) and *reason* for seeking genetic counseling.
2. Identify *two* things you said/did during the role-play that were effective and *two* things you could have done differently.

Give the recording, transcript/self-critique, and summary to the instructor who will provide feedback.

[*Hint*: This assignment encourages self-reflective practice regarding your clinical performance. The goal is not to do a perfect session. Rather the goal is to assess the extent to which you can accurately assess your psychosocial counseling skills. You will gain more from this exercise if you refrain from scripting what you plan to say as the counselor].

References

Abrams LJ, Kessler S. The inner world of the genetic counselor. J Genet Couns. 2002;11:5–17.

Anonymous. My story: a genetic counselor's journey from provider to patient: a mother's story. J Genet Couns. 2008;17:412–8.

Azar B. Defining the trait that makes us human. Am Psychol. 1997;28:1–15.

Barlow-Stewart K, Yeo SS, Meiser B, Goldstein D, Tucker K, Eisenbruch M. Toward cultural competence in cancer genetic counseling and genetics education: lessons learned from Chinese-Australians. Genet Med. 2006;8:24–32.

Barrett-Lennard GT. The empathy cycle: refinement of a nuclear concept. J Couns Psychol. 1981;28:91–100.

Bellcross C. A genetic counselor's story of birth, grief, and survival. J Genet Couns. 2012;21:169–72.

Bellet PS, Maloney MJ. The importance of empathy as an interviewing skill in medicine. JAMA. 1991;266:1831–2.

Brown D. Implications of cultural values for cross-cultural consultation with families. J Couns Dev. 1997;76:29–35.
Browner CH, Preloran HM, Casado MC, Bass HN, Walker AP. Genetic counseling gone awry: miscommunication between prenatal genetic service providers and Mexican-origin clients. Soc Sci Med. 2003;56:1933–46.
Charles S, Kessler L, Stopfer JE, Domchek S, Halbert CH. Satisfaction with genetic counseling for BRCA1 and BRCA2 mutations among African American women. Patient Educ Couns. 2006;63:196–204.
Chung RC, Bemak F. The relationship of culture and empathy in cross-cultural counseling. J Couns Dev. 2002;80:154–9.
Clark A. Empathy and sympathy: therapeutic distinctions in counseling. J Ment Health Couns. 2010;32:95–101.
Cohen SA. Lifetime continuing education: learning from my son. J Genet Couns. 2002;11:281–4.
Corker M. Deaf transitions: images and origins of deaf families, deaf communities, and deaf identities. London: Jessica Kingsley; 1996.
Danish SJ, D'Augelli AR, Hauer AL. Helping skills: a basic training program. New York: Human Sciences Press; 1980.
Duan C, Hill CE. The current state of empathy research. J Couns Psychol. 1996;43:261–74.
Duric V, Butow P, Sharpe L, Lobb E, Meiser B, Barratt A, et al. Reducing psychological distress in a genetic counseling consultation for breast cancer. J Genet Couns. 2003;12:243–64.
Egan G. The skilled helper. Pacific Grove/Monterey, CA: Brooks/Cole; 1994.
Eisenberg N, Eggum ND. Emprathic responding: sympathy and personal distress. In: Decety J, Ickes W, editors. The social neuroscience of empathy. Cambridge, MA: MIT Press; 2009. p. 71–83.
Elliott R, Bohart AC, Watson JC, Greenberg LS. Empathy. Psychotherapy. 2011;48:43–9.
Figley CR. Compassion fatigue: psychotherapists' chronic lack of self care. J Clin Psychol. 2002;58:1433–41.
Fine SF, Glasser PH. The first helping interview. Thousand Oaks, CA: Sage; 1996.
Fisher NL, editor. Cultural and ethnic diversity: a guide for genetics professionals. Baltimore, MD: JHU Press; 1996.
Geldard D, Anderson G. A training manual for counsellors: basic personal counselling. Springfield, IL: Charles C. Thomas; 1989.
Gladstein GA. Understanding empathy: integrating counseling, developmental, and social psychology perspectives. J Couns Psychol. 1983;30:467–82.
Gladstein GA. Empathy and counseling: explorations in theory and research. New York: Springer; 2012.
Glanzer PD. Psychological approaches to deep empathy. In: Walz GR, Bleuer JC, Yep RK, editors. Vistas: compelling perspectives on counseling 2006. Alexandria, VA: American Counseling Association; 2006. p. 125–7.
Glessner HD. Will my voice be heard? J Genet Couns. 2012;21:189–91.
Glickman NS. What is culturally affirmative psychotherapy? In: Glickman NS, Harvey MA, editors. Culturally affirmative psychotherapy with deaf persons. Mahwah, NJ: Erlbaum; 1996. p. 1–55.
Greenberg LS, Pascual-Leone A. Emotion in psychotherapy: a practice-friendly research review. J Clin Psychol. 2006;62:611–30.
Harvey MA. The influence and utilization of an interpreter for deaf persons in family therapy. Am Ann Deaf. 1982;127:821–7.
Hatten B. Pregnancy and genetic counseling: the other side of the fence. J Genet Couns. 2002;11:299–300.
Hill CE. Helping skills: facilitating exploration, insight, and action. 4th ed. Washington, DC: American Psychological Association; 2014.
Hoyt MF, Siegelman EY, Schlesinger HS. Special issues regarding psychotherapy with the deaf. Am J Psychiatry. 1981;138(6):807–11.

Imel ZE, Barco JS, Brown HJ, Baucom BR, Baer JS, Kircher JC, Atkins DC. The association of therapist empathy and synchrony in vocally encoded arousal. J Couns Psychol. 2014;61:146–53.
Izard CE. Human emotions. New York: Plenum; 1977.
Kao JH. Walking in your patient's shoes: an investigation of genetic counselor empathy in clinical practice. University of Minnesota. 2010. Retrieved from the University of Minnesota Digital Conservancy, http://hdl.handle.net/11299/96724.
Keilman K. Genetic counselor or patient—who am I today? J Genet Couns. 2002;11:289–92.
Kessler S. Psychological aspects of genetic counseling: XII. More on counseling skills. J Genet Couns. 1998;7:263–78.
Kessler S. Psychological aspects of genetic counseling: XIII. Empathy and decency. J Genet Couns. 1999;8:333–43.
Knafo A, Zahn-Waxler C, Van Hulle C, Robinson JL, Rhee SH. The developmental origins of a disposition toward empathy: genetic and environmental contributions. Emotion. 2008;8:737–52.
Martin DG. Counseling and therapy skills. 2nd ed. Prospect Heights, IL: Waveland Press; 2000.
McCarthy Veach P, LeRoy BS. Defining moments in genetic counselor professional development: one decade later. J Genet Couns. 2012;21:162–6.
McCarthy Veach P, Truesdell SE, LeRoy BS, Bartels DM. Client perceptions of the impact of genetic counseling: an exploratory study. J Genet Couns. 1999;8:191–216.
McCarthy Veach P, Bartels DM, LeRoy BS. Defining moments: catalysts for professional development. J Genet Couns. 2002a;11:277–80.
McCarthy Veach P, Bartels DM, LeRoy BS. Defining moments: important lessons for genetic counselors. J Genet Couns. 2002b;11:333–7.
McCarthy Veach P, Bartels DM, LeRoy BS. Coming full circle: a Reciprocal-Engagement Model of genetic counseling practice. J Genetic Couns. 2007;16:713–28.
Meiser B, Irle J, Lobb E, Barlow-Stewart K. Assessment of the content and process of genetic counseling: a critical review of empirical studies. J Genet Couns. 2008;17:434–51.
Miranda C, Veach PM, Martyr MA, LeRoy BS. Portrait of the master genetic counselor clinician: a qualitative investigation of expertise in genetic counseling. J Genet Couns. 2016;25: 767–85.
Neumann M, Bensing J, Mercer S, Ernstmann N, Ommen O, Pfaff H. Analyzing the "nature" and "specific effectiveness" of clinical empathy: a theoretical overview and contribution towards a theory-based research agenda. Patient Educ Couns. 2009;74:339–46.
Norcross JC, Wampold BE. Evidence-based therapy relationships: research conclusions and clinical practices. Psychotherapy. 2011;48:98–102.
Pedersen PB, Ivey AE. Culture-centered counseling and interviewing skills: a practical guide. Westport, CT: Praeger/Greenwood; 1993.
Pieterse AH, Ausems MG, Van Dulmen AM, Beemer FA, Bensing JM. Initial cancer genetic counseling consultation: change in counselees' cognitions and anxiety, and association with addressing their needs and preferences. Am J Med Genet A. 2005;137:27–35.
Pollard RQ Jr. Psychopathology. In: Marschark M, Clark MD, editors. Psychological perspectives on deafness, vol. 2. Mahwah, NJ: Erlbaum; 1998. p. 303–30.
Ridley C. Overcoming unintentional racism in counselling and counselling: a practitioner's guide to intentional intervention. Thousand Oaks, CA: Sage; 1995.
Ridley CR, Lingle DW. Cultural empathy in multicultural counseling. In: Pedersen PB, Draguns JG, Lonner WJ, Trimble JE, editors. Counseling across cultures. 4th ed. Thousand Oaks, CA: Sage; 1996. p. 21–46.
Ridley CR, Udipi S. Putting cultural empathy into practice. In: Pedersen PB, Draguns JG, Lonner WJ, Trimble JE, editors. Counseling across cultures. 5th ed. Thousand Oaks, CA: Sage; 2002. p. 317–32.
Rogers CR. The necessary and sufficient conditions of therapeutic personality change. J Consult Clin Psychol. 1992;60:827–32.
Rubin J. Empathy is not enough. In: Breggin PR, Breggin G, Bemak F, editors. Dimensions of empathic therapy. New York: Springer; 2002. p. 29–36.

Runyon M, Zahm KW, Veach PM, MacFarlane IM, LeRoy BS. What do genetic counselors learn on the job? A qualitative assessment of professional development outcomes. J Genet Couns. 2010;19:371–86.
Salzman M. Attributional discrepancies and bias in cross-cultural interactions. J Multicult Couns Devel. 1995;23:181–93.
Schema L, McLaughlin M, Veach PM, LeRoy BS. Clearing the air: a qualitative investigation of genetic counselors' experiences of counselor-focused patient anger. J Genet Couns. 2015;24:717–31.
Schirmer BR. Psychological, social, and educational dimensions of deafness. Boston, MA: Allyn & Bacon; 2001.
Selkirk CG, Veach PM, Lian F, Schimmenti L, LeRoy BS. Parents' perceptions of autism spectrum disorder etiology and recurrence risk and effects of their perceptions on family planning: recommendations for genetic counselors. J Genet Couns. 2009;18:507–19.
Siemińska MJ, Szymańska M, Mausch K. Development of sensitivity to the needs and suffering of a sick person in students of medicine and dentistry. Med Health Care Philos. 2002;5:263–71.
Slendokova B. Genetic counseling students' empathic understanding of a prenatal patient's reactions to the diagnosis of down syndrome: a simulation study. Unpublished master's paper, University of Minnesota, Minneapolis, MN; 2005.
Steinberg Warren N. A genetic counseling cultural competence toolkit. n.d.. www.geneticcounselingculturaltoolkit.com/. Accessed 21 Mar 2017.
Steinberg Warren N, Wilson PL. COUNSELING: a 10-point approach to cultural competence in genetic counseling. Perspect Genet Couns. 2013;Q3:6–7.
Stone HW. Brief pastoral counseling. J Pastoral Care Counsel. 1994;48:33–43.
Tluczek A, Koscik RL, Modaff P, Pfeil D, Rock MJ, Farrell PM, et al. Newborn screening for cystic fibrosis: parents' preferences regarding counseling at the time of infants' sweat test. J Genet Couns. 2006;15:277–91.
Valverde KD. Genetic counseling: a new perspective. J Genet Couns. 2002;11:285–7.
VandenLangenberg E. Empathy training in genetic counseling: an investigation of how genetic counselors learn to "walk in their patients' shoes". Retrieved from the University of Minnesota Digital Conservancy; 2012. http://hdl.handle.net/11299/96724.
Vincent S. Being empathic: a companion for counsellors and therapists. Oxford: Radcliffe; 2005.
Weil J. Psychosocial genetic counseling. New York: Oxford University Press; 2000.
Wells DM, Veach PM, Martyr MA, LeRoy BS. Development, experience, and expression of meaning in genetic counselors' lives: an exploratory analysis. J Genet Couns. 2016;25:799–817.
Williams CR, Abeles N. Issues and implications of deaf culture in therapy. Prof Psychol Res Pr. 2004;35:643–8.
Wispé L. The distinction between sympathy and empathy: to call forth a concept, a word is needed. J Pers Soc Psychol. 1986;50:314–21.
Zahm KW, Veach PM, Martyr MA, LeRoy BS. From novice to seasoned practitioner: a qualitative investigation of genetic counselor professional development. J Genet Couns. 2016;25:818–34.
Zanko A, Abrams L. Case report: concurrent Wilson disease and Huntington disease: lightning can strike twice. J Genet Couns. 2015;24:40–5.

Chapter 5
Gathering Information: Asking Questions

Learning Objectives
1. Distinguish among different types of questions.
2. Identify the functions of questions in genetic counseling.
3. Describe culturally sensitive ways to ask questions.
4. Develop questioning skills through self-reflection, practice, and feedback.

5.1 Obtaining Information from Patients

An essential component of genetic counseling is obtaining information about patient situations in order to assess their reasons for seeking genetic counseling; the decisions, if any, they wish to make; and factors that are relevant to their situations. Questioning also aids in diagnosis and risk assessment. Questioning is an important skill for eliciting these types of information. In the first part of this chapter, we define questioning skills and discuss effective and ineffective questioning strategies. Later in the chapter, we discuss a specific type of information-gathering activity—collecting information about patient histories.

5.1.1 Types of Questions

The most direct way to gather information from patients is by asking questions. Two broad categories of questions that are appropriate in genetic counseling are closed-ended and open-ended questions.

Closed-ended questions are questions patients can easily answer with a "yes," "no," or one- or two-word response. Typically closed questions begin with forms of the verb "to be": "When did…," "Is it…," "Do you…," and "Are they…?" (Danish

P. McCarthy Veach et al., *Facilitating the Genetic Counseling Process*,
https://doi.org/10.1007/978-3-319-74799-6_5

et al. 1980). Closed questions explore *specific details*, "Do you have any children?," or they ask about explicit or implied choices such as, "Are you going to have the test done?" (Hughes et al. 1997). Thus, closed questions constrain the patient's response. Closed questions are useful for several reasons including when you need a specific piece of information, when you wish to constrain a rambling or overly verbose patient who is not really answering a previous question, for silent patients, and for content that is uncomfortable or embarrassing for the patient (Brown 1997) (e.g., "What I'm really looking for in your family history is anyone with…"; "Because some conditions occur more frequently in certain ethnic populations, we always ask…").

Variations of closed questions include forced choice and rating questions (Brown 1997). Forced choice questions require a patient to respond to one of two options that you present (e.g., Do you want to do the CF carrier test only or have the full Jewish Ancestry panel carrier test?) rather than a simple yes or no (Brown 1997).

Rating questions ask patients to estimate their behaviors, feelings, beliefs, and/or attitudes on some sort of scale (Brown 1997). For example, you might ask "On a scale of 1(very uncomfortable) to 10 (very comfortable), how are you feeling about your decision to share this information with your family?"

Open-ended questions are questions patients cannot easily answer with a "yes," "no," or one- or two-word response. Typically, open questions begin with words such as "How," "What," "Tell me about," and "I'm wondering about." Open questions explore *processes*. They enrich the interview by inviting patients to freely express their views and experiences. Open questions encourage patients to fill in the gaps with respect to their feelings, thoughts, and situations. For example, you might ask, "How do you feel about the results of your test? Open questions can help patients disclose more fully; they can elicit concrete, detailed information and help you to better understand your patient's situation.

Sternlight and Robbennolt (2008) offer suggestions for lawyers when interviewing clients, and their recommendations are relevant for genetic counselors. For instance, they stress the importance of using open-ended questions. "Such questions are useful, from a psychological standpoint, for a variety of reasons. First, they allow clients to tell the story in the order that makes sense to them…This will encourage clients to tell a more complete story…aid clients' recall…allow clients to provide a level of detail with which they are confident…allow clients to explain their…concerns…and deter attorneys from putting their clients' stories into pre-existing schema…" (p. 540).

Open-ended questions are effective in guiding patient narratives. Djurdjinovic (2009) discusses the importance of giving genetic counseling patients the opportunity to tell their story in their own words. "It is the patient telling a personal story and our attuned listening that allows for assessment of concerns and emotional issues" (p. 136).

The following examples illustrate the types of open and closed questions you might ask patients during genetic counseling:

Closed question	Are you scared?
Open question	How do you feel?
Closed question	Are you concerned about what you will do if the test results are positive?
Open question	What do you think you might do if the test results are positive?
Closed question	Does your husband agree with your decision?
Open question	Tell me about how your husband feels about your decision (this response, although not grammatically a question, is still a question because it requests additional information)

Questions also vary with respect to the complexity of information they request. Sanders (1966) identified six types of questions that differ in their degree of cognitive and emotional complexity. His questions are based on Bloom et al.'s (1956) hierarchical taxonomy of educational objectives:

Memory questions. Require recall or recognition of information.

Example: When did you have the miscarriage?

Translation questions. Require an idea to be expressed in different words.

Example: Can you explain what you mean in another way?

Interpretation questions. Require generalizations of information.

Example: What does a one in ten chance mean for you?

Analysis questions. Require problem-solving through critical reflection about available knowledge.

Example: How can the ways that you've coped with loss in the past help you in this situation?

Synthesis questions. Require problem-solving through original thinking.

Example: Can you think of some ways to approach your family members about testing that you haven't tried yet?

Evaluation questions. Require value judgements.

Example: Which of the options we've discussed fits the best for you?

5.1.2 Functions of Questions in Genetic Counseling

As mentioned earlier, questions serve a variety of purposes in genetic counseling. They help with concrete exploration of a patient's situation, and they provide necessary information to allow you and the patient to determine goals (e.g., identifying what would be helpful for the patient) and taking action on those goals (e.g., patient decision-making). The more information you have about patients' concerns, feelings, motivations, and factors that affect decision-making, the more valid your assessment will be of their goals, and the more helpful you will be in assisting patients in their decision-making processes. In genetic counseling, effective use of questions is also important for gathering information for diagnosis and genetic risk assessment, such as collecting family and medical history.

Wubbolding (1996) lists four functions of questions:

1. To enter the patient's world by asking about their wishes, desires, perceptions, behaviors, etc.
   Example: How are you dealing with your fears about possibly having the breast cancer gene?
2. To gather information.
   Example: Have you had any previous pregnancies?
3. To give information. Sometimes questions subtly communicate information.
   Example: Tell me how you will talk with your child's teachers about his PKU diet challenges. (This question suggests the patient has the knowledge and resources to advocate for her child.)
4. To help patients gain more effective control.
   Example: Please talk about who will be supporting you at home. (This question encourages the patient to formulate an action plan.)

Questions to Obtain Medical and Family History

Questions are most useful when you use them strategically, with a purpose that is clear to you and to your patient. Strategic questioning is particularly appropriate during the family and medical history taking and pedigree construction phase of genetic counseling. This is a highly structured phase of the session in which you use questions to gather specific information from your patients. In order to manage patient expectations, you should explicitly tell patients you will be asking a series of questions to help you understand their medical and family history. For a comprehensive overview of gathering family history, pedigree construction and risk assessment based on family history, see Bennett (2010).

Family history taking is an essential component of genetic counseling because it provides "a basis for making a diagnosis, determining risk, and assessing the needs for patient education and psychosocial support" (Schuette and Bennett 2009, p. 37).

Family history taking is also a good way to begin to establish rapport with a patient. There are several process functions of taking a pedigree:

- Pedigree taking can foster counselor empathy and lead to greater rapport between the genetic counselor and patient(s) (Bennett 2010; Erlanger 1990; Schuette and Bennett 2009).
- Constructing a pedigree puts the patient in the role of expert and the counselor in a one-down position; this can be especially important if patients feel out of control of their situations or are mistrustful of health-care professionals (Erlanger 1990). Patients may be more likely to view themselves as active participants in the etiology and management of their conditions (Stanion et al. 1997).
- Some research suggests patients view pedigree construction positively; for instance, they like to provide information, it makes them feel listened to, and the process eases their anxiety (Erlanger 1990; Rose et al. 1999).
- Pedigree construction can help patients who are uncomfortable with open-ended questions to respond because questions are asked in a more systematic, *matter-of-fact* way (Paradopoulos et al. 1997).
- The pedigree provides a mechanism for considering information about patient risk and serves as a stimulus for discussing genetic risks, relevant tests, and further actions (Bennett 2010; Rose et al. 1999; Schuette and Bennett 2009).
- A pedigree provides an immediate illustration of the family's medical history that can be more easily updated, and important information can later be located more easily as compared to a narrative report (Paradopoulos et al. 1997; Stanion et al. 1997).

Questions to Meet Genetic Counseling Goals

Research shows that genetic counselors use questions to achieve the Reciprocal-Engagement Model (REM) goals associated with promoting understanding and appreciation of the patient, providing support and guidance, facilitating decision-making, and providing patient-centered education (Redlinger-Grosse et al. 2017). Examples include open-ended and closed-ended questions about how much information patients would like and their prior knowledge, emotional impact of genetic information, anticipated feelings about information, patients' communication with family members, family members' decision-making and reaction to crisis, cultural context in decision-making, patients' support persons and experience with crisis situations, and impact of options on family.

Miranda et al. (2016) interviewed a sample of master genetic counselors and found all but one described the importance of "attunement to their patients' emotions" (p. 772). They achieved this attunement "by using intuitive and perceptive skills (e.g., 'There's this internal dialogue: What else is going on here? What do I need to do to get to that place with them?'), life experience, immediacy, and *strategic questioning* [emphasis ours] to connect and provide an opening for emotional conversation" (p. 772). Note, their use of questions includes internal ones that you should ask yourself, while others are questions you would ask patients.

Ellington et al. (2005) content analyzed 167 cancer genetic counseling pretest sessions conducted by one of three genetic counselors. They found that the sessions included "both closed and open-ended questions of any nature (e.g., medical, psychosocial, and family history)" (p. 379). The genetic counseling sessions ranged in length from about 73–81 min, and the number of questions counselors asked ranged from 9 to 206 (mean = 84). The researchers concluded, "Despite counselors devoting the major portion of the sessions to presenting information, the number of questions the counselors asked…indicates that they were also eliciting a substantial amount of information" (p. 383).

Questions that Encourage Reflection

Sarangi et al. (2004) studied genetic counselors' use of reflective frames with patients during Huntington disease (HD) counseling sessions. They defined reflective frames as "exploring the psychosocial and the social relational dimension of decision making about predictive testing and its future implications" (p. 137). Reflective frames invite patients "…to offer a display of their understanding of the decision-making procedure as well as their readiness to adjust to favorable, unfavorable, or indeterminate results arising out of testing. From the genetic counseling perspective, clients need to think through the intended and unintended consequences of having a test and do so in the clinical context of 'here and now'" (p. 138). They identified six types of reflective questions that occurred across initial and second appointments with patients (pp. 141–142):

1. *Nonspecific invites*—open-ended questions that invite patients to describe their agenda and to raise any issues of concern (e.g., "When you came here today, what were the issues you wanted to raise?").
2. *Awareness and anxiety*—questions that explore patients' and their family members' experiences of living at risk (e.g., "How much do you worry about HD?" "What is your intuition about your HD status?").
3. *Decisions about testing*—questions that explore how they reached their testing decision and their primary motivations, whether timing of the decision is right, and how other family members feel about the patients' decision to have the test (e.g., "What has made you think about having the test now?").
4. *Impact of result*—questions assessing patients' coping strategies and consequences for them and their family members if the result is positive or negative (e.g., "How do you think you would deal with knowing…?").
5. *Dissemination*—questions that explore who the patient may wish to tell, when, and how (e.g., "Who do you think you will tell?" "How will you go about telling them?").

6. *Other*—questions that tend to explore patients' personality and general coping strategies as well as general family dynamics and future aspirations (e.g., "What are your feelings about having children?).

Sarangi et al. (2005) conducted further research on patients' reactions to genetic counselor use of reflective frames during HD counseling sessions. They found some patients "take up the opportunity to engage in self-reflection, and thus endorse the legitimacy of the reflective frame. At the other extreme, clients may implicitly or explicitly challenge the relevance of self-reflection" (p. 29). The researchers concluded that some patients have a greater need to "prove their readiness" for predictive testing and thus are more responsive to reflective frames. These findings illustrate the importance of assessing and respecting individual and cultural differences with regard to the type and number of questions you ask.

Exploring Perceptions and Values Clarification

Genetic counselors can use questions to assess patient perceptions about genetic conditions or genetic risk. Questions can also be used to help patients better understand their perceptions and values and to facilitate decisions. Farrelly et al. (2012) content analyzed 93 transcripts of simulated prenatal patient genetic counseling sessions. The results of this study illustrate the importance of using questions strategically to facilitate patient and counselor understanding of patient perceptions and values. For example, many counselors asked patients about their personal experiences with disability, and half of the counselors asked patients if they had thought about how they might use the results of prenatal screening.

Regarding questions about patients' personal experiences with disability, the researchers found that "The majority of genetic counselors (86%) asked the simulated client very general level questions, such as 'Have you heard of Down syndrome?' or 'Are you familiar with Down syndrome?'" A smaller number of genetic counselors (38%) asked personal questions, such as "Do you know someone with Down syndrome?" Of note, most of the transcripts that demonstrated the genetic counselor asking about the simulated client's experience with disability showed the genetic counselor asking the question, only to move forward without acknowledging or further exploring the client's response. [Examples from this paper follow:]

> Genetic counselor: So, are either of you familiar with what happens with Down syndrome? Or are you familiar with Down syndrome at all?
> Client: I met some kids with Down syndrome so that's really about it.
> Genetic counselor: OK. Well this is what happens in Down syndrome, why this test, the amniocentesis, can really give you an answer as to whether the baby has it or not...

In some of the transcripts, genetic counselors did explore the patient's experiences and how those experiences informed the patient's knowledge of Down syndrome:

> Genetic counselor: Are you familiar at all with Down syndrome?
> Client: Yeah, I drive a bus and some of the kids on my school bus have Down syndrome.
> Genetic counselor: And so kind of tell me about the kids…" (pp. 818–819).
>
> The researchers noted, however, that "Only a small fraction of these genetic counselors directly asked if the client had thought about what life might be like if they had a child with disabilities. These questions have different aims. Questioning a client about what she will do with the results from prenatal testing is aimed at the outcome: will an affected pregnancy be terminated or will the patient continue with the pregnancy, keeping the child or offering the child up for adoption? Such a question may provide insight about the client's perception of disability, but it does not necessarily facilitate informed decision-making. Instead, by asking if the client has thought about what it would be like to raise a child with disabilities, genetic counselors will position themselves to directly address questions or misinformation about disability" (p. 821).

5.1.3 Asking Questions Effectively

Know **When** *to Ask a Question*

There are three times when a question can be particularly effective:

- *When you have a clear reason for asking a question.* The ultimate test of a question is whether it will be helpful to your patient (Hill 2014). Before asking a question, consider whether you would know what to say if your patient asked why you want to know.
- *When you want to gather more information and/or clarify patient meaning*. You may not have the same definitions as your patients for certain words and experiences.
- *When you don't understand.* One of the biggest mistakes you can make is to assume you understand without checking out those assumptions with your patient (Spitzer Kim 2009). Questions help to clarify your misperceptions.

Know **How** *to Ask a Question*

- *Use questions strategically.* Questions lead the patient, and therefore they are very directive. For example, if your patient says, "My husband doesn't agree with my decision about prenatal testing." You could respond, "Tell me more about the discussions you had with your husband about this," "Is this upsetting to you?," "How do you usually handle disagreements?," and "What is your understanding of his reasons for not wanting you to have this test?" Each of these questions would take the conversation in a very different direction. Be sure you know which direction you want to go. Also, the indiscriminate use of questions may cause patients to withdraw (Guimarães et al. 2013). It's tempting to ask questions because they fill silences (something beginning counselors are uncomfortable with), and they *demand* that patients respond (Martin 2015). You should be careful about relying too much on them. As you gain experience, you will appreciate the value of interspersing empathy and silence with questions.

- *Be specific and comprehensive.* When gathering information, ask about your patient's thoughts, feelings, behaviors, and social systems (family, culture, peers, etc.) (Hackney and Bernard 2017). You should also request *concrete examples* (Hill 2014). For instance, a genetic counselor might ask: "What are your thoughts about genetic testing?," How do you feel about your risk for developing breast cancer?," "How do you usually make decisions?," and "When you need support, who do you call?"
- When discussing important topics, Fontaine and Hammond (1994) recommend that you "...remember three Cs: Be concrete in getting specific details about the events, ask about the context of the event, and look for conceptual themes in the client's stories about his or her life...Don't be afraid to ask for more facts. It is often in the retelling that important information is revealed or emotional connections are made" (p. 225). For example, a patient is referred for carrier testing for Duchenne muscular dystrophy (DMD). As you are obtaining the family history, the patient begins to cry. Questions you might ask include "How old were you when your brother died?" (concrete), "Tell me about your relationship with your brother?" (context), and "What was it like you for growing up with a brother with muscular dystrophy?" (conceptual themes).
- *Be systematic.* Stay with one topic before jumping to others. Follow up on content from your patient's previous statement, or bring your patient back to a topic if the patient is *topic-hopping*. Begin with more general questions and ones that are easier and less threatening to answer. Gradually move to more specific questions concerning more complex or more threatening issues. For example, a genetic counselor might begin by asking "What is your understanding of why your doctor referred you for genetic counseling?" (general) and "What do you already know about your screening test results?" (more specific). "How do you feel about your increased risk?" (more complex and potentially threatening)
- *Keep questions simple.* Ask one question at a time. Patients will be confused if you string several questions together in one response. For example, "What do you think about your risk for being a CF carrier, and do you think you might be interested in carrier testing, or prenatal diagnosis?" You should separate these into a series of questions.
- *Avoid interrogating.* Questions may imply you are interrogating or judging the patient (especially *Why* questions). Intersperse other types of responses with questions. For instance, follow up a question with an empathy response that clarifies or summarizes your patient's answer to your question.

Know **What Type** *of Question to Ask*

- *Use both open and closed questions.* Open-ended questions allow patients to express themselves more autonomously. As mentioned earlier, patients can choose to express things that are most important to them. Open questions can be especially effective when first introducing a topic (Spitzer Kim 2009). Closed questions, as stated earlier, allow you to gather precise information (e.g., details about family history), and they can keep the session from wandering off-track.
- *Be sure to ask the type of question you intended to ask.* It's generally a mistake to ask closed questions when you want extended answers and to ask open questions when you want precise answers. Also, you need to clearly understand the difference between open and closed questions.
- *Use follow-up questions.* If a patient provides little or no response to your question, consider saying "Tell me more about that." If a patient is unable or unwilling to answer an open question, you can ask a closed question as a way of drawing the patient out. For example, if in response to the question "How is your pregnancy going," a patient says "Fine," a genetic counselor may follow up with some closed-ended questions, such as "Have you had any bleeding or cramping?" Or, if in response to the question "How do you feel about having this test?," the patient says "OK, I guess," the counselor might say, "Do you think you want to proceed with this test today, or do you need time to talk with your family first?" (forced choice). Or, if in response to the question "How do you feel about pursuing another pregnancy," the patient says, "I want to have another child, but I worry about having yet another miscarriage," the genetic counselor might respond "Tell me how your fear of another miscarriage compares to your desire of adding a child to your family?" (ranking question).

Additional Guidelines for Effective Questioning

- Listen to determine whether the patient answers your question and what the answer is. Ask again later or in a different way if the patient does not answer. Questioning skills take time and practice to develop. Initially you will learn how to ask questions (question format) and then learn what topics to focus on in your questions (content and context). Next you will learn to concentrate on listening to the answer, and then you will gain further skills for determining where to go next based on the patient's answer.
- Avoid interrupting. Unless patients ramble excessively, allow them to finish their sentences and thoughts. Ask patients to complete unfinished sentences.

  Sternlight and Robbennolt (2008) provide similar recommendations for lawyers: "In order to both listen effectively and appear to clients to be listening effectively, lawyers should typically let their clients tell their initial stories without interruptions…follow up their accounts with clarifying questions…and then provide feedback and legal information that reflects that the attorney was listening carefully…Studies of interviewers, including lawyers…police interviewers…and physicians, have found that interviewers are prone to interrupt early and often. Research shows that interjecting a large number of specific questions can make it difficult for the interviewer to listen to the answers provided by the interviewee…Directing those limited mental resources to formulating many questions—rather than listening intently to the witness's narrative response to open-ended questions—ought to increase the difficulty of understanding or notating the witness's responses…." Furthermore, psychological research has documented the benefits to memory that come from listening to interviewees and not interrupting their answers to questions…" (pp. 492–493).

- Allow patients to interrupt you. Usually, what they have to say is important and indicates they are engaged in the process and willing to share with you.
- You can always *back track*. If the discussion shifts before you have gathered all the information you need, remember you can always *redirect* your patient. For instance, you could say, "Earlier, you were saying…Can I ask you more about that?"
- Re-invite patients to share an experience. If your patient provides a minimal response to your open question, ask the question again. It's important to consider that this may be the first time a patient has had the chance to share the whole story with a health-care professional.
- Be transparent. When you repeat questions, shift topics, or introduce new topics, patients will be more open to answering your questions if you explain why you are doing so. For example, "Part of my role is to ask you to talk about how you made this decision. I'm doing this to be sure you have all the relevant information I'm able to give you. I'm *not* trying to judge or change your decision."
- Use silence. Silences allow patients the time and space to consider your question and to formulate thoughtful responses. As we mention in Chap. 4, silence can be difficult to gauge. Try counting silently to 10 or 15 in order to allow sufficient time.
- Try other ways to obtain information. Remember that a good empathic reflection can encourage patients to disclose a great deal of information (Martin 2015). Their disclosure may not be as *systematic* as in response to a question, but patients do have more autonomy and control over the discussion when you use a less leading response such as empathy. Monitor your questioning behavior to see if you're resorting to questions because you don't know what else to do, or you're trying to avoid patient feelings. If this is the case, try to use other types of responses.
- Follow up with primary empathy. Summarize your patient's response to your question (see Chap. 4 for a discussion of primary empathy). Primary empathy not only shows you heard and understood the patient's answer, it also allows the patient to "hear" what she or he said.

Remember that not every response you give in a questioning tone is necessarily a question. The primary goal of a question is to gather additional information. Empathy responses often are stated in a questioning tone, but their intent is to reflect the patient's experience, not to gather new information.

5.1.4 Limiting Your Use of Open and Closed Questions

We cautioned earlier about the indiscriminate use of questions and stressed the importance of not interrogating patients. We elaborate on these points in this section because we believe it is very important for beginning counselors to recognize both the potential benefits and limitations of questions. Two specific reasons to ask questions are to learn about patients and to cue patients about the types of information you need. When you want your patient to elaborate, an open question may be more effective (e.g., "What types of options do you believe you have open to you?"). If you need to efficiently gather specific information, then a closed question may be more effective. Closed question are particularly useful for gathering information for family and medical histories (e.g., "How many siblings do you have?").

Before asking questions, consider their potential impact. Open and closed questions may have different effects on patients and the counseling process. As noted by Spitzer Kim (2009), "Closed ended questions are questions that typically can be answered with one or two words (yes or no). These questions are useful for obtaining specific information. They tend to keep the discussion to a minimum and do not encourage expression of emotion. Open ended questions invite a client to say more about a subject and give a more nuanced response" (p. 84).

Too many questions can lead to an *interrogation* in which you control the process, with the patient becoming *less* rather than *more* communicative. Excessive questions may also result in patient passivity (e.g., "I will just sit here and wait for my genetic counselor to ask me the next question"). Bertakis et al. (1991) found that patient satisfaction was highest when physicians communicated interest and friendliness and avoided behaviors that were dominating, such as excessive questioning. Over-reliance on closed questions has been found to lead to lower patient satisfaction during medical appointments with physicians (Bertakis et al. 1991), during mental health counseling sessions (Hill 2014), and during genetic counseling (Guimarães et al. 2013).

Guimarães et al. (2013) interviewed 22 patients in Portugal undergoing presymptomatic testing for Huntington disease, spinocerebellar ataxias, or familial amyloid polyneuropathy. They explored patients' perceptions of the testing process, the extent to which their personal expectations and needs were met, their views of the decision-making process, and the counselors' engagement and counseling skills. They found excessive questioning was negatively associated with patient satisfaction. They cautioned against excessive questioning, especially if the questions are challenging and/or redundant. They also noted the potential for patients to become defensive in reaction to numerous questions about life changes, possible advantages and disadvantages of performing presymptomatic testing, and/or potential consequences of the test results: "Under these circumstances, the counsellor will be perceived as a 'gate keeper,' a barrier in front of the decisional process, and not as a facilitator. This may be overcome by the appropriate use of counselling skills, such as the ability to create empathy, the use of open questions and responses…in a flexible way, adapted to each counselee needs and expectations" (p. 444). This study serves as a reminder about the importance of strategic and sparing use of questions in combination with primary empathy.

You must be sure that your questions are focused on your patient's needs and reasons for seeking genetic counseling and not from your own personal interest. For example, "So, what's it like to have a baby with a birth defect?" sounds like a question intended to satisfy your own curiosity. Compare this question with the following: "Please tell me how you're dealing with raising a child with cystic fibrosis." The latter question is more appropriately focused on the patient's situation and needs. Similarly, when asking patients about their cultural backgrounds, it should be on a "need-to-know" basis, namely, for its relevance to the genetic counseling goals. Avoid being a "cultural tourist." Consider the difference between these two questions: "Why do people in your culture think that having a child with a cleft lip and palate is caused by something the mother did during her pregnancy?" versus "Tell me how the beliefs in your culture might affect your family's reaction to your child's cleft lip and palate?" The latter question invites the patient to share her or his own cultural experience. If the patient tells you that this is an issue, then you might follow up by asking, "How can I help?"

Patients can become defensive if they are bombarded with a string of questions, especially if the questions appear to challenge something they have just said (Wubbolding 1996). Consider the following example of excessive and challenging questions. In this example, the questions imply judgment:

Pt: I don't want to have a baby with Down syndrome.
Co: What do you mean?

PT: I just don't think I could handle it.
Co: Are you telling me that you'd want to terminate the pregnancy?

PT: Well, I'm not sure…
Co: Where does this feeling that you "couldn't handle it" come from?

Cl: I don't know what you mean.
Co: Well, is it coming from you or from your family?

Cl: Well, I guess from them.
Co: Do they have to live with the consequences of this decision or do you?

Cl: Well, it will affect them, too.
Co: But can they really tell you what to do?

Cl: No, I guess not.
Co: So, let me ask you, what do *you* want to do?

In this example, the counselor overwhelmed the patient with a series of questions that were quite presumptive and seemed to *demand* a certain answer. These questions raised a barrier between the counselor and patient as the patient became increasingly defensive and distressed.

Compare the previous example to this more appropriate interchange:

Cl: I don't want to have a baby with Down syndrome.
Co: Tell me more about that.

Cl: I just don't think I could handle it.
Co: You're afraid that you couldn't manage?

Cl: Right...I have to work fulltime, and I'd have no one to watch the baby. And I'm not sure I could give it all of the special care it would need.
Co: What are your impressions of what a child with Down syndrome is like?

Cl: [Patient describes her perceptions]
Co: [Counselor affirms or correct patient perceptions, including a discussion of different levels of severity and then says] What options have you considered if the test results indicate Down syndrome?

Wubbolding (1996) cautions against the use of questions that "mask" the counselor's opinions. For example, "Do you think you should be making this decision alone?" "Do you think you should talk to your mother and find out more about her health history before having this test?" "Have you tried talking with your child about the importance of following the recommended diet for PKU?"

Although it may be appropriate at times to express your opinions and offer advice (see Chap. 10), you should not disguise them as requests for more information.

5.1.5 Questions You Generally Should or Should Not Ask

Questions to Ask

Although every patient and genetic counseling situation differs, there are a few critical questions you should consider asking most patients early in the session: "What brought you to genetic counseling?" and "What's brought you here now?," as well as either "How can I be helpful to you?" or "Can you tell me what you're hoping to get out of genetic counseling?" Patients' responses to these questions can indicate their major goals for the genetic counseling session as well as give you some idea about how much they understand about genetic counseling. There can be risks with these questions, however. Some patients may be overwhelmed if you ask these questions right away. They are not always sure of what they want, and they may not even know why they are seeking genetic counseling (especially likely if they were referred). So, these questions will not be a *magical* way to get patients to open up to you. You may need to first spend time describing what genetic counseling is and what they might be able to get from the session, and then ask your question again in a different way. For example:

Co: What brought you to genetic counseling?
Pt: I really don't know. Dr. Smith told me I should come.
Co: Well, I see you have some family history of…We can discuss your risks for…and options for…Would you like to do that?

Additional "gold standard" types of questions to consider used throughout the session are as follows: "Please tell me more." "Please give me an example." "What are you thinking about right now?" and "What are you feeling right now?" These questions may be particularly helpful for quiet patients and/or patients who are speaking in generalities.

Questions to Avoid Asking

As we mentioned earlier, one type of question you generally should avoid is "Why?" questions. "Why" questions ask for a rational explanation of a person's behaviors, thoughts, or feelings. As such, they imply the person is reacting rationally. In reality, a great deal of human behavior is based on irrational, unplanned, and *unconscious* forces or is due to habit or ritual; your patient will probably *make up* a reason, when there isn't a rational one (Krueger and Casey 2014). Furthermore, *why* questions imply judgment (e.g., "Why didn't you talk to your doctor about having the test?"), and the patient may become defensive, feel guilty, or be offended (Geldard and Anderson 1989; Hill 2014). Any response to this type of question will be a rationalization or excuse (e.g., "Well, I didn't have the time to call and schedule an appointment with her") (Geldard and Anderson 1989). Asking your patient, "'Why do you feel that way?' can't be answered, doesn't go anywhere, and may well make your patient defend himself…If a why question is necessary, we find that the client feels better if you tell him why you are asking him why…" (Fine and Glasser 1996, p. 69) (e.g., I'm asking you why you didn't have prenatal testing done because it might relate to your decision about this pregnancy). You can try to rephrase why questions, for example, "Could you tell me about your decision not to talk to your doctor about having the test?" Be aware, however, that rephrased questions may still sound judgmental.

5.2 Other Considerations

Goodenberger et al. (2015) present several hypothetical scenarios illustrating the importance of psychosocial counseling skills, including questions, used by genetic counselors working in diagnostic laboratories. For example, when speaking with physicians, genetic counselors would use "open and closed-ended questions…to gather information. The counselor initiates the information gathering part of the interaction by stating her reason for calling. This statement sets the expectation for the call and provides the physician (her client) with something to react and respond to… [An open question] allows the counselor to not only gain an understanding of why the test was ordered but also to assess whether the physician is aware that the test could be uninformative. Subsequently, by asking closed-ended questions about the patient's symptoms, age, and father's diagnosis, the genetic counselor relieves the physician of the responsibility of interpreting what information is relevant to the counselor" (p. 8). Similarly, when counseling patients about how to obtain information from their physicians, genetic counselors facilitate that process by identifying questions patients should ask their doctors and by providing guidance for speaking with the physician: "It sounds like you will need to be direct and ask your questions quickly'" (p. 10). The authors further note that given the brief nature of typical laboratory genetic counselor/client interactions, "genetic counselors must carefully articulate the questions that are of most immediate importance" (p. 13).

Goodenberger et al. (2015, p. 14) provide examples of questions laboratory genetic counselors might ask. These include:

- *Closed-ended or focused questions* to obtain clinical or order-specific information, and focus the conversation to ensure relevant information is discussed. For example, "Has the patient's father had genetic testing for Lynch syndrome?" "Based on the paperwork submitted with the sample, I understand that this child has asthma. Is there another reason why chromosomes were ordered?"
- *Open-ended questions* to elicit a patient's medical and/or social history, understand provider's concerns, learn what information the person on the other end has available, and assess the provider's/lab staff's understanding of the clinical, genetic, and technical concepts. For example, "How was this patient first diagnosed with Marfan syndrome?" "What information were you given when you were asked to order this test?" "What is your past experience with microarray testing in children with autism?"

Burgess et al. (2016) surveyed genetic counselors about their perceptions of the similarities and differences between telephone genetic counseling and in person genetic counseling. With respect to questioning skills, a large majority of their respondents viewed these question-asking skills as similar: "Tailor questioning for the individual case…. Assess client emotion and/or behavior [with questions]" (p. 120). Some participants noted differences that included "…[using] more direct questioning in telephone genetic counseling than they would typically use in an in person genetic counseling [session]. One participant illustrated this well by stating: 'When there is a silence on the end of the line I have no visual cues to guide me as to why. I have to be more direct and I cannot verify my best guesses with visual corroboration…'" (p. 121). Some counselors also commented that with respect to family history and pedigree taking, the lack of visual information required them to "modify questioning due to the inability to make any kind of visual assessment of ethnicity. For instance, one participant expressed that "'Ethnicity can be easier to determine when you can see the patient/client; you may phrase the ethnicity question differently in these cases, such as 'would you consider yourself to be African American?' versus just blatantly asking. It may be more difficult to draw these conclusions from telephone counseling, so the question may be more pointed'" (p. 122).

5.3 Cultural Considerations

Adapting your questioning to your patient's needs and cultural background is critical. Questions may seem rude and intrusive to patients from some cultures (Oosterwal 2009). Explain at the beginning of the session that you will need to obtain certain information and why you need to do so. Fisher (1996) offers these examples of cultural views of questions:

- Some Southwest Native American tribes believe that "speaking about a deformity may give it the power to manifest itself in human form" (p. 78).
- Some members of the Navajo tribe and others may not answer questions immediately (p. 83).
- Some Southeast Asian patients will more readily answer questions such as the date of the last menstrual period when you are the same gender as they are (p. 118).

Glessner et al. (2012) surveyed GLBT patients about their experiences in genetic counseling and genetic counselors about their attitudes and practices when counseling GLBT patients. Some counselors reported treating GLBT patients differently during sessions. Pertinent to using questioning skills to gather information, one participant commented "I may ask how they would prefer that I refer to their partner or may ask more detailed questions about their reproductive plans" (p. 331). Based on responses from both samples, Glessner et al. (2012) recommended "As in any counseling situation, [genetic counselors] should talk directly to patients and their partners about their experiences in a non-judgmental way in order to build rapport. During verbal communication, they could use open-ended questions containing gender neutral terms, especially when inquiring about family…attend to their patients' use of language and self-identification, and use similar terms; when in doubt, they could ask patients what terms they prefer…" (p. 335). They further recommended that when patients openly disclose their sexual orientation, counselors ask follow-up questions such as "'Do you have a partner?'...[and] It is also important for providers to ask patients how they would like them to refer to their partner and how that relationship should be documented in their medical file. It may be helpful to explain to patients why such personal questions are being asked…" (p. 335).

In a follow-up study VandenLangenberg et al. (2012) interviewed lesbian and gay individuals about their experiences as genetic counseling patients. Their participants recommended that genetic counseling service providers ask about a patient's orientation if medically relevant and, during the remaining discussion, take orientation into consideration and ask further about orientation in safe and appropriate ways. The researchers suggested that providers "should proceed cautiously…[for example] prior to asking questions about sexuality, it is important for genetic counselors to have established a safe environment and supportive relationship. Further, inquiring in such a way that a person could decline disclosing if he or she does not feel safe or comfortable may be an effective strategy" (p. 746). They further recommended asking questions with gender-neutral language. For example, some genetic counselors have told us that when patients bring people to the session, they begin by asking the patient "And who have you brought with you today?" This neutral question avoids stereotypic assumptions about relationship status based on peoples' apparent gender identity, age, and so forth.

The results of Glessner et al. (2012) and VandenLangenberg et al. (2012) provide excellent examples of "culturally educated questioning" skills, as described in Rodriguez and Walls (2000). Rodriguez and Walls (2000) advocate that counselors conduct cultural assessments to gather "clinically relevant cultural data" (p. 89). Culturally educated questioning is based on four assumptions; "First, the client, the counselor, and the counseling process all exist within a multicultural context. It is widely accepted that culture is inseparable from human experience…and, therefore, from counseling interactions. Second, client cultural identification or experience may or may not relate significantly to presenting problems. Indeed, the challenge for counselors…is to consider cultural influences without unduly emphasizing their importance…[Third,] effective multicultural counseling requires that the salience of the cultural context within which the presenting problem exists be assessed, not assumed…Finally, client self-report is the most reliable source of information regarding relevance of cultural factors" (pp. 92–93).

5.4 Closing Comments

Questions are the most direct way to elicit information from patients. They are useful throughout genetic counseling sessions as they assist in rapport building, goal-setting, exploration of the patient's situation, decision-making, and follow-up. Questioning requires a great deal of skill in order to ask the correct questions and to actively listen to what patients are telling you about themselves and their families. Skillful questioning requires you to be aware of what you want to know and why you want to know it, and to anticipate when and how best to ask each question to obtain desired information without unduly stressing patients or causing them to feel judged. We caution you to only ask questions as necessary and to follow up with reflections/summaries of what you hear to ensure that you and the patient are "on the same page."

Questions can be particularly useful for gathering relevant family and medical histories. As the family history is often one of the first activities to take place in a genetic counseling session, it provides an excellent opportunity to learn more about the patient's concerns, perceptions, family relationships, and support systems. Pedigree construction is also a wonderful vehicle for establishing rapport. Moreover, particularly revealing patient responses, made during this phase, can be revisited later in the session and can greatly enhance genetic counseling. Although family history gathering tends to become routine, it is a process that can set the tone and the framework for the session.

5.5 Class Activities

Activity 1: Asking Questions (Think-Pair-Share Dyads)

Students individually consider the following questions and then discuss them with a partner:

- What is the role of questioning in genetic counseling?
- What are potential benefits of asking questions?
- What are potential risks of asking questions?
- Are there certain types of patients with whom you would be particularly cautious about asking questions?
- What are some reasons patients might not answer your questions?

Estimated time: 10 min.

Process
Dyads report on their discussion. The instructor summarizes major themes and presents any ideas that did not emerge from the dyads.

Estimated time: 15 min.

Activity 2: Brainstorming Questions

Present students with a brief genetic counseling patient description/statement, and ask them to generate all the questions they can think to ask this patient. This activity can be repeated several times with different patient descriptions.

Patient Statements
- I'm afraid I'm going to get breast cancer.
- I was hoping that you could tell me my chances of having another miscarriage.
- My sister has a child with CF. I don't want that to happen to me.
- I want every test there is to make sure my baby is OK.
- My cousin has NF and I have some spots. My doctor thinks I have it, too.

Estimated time: 15 min per patient description.

Activity 3: Small Versus Big Questions

Provide students one of the following hypothetical scenarios.

- Patient is referred for evaluation of a family history of colon cancer. The patient's father, brother, and sister all had colon cancer diagnosed in their 40s. The patient is 35 years old, recently married, and wants to start a family.
- You are seeing a Latino couple whose infant has multiple congenital anomalies. The baby is in the ICU and is being evaluated for a chromosomal disorder.
- A couple is referred for genetic counseling following a positive newborn screen for cystic fibrosis in their daughter.
- Your patient is a 36-year-old African American female referred for genetic counseling during her first pregnancy. She and her husband are newly married. The pregnancy is unplanned. She is 8 weeks pregnant. She has a brother with unexplained intellectual disability. Her mother had two miscarriages. Her maternal aunt had a stillborn baby with "multiple birth defects."

Tell students to imagine they could ask the patient only six questions (excluding family history questions). What would they ask? Have students write down their six questions.

Next students exchange papers with one or more classmates and review each other's questions.

Estimated time: 20 min.

Process

Ask students to read their six questions, and have a general discussion about the similarities and differences in questions and whether questions were primarily open-ended or closed-ended. Finally, refer students to Sarangi et al.'s (2004) descriptions of six types of reflective frames described in this chapter, and ask them to identify which of their questions correspond to each of the frames.

As a conclusion to this activity, point out to students that having a framework for the "big questions" is an important part of case preparation, and it helps them structure the genetic counseling session.

Estimated time: 50 min.

Activity 4: Constructing Culturally Educated Questions (Dyads or Small Groups)

Introduce this activity with the following information: Charles et al. (2006) compared culturally tailored genetic counseling versus standard genetic counseling in a sample of African American women at risk for BRCA 1/2 mutations and found women who received the culturally tailored counseling reported greater satisfaction and a greater reduction in their worries than women who received the standard counseling. Specific to cultural empathy, the culturally tailored approach included questions that invited discussion of the women's cultural beliefs and values and how they apply to health-care decisions and coping with medical concerns. The questions addressed three aspects of worldviews common in the African American community—communalism, spirituality, and a flexible temporal worldview.

Next, assign dyads or small groups of students a specific cultural group. Task them with generating a series of questions aimed at exploring common worldviews of their assigned cultural group and how members of that cultural group might apply those worldviews to their health-care concerns and decision-making. Next have each dyad or small group present their list of questions to the class. Then lead the class in a discussion of the similarities and differences in their lists.

Estimated time: 60 min.

Instructor Note

- For this activity to be effective, students must first investigate common worldviews of specific cultures. For example, they could be assigned one or more readings on their cultural group in advance of this activity.
- This activity could be done individually as a written exercise for one or more cultural groups.
- Students could use the lists as prompts for the "counselors" in subsequent role-plays with "patients" representing members of the various cultural groups.

Activity 5a: Low-Level Questioning Skills Model

Instructor and a volunteer genetic counseling patient engage in a role-play in which the counselor demonstrates poor questioning skills (e.g., closed questions, why questions, strings several questions into one response, repeats questions unnecessarily, implies an opinion or advice—"Don't you think that you should…"). Students should observe and take notes of examples of poor questioning.

Estimated time: 10 min.

Process

Students share their examples of poor questioning skills. Then they discuss the impact of the counselor's poor skills on the patient.

Estimated time: 10–15 min.

Activity 5b: High-Level Questioning Skills Model

Instructor and a volunteer genetic counseling patient engage in the same role-play, but this time the counselor demonstrates good questioning skills, as well as good empathy and attending. Students should observe and take notes of examples of good questioning, empathy, and attending.

Estimated time: 10 min.

Process
Have students share their examples of good counseling skills, especially focusing on question asking. Then discuss with students the impact of the counselor's good skills on the patient.

Estimated time: 10–15 min.

Activity 6: Triad Role-Play

Three students practice using questions, primary empathy, and attending skills in 10–15-min role-plays taking turns as counselor, patient, and observer. Allow 10 min of feedback for each role-play.

Criteria for Evaluating Counselor Questions
Concrete and specific (asks for examples)
Systematic (questions seem planful)
Comprehensive (covers thoughts, feelings, behaviors)
Uses silence
Avoids interrupting
Avoids use of "why" questions
Follows-up questions with primary empathy
Uses open questions where possible
Estimated time: 60–75 min

Process
In the large group, discuss what students learned from the role-plays, what concerns or confusion they still have about questioning skills, and what they think about the utility of questioning skills in genetic counseling.

Estimated time: 15 min.

Activity 7: Brainstorming Family History Content Areas

Students generate areas in which genetic counselors would question a patient to obtain a family history and construct a pedigree. Instructor records their ideas on the board and fills in any areas which they miss.

Estimated time: 15–20 min.

Activity 8: Constructing a Pedigree Model

Instructor interviews a volunteer from class (or from outside of class) to gather a *simulated* family history and draws a pedigree on the board as the volunteer provides information. Instructor explains why she/he is using certain symbols, notations, lines, etc. as the interview progresses.

Estimated time: 45–60 min.

Activity 9: Family History Taking Model

Instructor and a volunteer from outside of the class engage in a *simulated* genetic counseling session in which the instructor gathers family history. Students observe and take notes on family history. They also record examples of the genetic counselor using good question-asking skills, empathy, and attending. This session should be audio-recorded for students to use in written Exercise 5: Constructing a Pedigree.

Estimated time: 30 min.

Process 1

In small groups, students summarize the family history information per major categories (identified in the previous brainstorming Activity #5) or using categories provided by the instructor. Possible categories include:

- Biological relationships
- Significant life events (births, deaths, marriages, divorce, etc.)
- Role of extended family members (close and supportive, distant and uninvolved)
- Experience with health-care delivery (close family member with chronic illness vs. no health issues in close family members)
- Experience with diseases
- Educational level

Estimated time: 20 min.

Process 2

In large group, instructor has students provide their group summaries for each category (a different small group can provide information for each area, and the other small groups can add to or modify the summary).

Estimated time: 20 min.

Process 3

In large group, discuss student observations about the genetic counselor's use of good questions, empathy, and attending.

Estimated time: 15 min.

Activity 10: Pedigree Construction (Dyads)

Pairs of students practice constructing pedigrees for each other. [Tell students they are not required to share personal information that they are uncomfortable disclosing. They can provide their own family history or use a fictitious family.]

Estimated time: 50 min.

Process

In large group discuss any confusion students have, clarify pedigree construction process, etc. Talk about what they perceive to be the benefits of constructing a pedigree.

Estimated time: 25 min.

Instructor Note

- History taking comprises a major component of initial genetic counseling sessions. This activity provides practice in data gathering and summarization.
- This activity can be extended such that each student takes pedigrees from several other students. Given time constraints, it could be done as an "outside" exercise rather than an "in class" activity.
- Encourage the students to consider cultural issues and develop culturally appropriate questions.

Activity 11: Constructing and Interpreting Pedigrees (Dyads)

Students construct their own pedigrees. Dyads exchange pedigrees in class. Next, each student attempts to write a narrative of the family history based on the pedigree. The dyad members discuss the narratives and pedigrees until both are clear and accurate.

Estimated time: 60 min.

Instructor Note

- The pedigree construction portion of the activity could be done outside of class.

5.6 Written Exercises

Exercise 1: Formulating Questions[1]

Rewrite each of the following counselor closed-ended questions, turning them into open-ended questions.

- Do you understand this information?
- Do you have any questions?
- Are you upset?
- Are you OK with having a child with Down syndrome?
- Does this test make sense to you?
- Do both of you agree about having this test?
- Does your fiancé know about this disease in your family?
- Do you want any more children?

Exercise 2: Using Questions Appropriately

Refer to the counselor-patient dialogue in this chapter where the counselor's excessive use of questions led to the patient feeling defensive. Create a similar dialogue

[1]Adapted from Geldard and Anderson (1989).

between a genetic counselor and patient. First write the interchange with the counselor asking excessive and challenging/judgmental questions. Then rewrite the interchange, using a combination of counselor questions, primary empathy responses, and silence, as appropriate.

[*Hint*: (1) Patient responses naturally would be expected to change in response to the more effective counselor interventions.]

Exercise 3: Strategic Questioning[2]

Write one question for each of Sanders (1966) six types of questions. Write your questions as if you are actually asking them during a genetic counseling session.

Memory question:

Translation question:

Application question:

Synthesis question:

Analysis question:

Evaluation question:

Exercise 4: Pedigree Role-Play

Audio-record an interview in which you gather a family history from a volunteer. Next, construct a pedigree based on the information obtained in the interview. Submit your tape and pedigree for evaluation.

Exercise 5: Pedigree Construction

Construct a pedigree using the audio recording and notes from the simulated history taking session (see Activity #9) conducted by the instructor.

References

Bennett RL. The practical guide to the genetic family history. 2nd ed. Hoboken, NJ: Wiley-Blackwell; 2010.

Bertakis KD, Roter D, Putnam SM. The relationship of physician medical interview style to patient satisfaction. J Fam Pract. 1991;32:175–82.

Bloom BS, Engelhart MD, Furst EJ, Hill WH, Krathwohl DR. Taxonomy of educational objectives, handbook I: the cognitive domain. New York: David McKay Co; 1956.

[2] Adapted from Pedersen and Ivey (1993).

Brown D. Implications of cultural values for cross-cultural consultation with families. J Couns Dev. 1997;76:29–35.
Burgess KR, Carmany EP, Trepanier AM. A comparison of telephone genetic counseling and in-person genetic counseling from the genetic counselor's perspective. J Genet Couns. 2016;25:112–26.
Charles S, Kessler L, Stopfer JE, Domchek S, Halbert CH. Satisfaction with genetic counseling for BRCA1 and BRCA2 mutations among African American women. Patient Educ Couns. 2006;63:196–204.
Danish SJ, D'Augelli AR, Hauer AL. Helping skills: a basic training program. New York: Human Sciences Press; 1980.
Djurdjinovic L. Psychosocial counseling. In: Uhlmann WR, Schuette JL, Yashar B, editors. A guide to genetic counseling. 2nd ed. New York: Wiley; 2009. p. 133–75.
Ellington L, Roter D, Dudley WN, Baty BJ, Upchurch R, Larson S, et al. Communication analysis of BRCA1 genetic counseling. J Genet Couns. 2005;14:377–86.
Erlanger MA. Using the genogram with the older client. J Ment Health Couns. 1990;12:321–31.
Farrelly E, Cho MK, Erby L, Roter D, Stenzel A, Ormond K. Genetic counseling for prenatal testing: where is the discussion about disability? J Genet Couns. 2012;21:814–24.
Fine SF, Glasser PH. The first helping interview. Thousand Oaks, CA: Sage; 1996.
Fisher NL, editor. Cultural and ethnic diversity: a guide for genetics professionals. Baltimore, MD: JHU Press; 1996.
Fontaine JH, Hammond NL. Twenty counseling maxims. J Couns Dev. 1994;73:223–6.
Geldard D, Anderson G. A training manual for counsellors: basic personal counselling. Springfield, IL: Charles C. Thomas; 1989.
Glessner HD, VandenLangenberg E, Veach PM, LeRoy BS. Are genetic counselors and GLBT patients "on the same page"? An investigation of attitudes, practices, and genetic counseling experiences. J Genet Couns. 2012;21:326–36.
Goodenberger ML, Thomas BC, Wain KE. The utilization of counseling skills by the laboratory genetic counselor. J Genet Couns. 2015;24:6–17.
Guimarães L, Sequeiros J, Skirton H, Paneque M. What counts as effective genetic counselling for presymptomatic testing in late-onset disorders? A study of the consultand's perspective. J Genet Couns. 2013;22:437–47.
Hackney HL, Bernard JM. Professional counseling: a process guide to helping. 8th ed. London: Pearson; 2017.
Hill CE. Helping skills: facilitating exploration, insight, and action. 4th ed. Washington, DC: American Psychological Association; 2014.
Hughes JN, Erchul WP, Yoon J, Jackson T, Henington C. Consultant use of questions and its relationship to consultee evaluation of effectiveness. J Sch Psychol. 1997;35:281–97.
Krueger RA, Casey MA. Focus groups: a practical guide for applied research. Thousand Oaks, CA: Sage; 2014.
Martin DG. Counseling and therapy skills. 4th ed. Long Grove IL: Waveland Press; 2015.
Miranda C, Veach PM, Martyr MA, LeRoy BS. Portrait of the master genetic counselor clinician: a qualitative investigation of expertise in genetic counseling. J Genet Couns. 2016;25:767–85.
Oosterwal G. Multicultural counseling. In: Uhlmann WR, Schuette JL, Yashar B, editors. A guide to genetic counseling. 2nd ed. New York: John Wiley & Sons; 2009. p. 331–61.
Paradopoulos L, Bor R, Stanion P. Genograms in counselling practice: a review (part 1). Couns Psychol Q. 1997;10:17–28.
Pedersen PB, Ivey AE. Culture-centered counseling and interviewing skills: a practical guide. Westport, CT: Praeger Publishers/Greenwood Publishing Group; 1993.
Redlinger-Grosse K, Veach PM, LeRoy BS, Zierhut H. Elaboration of the Reciprocal-Engagement Model of genetic counseling practice: a qualitative investigation of goals and strategies. J Genet Couns. 2017;26:1372–87.
Rodriguez RR, Walls NE. Culturally educated questioning: toward a skills-based approach in multicultural counselor training. Appl Prev Psychol. 2000;9:89–99.

Rose P, Humm E, Hey K, Jones L, Huson SM. Family history taking and genetic counselling in primary care. Fam Pract. 1999;16:78–83.

Sanders NM. Classroom questions: what kinds? New York: Harpercollins College Div; 1966.

Sarangi S, Bennert K, Howell L, Clarke A, Harper P, Gray J. (Mis) alignments in counseling for Huntington's disease predictive testing: clients' responses to reflective frames. J Genet Couns. 2005;14:29–42.

Sarangi S, Bennert K, Howell L, Clarke A, Harper P, Gray J. (2004). Initiation of reflective frames in counseling for Huntington's disease predictive testing. J Genet Couns. 2004;13:135-55.

Schuette JL, Bennett R. The ultimate genetic tool: the family history. In: Uhlmann WR, Schuette JL, Yashar B, editors. A guide to genetic counseling. 2nd ed. New York: Wiley; 2009. p. 37–69.

Spitzer Kim K. Interviewing: beginning to see each other. In: Uhlmann WR, Schuette JL, Yashar B, editors. A guide to genetic counseling. 2nd ed. New York: Wiley; 2009. p. 71–91.

Stanion P, Papadopoulos L, Bor R. Genograms in counselling practice: constructing a genogram (part 2). Couns Psychol Q. 1997;10:139–48.

Sternlight JR, Robbennolt JK. Good lawyers should be good psychologists: insights for interviewing and counseling clients. Ohio State J Disput Resolut. 2008 May 5; 23:437; UNLV William S. Boyd School of Law Legal Studies Research Paper No. 08-24; U Illinois Law & Economics Research Paper No. LEC08-024.

VandenLangenberg E, Veach PM, LeRoy BS, Glessner HD. Gay, lesbian, and bisexual patients' recommendations for genetic counselors: a qualitative investigation. J Genet Couns. 2012;21:741–7.

Wubbolding RE. Professional issues: the use of questions in reality therapy. J Real Ther. 1996;16:122–7.

Chapter 6
Structuring Genetic Counseling Sessions: Initiating, Contracting, Ending, and Referral

Learning Objectives
1. Describe activities for initiating the genetic counseling session.
2. Define contracting and describe steps in the goal-setting process.
3. Describe genetic counselor activities for ending the session and the relationship.
4. Identify referral strategies for effective follow-up.
5. Develop skills at initiating, contracting, ending, and referral through self-reflection, practice, and feedback.

This chapter discusses four of the components of a genetic counseling session: initiating the session, introductions and contracting (setting goals), ending the session/relationship, and making referrals. The components described in this chapter correspond to several of the categories identified by the Accreditation Council for Genetic Counseling (ACGC 2015) for logbook case documentation.

6.1 Initiating the Genetic Counseling Session

Close your eyes and imagine that you are about to see your first genetic counseling patient. What are you feeling? What are you doing to prepare for your first encounter? Do you have a clear picture of how you will begin? What is the first thing you will say or do? Now ask yourself how your patients may feel about coming to genetic counseling and what they might say or do.

Many people have never heard of genetic counseling prior to becoming genetic counseling patients. They may be anxious, confused, frightened, and disoriented about the relationship they are about to enter with you. It is important that you try to alleviate their discomfort by providing guidance about what will happen in this relationship.

P. McCarthy Veach et al., *Facilitating the Genetic Counseling Process*,
https://doi.org/10.1007/978-3-319-74799-6_6

You can take several steps to set the stage for genetic counseling. These include case preparation, introductions and orientation to the session, contracting, and goal setting.

6.1.1 Preparation

Review Patient Records

Review any available patient records prior to the genetic counseling session. If information from a referring physician is missing, you should attempt to acquire it prior to seeing the patient. Reviewing the records not only better prepares you to assess patient goals for genetic counseling, it also indicates to the patient that you are interested and respectful enough to take the time to do this preparation. Uhlmann (2009) presents a detailed approach to case preparation and management in clinical genetic counseling.

Arrange the Counseling Environment

Surroundings are an important aspect of setting the overall tone. Keep your office or working space neat, uncluttered, and inviting.

- If possible, have chairs of approximately equal size and comfort available (Martin 2015).
- Position your chair so you face your patients and if possible move any desks so they are not between you. Have a box of tissues available.
- If you carry a pager or cell phone, turn it to vibrate mode and warn your patient if you expect someone to contact you during the session.

Prepare Yourself to Begin

- Minimize distraction. Be sure your manner of presentation is not distracting. Think about the type of impression you wish to convey, and then dress and behave accordingly. Wear clothes that are appropriate for your setting and for the patients with whom you are working. In genetic counseling, it is not appropriate to wear casual clothing such as jeans, hiking boots, and shorts. You should avoid clothing that could be regarded as provocative—short skirts, sheer blouses, low-cut shirts, thong-type sandals, and tight clothing. Cover up any tattoos. Also, as we discussed in Chap. 3, work on reducing or eliminating personal habits that might be distracting (e.g., twisting your hair, playing with jewelry, excessive use of filler words such as OK, right, uh-huh, you know).
- If you wear any obvious religious symbols (e.g., crucifix, yarmulke, burka), expect that some patients may react or even comment on them. Think about how you could respond if they do.

- If you have time between sessions, take a moment to psychologically prepare for the next session. Sit in a quiet room, take some deep breaths to calm yourself, try to put aside extraneous thoughts, and focus on the patient(s) whom you will meet in a few minutes. Visualize how you will greet your patient and what you might say at the beginning and end of the genetic counseling session.
- Begin on time, if possible, so as not to keep patients waiting. If your clinic is running behind schedule, explain the reasons for the delay.
- At any time during the session, if someone comes to the door, step outside and close the door to protect patient privacy. Handle the interruption quickly, come back to your patient, apologize, and briefly summarize what you were talking about before being interrupted (Fine and Glasser 1996).

6.1.2 Introductions and Orientation

Introductions

- Greet your patients and, if possible, escort them to the room. Remember there are cultural variations regarding touch. For example, some individuals from the Middle East do not shake the hands of members of the opposite sex. We recommend that you shake hands only if the patient initiates this behavior.
- Introduce yourself by first and last name. There is no clear protocol about how to address patients, but your institution may have one. For instance, in calling someone from the waiting area, you may be required to use only a first name. "At the start of the session, the counselor will want to greet everyone present, establish how they are related to the patient, and determine what each person wants to be called" (Spitzer Kim 2009, p. 73). There are cultural differences in how individuals wish to be addressed. For example, some older immigrants from Asia or from conservatively stratified societies may wish to be treated more formally rather than being called by their first names (Ishiyama 1995; Spitzer Kim 2009; Sue and Sue 2012). Also, when patients are older than you, it may be appropriate to address them more formally (Mr., Ms., etc.). Generally speaking, you should address people more formally until they invite you to do otherwise.
- Do not insist that patients address you in a certain way. For example, some patients may not be comfortable using your first name. Pay attention to any changes in the way a patient addresses you, as they may indicate a change in your relationship, either toward or away from trust and comfort (Fine and Glasser 1996; Spitzer Kim 2009).
- Allow your patients to choose the chairs in which they sit, and wait for them to be seated first so you don't suggest you are rushing or directing them (Fine and Glasser 1996). When your patients are couples or families, where and how they position themselves provide important clues, for instance, about power dynamics and degree of closeness among family members (Schoeffel et al. 2018). Pay attention to who directs the action, who takes the most prominent seat, who sits closest to you, who sits next to whom, who speaks first and who speaks after

whom, whether individuals introduce themselves or are introduced by others, and how they refer to each other (Fine and Glasser 1996; Schoeffel et al. 2018). Additionally, you can gain important clues about individual patients by how they position their chair. For example, do they move it closer to or further away from you? Do they pick a chair that is closer to or farther away from yours?
- In general, you should limit your small talk to an amount that helps your patient relax a bit. Small talk also helps you to begin, "…assessing the client's level of comfort, mood, language skills, and a variety of other factors that can influence the subsequent interaction" (Spitzer Kim 2009, p. 72). A small amount of social conversation can be especially beneficial for individuals from certain ethnic backgrounds. For instance, some Asians, Native Americans, Hispanics, and African Americans may prefer a brief period of social conversation before proceeding to more intimate topics (Fine and Glasser 1996). In our experience, this is true of most patients regardless of their ethnic background. Too much small talk, however, is usually due to your own discomfort rather than for the patient's benefit.

Orientation

- First assess patients' understanding of the purpose of the visit. As part of this process, you could ask patients to describe their understanding of what will happen in the session. For example, "What was your doctor able to tell you about your appointment today?"
- Explain the genetic counseling process. Provide an overview of what will happen during the session (e.g., obtaining family history, reviewing medical history, physical examination, etc.) and who will be involved. Patients typically enter genetic counseling without knowing exactly what to expect or what will be expected of them. They may feel uncertain, vulnerable, or even embarrassed. By describing what will happen and by conveying a caring attitude, you can help them adapt to the situation (Spitzer Kim 2009).
- Bernhardt et al. (2000) found that patients often had few identified goals prior to a session due to their lack of familiarity with genetic counseling. They were unsure what the role of the genetic counselor was meant to be or how the session(s) would be structured. They appreciated receiving an orientation to genetic counseling.
- If you intend to take notes during the session (either with pen and paper or electronically), explain why you are doing so. Be aware that you may lose valuable nonverbal cues because you are not able to consistently look at your patients. Taking notes unobtrusively, while simultaneously paying close attention to your patient, is a skill that requires a fair amount of practice. You may wish to practice this type of note-taking outside of the genetic counseling session (e.g., role-playing with a friend). You will need to become proficient enough that your patients feel as if they have your full attention throughout the genetic counseling session.
- Consider developing and using an interview checklist outlining the topics you wish to cover during a session. A checklist may help you proceed in an unhurried but efficient manner, and it may be helpful for constructing post-session notes. A checklist may also serve as a stimulus for supervision (i.e., discussion of aspects

of the session that were difficult for you). When using a checklist, remember you will likely vary the order in which you raise topics, and you may not cover all topics with all patients. Also, as with note-taking, you should explain why you are using a checklist and allow the patient to see it. Finally, you can review your prepared checklist toward the end of the session to be sure you covered important topics (e.g., "I made a list of things I want to be sure we discussed during this appointment. Let me take a look to be sure we covered everything."). This review can communicate to your patient that you prepared for the session. A *mental* checklist is always an option as well.

- If you plan to record a session, ask your patient's permission, and request that she/he give permission in writing. Present the purpose of recording in a matter-of-fact way (e.g., "I'm doing this in order to receive supervision on my genetic counseling skills"), and assure your patients of the confidentiality of the recording (Martin 2015). We recommend telling patients that you will erase the recording at the end of your clinical rotation. If a patient is resistant to recording, offer to turn off the equipment if she/he wishes you to do so, at any point during the session. Note that you should always check clinic policies before recording a session, even with permission of a patient.
- Think about how you will respond if a patient wishes to record the session.
- Consider cultural factors in providing an orientation for patients, in particular, variations in how people communicate, possible culturally related obstacles, and how to overcome them (Oosterwal 2009). "The following factors need to be considered:

  - How do you greet and address each other, formally or informally, by first name or family name, looking each other in the eye or not?
  - What kind of relationship is expected between the [patient] and the counselor: paternalistic and hierarchical, or a more equal partnership?
  - When listening, is it acceptable to interrupt?
  - What types of questions are culturally appropriate?
  - How much time is available for the various activities that make up the process of counseling?

All of these issues are very different from one culture to another. What is appropriate or respectful in one culture may be offensive in another" (Oosterwal 2009, p. 352).

6.2 Contracting and Goal Setting

6.2.1 Contracting

Imagine yourself starting out on a vacation with a friend. The two of you are driving down the road, engaged in a lively conversation, as you head for Canada. About 30 min or so into the conversation, your friend looks around at the road signs and says, "Wait! I thought we were going to Florida!" You slam on the brake. What happened in this situation? Evidently the two of you failed to discuss your intended destination. You did not develop a road map for your journey. A similar situation is likely to arise when you and your patients do not identify explicit and compatible goals for your session/relationship. Without a road map, sooner or later you'll have to pull over to the side of the road. In genetic counseling, the term "contracting" describes the process by which the genetic counselor and patient mutually reach agreement about the goals of the session. In this section, we will describe the contracting process and discuss goal setting in genetic counseling.

The Accreditation Council for Genetic Counseling (ACGC) defines contracting as "the two-way communication process between the genetic counselor and the patient/client which aims to clarify both parties' expectations and goals for the session" (ACGC 2015, p. 8). Genetic counselors "establish a mutually agreed upon genetic counseling agenda with the client" by doing the following:

1. Describe the genetic counseling process to clients.
2. Elicit client expectations, perceptions, knowledge, and concerns regarding the genetic counseling encounter and the reason for referral or contact.
3. Apply client expectations, perceptions, knowledge, and concerns toward the development of a mutually agreed-upon agenda.
4. Modify the genetic counseling agenda, as appropriate by continually *contracting* to address emerging concerns" (ACGC 2015, p. 4).

The first step in contracting and goal setting is to establish a "working agreement" or shared vision for the session with your patient (Spitzer Kim 2009, p. 76). This process begins by inviting patients to describe their understanding of why they were referred or the reasons they sought genetic counseling. Use your attending skills (Chap. 3), empathy skills (Chap. 4), and questioning skills (Chap. 5) to engage the patient in a conversation that will help you understand their reasons for seeking genetic evaluation/counseling. What do they hope to learn? What are their questions or concerns?

Invite patients to express their concerns about the visit. It can be very helpful to start by asking what questions or concerns are most pressing and addressing those first, if possible. Also, use this opportunity to tell them that the aim of genetic counseling is to be able to address those concerns. For example, the parents of a pediatric patient may start by saying "We're very concerned about our child's developmental problems and really need some answers!" In response, you could explain that this is a primary aim of a pediatric genetics evaluation, and describe the steps you will take to help achieve this goal.

An increasing body of literature addresses genetic counseling contracting and goal setting. Below, we briefly describe the findings and conclusions of several investigations of one or more aspects of contracting and goal setting.

Case et al. (2007) asserted that, "Informed decision-making, the foundation of prenatal counseling, rests on the practice of contracting with patients (the process of finding out what a patient knows and what attitudes she may hold and adapting information presented to that [patient's] knowledge)…" (pp. 655–656). They interviewed pregnant and nonpregnant women and found tremendous variability in their knowledge and beliefs about genetic counseling. They concluded that this variability "…confirms the importance of contracting and taking time to understand an individual's personal beliefs, knowledge and attitudes about prenatal diagnosis" (p. 661).

Lafans et al. (2003) asked genetic counselors how they manage fathers' involvement in prenatal sessions. Their participants identified several strategies, including orienting and contracting (e.g., "...I usually start with defining what I am, and the process. Part of the contracting is to say, 'I'm not here to tell you what to do; and ... Usually the woman is the spokesperson, and she...has an agenda; she kind of tells him what it is, and he usually sits there and so, I turn to him and say 'Okay, so your wife says she wants to talk about this, this, and this. What about you? Do you have the same agenda, or is yours a little bit different?'…" (p. 230).

Andrighetti et al. (2016) surveyed parents of children affected with obsessive-compulsive disorder (OCD) about their recommendations for genetic counselors. Their recommendations included, "thorough contracting with families upfront about what genetic counseling for OCD entails, as well as whether they are interested in knowing specific recurrence information" (p. 919). For example, counselors could ask parents, "'How involved do you want us to get? Do you want it right down to, 'these are the odds of it happening again' or do you just want to understand more of how it happens and why it happens?'" (p. 919).

Griswold et al. (2011) interviewed genetic counselors about how they counsel adolescents compared to how they counsel adults. Their participants reported "spending more time on case preparation, contracting, and psychosocial assessment with adolescents and more time on inheritance/risk counseling, pedigree, and discussing testing options/results with adults" (p. 187). The authors speculated that counselors may spend more time on case preparation when anticipating an adolescent patient in order to identify additional support and resources for them. Also, adults tend to have more questions and are more open to discussion with the counselor than adolescents because they may have given more thought to their options. In contrast, adolescents may be more focused on the here-and-now and less able to think about long-range outcomes (Berger 2005). Thus, discussions about inheritance and testing results may be more difficult with adolescents, and they may seem shorter. It also may be more difficult "...to engage adolescents in a conversation about emotions, and be more difficult for counselors to assess the needs of adolescents who are pregnant because adolescent girls are more likely to internalize problems…" (p. 187). It may require more time for genetic counselors to accomplish these goals. The authors concluded that contracting with adolescents and psychosocial assessment may be more difficult than with adult patients.

Pieterse et al. (2005) developed a measure of cancer genetic counseling patients' needs and preferences. They found that patients generally rated as most important the information about risk and prevention strategies and information about the counseling process (what happens and how) and, to a lesser extent, receipt of emotional support and discussion of feelings. The authors concluded that, "A primary goal of genetic counseling and testing is to educate individuals about cancer risk and cancer prevention, with the aim of reducing morbidity and mortality" (p. 361).

Importantly, however, you should always consider individual differences in patient needs and preferences and proceed accordingly.

6.2.2 *Setting Genetic Counseling Session Goals*

Goals are the road maps that bring focus and direction to the session and help to structure the relationship. Setting genetic counseling session goals is part of the contracting process. Goals are "…mental representations of desired outcomes to which people are committed…" (Mann et al. 2013, p. 488). They help counselors and patients identify precisely what they can and cannot achieve in genetic counseling (Hackney and Bernard 2017). Goals help you determine what information to present, how to structure the session, and the types of interventions to use. Goal setting encourages patients to be clear about what they want to accomplish in a genetic counseling session. Furthermore, goals can help patients feel motivated to take action, and they allow both you and your patients to evaluate the effectiveness of the genetic counseling session and relationship.

The importance of explicitly stated and agreed-upon goals is illustrated in a study of concordance between genetic counselors' and patients' views of the nature/type of patient concerns and the level/severity of their concerns. Michie et al. (1998) found that genetic counselors were sometimes inaccurate in judging patient concerns: "When there was not concordance, counselors were more likely than patients to think the patients' main concern was to get information or to find out about their risk status" (p. 228). Concordant sessions tended to emphasize more emotional issues and resulted in greater patient satisfaction with the information received and greater satisfaction with the extent to which their expectations were met.

6.2.3 *Goals of Genetic Counseling*

Genetic counseling is "the process of helping people understand and adapt to the medical, psychological and familial implications of genetic contributions to disease" (Resta et al. 2006, p. 77). Consistent with this definition, the Reciprocal-Engagement Model (REM) of genetic counseling practice (McCarthy Veach et al. 2007) identifies three overarching outcome goals. Specifically, the patient understands and applies information in order to make decisions, manage conditions, and adapt to her or his situation. To achieve these broad outcomes, there are 16 goals for genetic counseling sessions that reflect 4 major factors: *Understanding and Appreciation, Support and Guidance, Facilitative Decision-Making, and Patient-Centered Education* (Hartmann et al. 2015). The following list displays the REM goals associated with each factor (Hartmann et al. 2015):

Goals of Reciprocal-Engagement Model (REM) of Genetic Counseling

Factor I: Understanding and appreciation
Counselor and patient reach an understanding of patient's family dynamics and their effects on the patient's situation
Counselor promotes maintenance of or increase in patient self-esteem
Counselor facilitates the patient's feelings of empowerment
Counselor integrates the patient's familial and cultural context into the counseling relationship and decision-making
Counselor works with patient to recognize concerns that are triggering the patient's emotions
Counselor establishes a working contract with a patient
Factor II: Support and guidance
Counselor recognizes patient strengths
Counselor and patient establish a bond
Counselor's characteristics positively influence the process of relationship-building and communication between counselor and patient
Counselor helps the patient to gain new perspectives
Counselor helps patient to adapt to his or her situation
Counselor helps the patient to feel in control
Factor III: Facilitative decision-making
Counselor helps the patient to feel informed
The counselor knows what information to impart to each patient
Counselor facilitates collaborative decisions with the patient
Factor IV: Patient-centered education
Counselor presents genetic information in a way that the patient can understand
Good counselor-patient communication occurs

McCarthy Veach et al. (2007) distinguish between process goals and outcome goals in the REM of genetic counseling practice. "Process goals refer to the conditions that must be present during genetic counseling sessions in order to achieve desired genetic counseling outcomes…Outcome goals refer to the results of genetic counseling…" (p. 719). Process goals refer to the conditions necessary to establish the relationship (e.g., promoting patient autonomy, demonstrating good attending behaviors). Within genetic counseling, process goals tend to be fairly general, applicable to all genetic counseling relationships. They are primarily your responsibility to accomplish, and they are not necessarily verbalized to patients.

In contrast, outcome goals are unique to each patient and each situation. They are more specific, and you and your patients share a mutual responsibility for their establishment, through the contracting process. Outcome goals may change as the genetic counseling relationship progresses; therefore, a certain amount of flexibility is necessary in setting and sticking to goals. Although process goals are generally applicable to all genetic counseling relationships, outcome goals vary in their relevance for a given patient. Therefore, it is critical that you identify individualized genetic counseling goals with each patient.

6.2.4 Characteristics of Effective Goals

Greenberg et al. (2006) note that "… people will strive toward a goal, as long as they believe that the goal is within their reach" (p. 664). What makes a goal feasible? A feasible goal is specific, realistic, and mutually agreed upon; it defines the conditions necessary for reaching a desired outcome (e.g., making a decision, gaining genetic information); it is compatible with patient and counselor values; and it is qualified, that is, it tends not to have an all-or-nothing quality (Cavanagh and Levitov 2002; Stone 1994). For instance, a patient might say, "I want to know for certain that my child is OK." This is a very difficult, if not impossible, goal. Usually this type of certainty in genetic counseling cannot be achieved because of the complexity and the limits of genetic knowledge and testing (McCarthy Veach et al. 2001). A feasible goal is also open to revision as you and your patients reach new understandings (Martin 2015).

The goals that are established cannot be more specific than either the counselor's or the patient's understanding of the problem (Hackney and Bernard 2017). So, effective goal setting requires not only solid attending and empathy skills and good information-gathering skills, it also requires good inferential skills (i.e., advanced empathy—see Chap. 8). You may have to "look beneath" what patients are saying on the surface to identify more specific goals. Most patients will be general and will tend to talk about goals in problem language. Your challenge is to reframe these statements into specific, positive goal statements. For example, a patient says, "I don't want to make the wrong decision." You can reframe this goal as, "You want to learn about genetic risk factors, weigh your available options, and reach a decision based on that knowledge." Or, a patient says, "Because my mother had breast cancer, I'm afraid that I will develop breast cancer, too." You might reframe this goal as, "You want to pursue genetic evaluation in order to find out if you are at increased risk for an inherited form of breast cancer."

Sometimes you will need to use mild confrontation in addition to advanced empathy (see Chap. 8) to help patients set realistic goals. For example, it is not a realistic goal when a tearful prenatal patient who wanted the pregnancy says, "I want to feel good about my decision to terminate my pregnancy." You might say, "I wonder if it would ever be possible for you to feel good about this. Perhaps you're saying you want to feel confident that you made the best decision possible with the information we have?" Indeed, as Anonymous (2008) poignantly writes about the decision she and her husband made to terminate a pregnancy due to multiple serious anomalies, "My husband and I do not feel we made the wrong decision, but we are not entirely sure we made the right one either. We have to live with the decision we made" (p. 417).

6.2.5 Strategies for Setting Goals and Attaining Goals

Setting Goals

- Be responsive to the patient's concerns. Levack et al. (2011) take a patient-centered view of health care that values patient participation in decision-making, considers patients' unique life contexts, and respects them as individuals. They recommend that anything patients or families raise when talking about goals "should at least be considered for discussion. This might require clinicians to consider goals outside of their traditional scope… [of practice]. It may also require clinicians to consider goals that they consider to be 'unrealistic'" (p. 212). Acknowledging a patient's goals does not mean you have to fully address them in genetic counseling. Through sensitive provision of information, you can help patients see how some of their goals may be unrealistic. For example, a patient might ask if you can provide counseling to help with some marital problems. For goals outside your scope of practice, you can make a referral (described in more detail later in this chapter).
- Notice patient nonverbals and try to use that information to understand the patient's emotional state.
- Translate patient questions or concerns into specific statements of goals toward which you can orient the genetic counseling session.
- Try for patient agreement to work on these goals.
- Try to establish both immediate and longer-range goals, if appropriate. For example, an immediate goal would be, "To learn the risk for a genetic condition." A longer-range goal would be, "To make a decision about whether to be tested."
- Try to establish goals that build on the patient's resources and assets (Hackney and Bernard 2017; Stone 1994). As Stone (1994) says with respect to brief pastoral counseling, "It has been my experience that people who are going through difficult times tend to ignore their own strengths and resources… the focus of brief pastoral counseling is not to break down people's defenses; rather it is to build upon the counselees' own coping resources and strengths, latent though they may be. One of the quickest ways to help individuals begin to feel better about themselves, thus enhancing self-esteem, is to get them to use some of those latent strengths. Breaking down defense mechanisms, or gaining insight into one's own defenses, is generally not necessary for the management of a problem. It almost always is quicker to help people develop their own resident strengths than it is to break down their defenses-but even more importantly, it is more humane…" (p. 42). For example, a woman who is pregnant with a baby with anencephaly might say she's praying for a miracle and that maybe her baby will live. A genetic counselor might respond to say, "It's clear that your faith is important to you. Tell me about the support you might get from your church commu-

nity." Sometimes patients express doubt in their ability to make a good decision. It can be helpful to ask patients to talk about other major decisions they made and think about how they approached those decisions. Their responses can help patients recognize both their strengths and their resources.

- Focus, when appropriate, on *approach goals*. Mann et al. (2013) state that "Goals can be oriented not only toward securing desired outcomes (approach goals) but also to avoiding unwanted outcomes…Because approach goals tend to be more effective than typical avoidance goals, one intervention strategy may be to reformulate avoidance goals into approach goals (e.g., 'avoid being sedentary' can be transformed into 'take regular walks')" (p. 490). So, for example, a genetic counselor might point out that if a patient's goal is to avoid getting cancer, a positive BRCA test could be viewed as an opportunity to pursue surveillance for early diagnosis and management if cancer occurs (approach goal).
- Use an established framework for setting goals. Latham (2003) demonstrated the utility of SMART goals in organizational settings. SMART stands for specific, measurable, attainable, realistic, and timely. These may be especially relevant in management of genetic risks or conditions for which there is treatment, such as metabolic disorders.
- Keep in mind that not all patients will be forthcoming about their situations (Schema et al. 2015). In Chaps. 3 and 4, we discussed ways in which you can use attending and empathy skills to build rapport and trust that facilitates greater patient self-disclosure.
- Genetic counselors are frequently involved in evaluations to identify a genetic diagnosis and/or risk assessment. Yet, as genetic counseling becomes more integrated with other areas of medicine (such as cardiology, cancer), genetic counselors will increasingly help patients set goals for disease risk management through surveillance, adherence to treatment recommendations, and/or lifestyle modifications. Thus, you can play a role in helping patients determine action steps necessary to attain their goals. Mann et al. (2013) recommend that in order:

> "To promote health behavior, people ideally should commit to health goals that are consistent with other personal goals, and they should give careful consideration to the desirability and feasibility of these goals…Once committed to a health goal, people need to think about how to implement these goals in the near and distant future. Attention should be paid to identifying goal-relevant opportunities and planning appropriate goal-directed behavior that capitalizes on these opportunities. Individuals should also think about obstacles, distractions, and temptations that may undermine goal-directed behavior and take prospective action to prevent their interference" (p. 494).

For example, a patient who is at risk for colon cancer avoids having a colonoscopy because it is unpleasant. A genetic counselor might help this patient recognize the long-term benefits of colonoscopy, early detection, and treatment, such as being around to watch his children grow up.

6.3 Obstacles to Goal Setting and Goal Attainment

Tryon and Winograd (2011) assert that, "Patients, particularly those who are new to psychotherapy, may have an inaccurate perception of the role they are expected to play in the treatment process. In their experiences with other health professionals such as physicians, patients tend to play a relatively passive, submissive role, presenting their symptoms and receiving treatment. The goals of such treatment typically do not involve much discussion, and there may be little collaboration regarding treatment beyond patient compliance in following professional directives" (p. 55). This is arguably true for genetic counseling. Thus, a common obstacle to patients' active engagement in setting goals is their misperceptions about the nature of genetic counseling.

Danish and D'Augelli (1983) identify four major obstacles or roadblocks to patient goal setting and attainment, which we define in Table 6.1, along with examples and possible genetic counselor interventions. These obstacles, either alone or in combination, can prevent patients from achieving their desired outcomes. So, you need to assess patient roadblocks and take steps to reduce or remove them.

Here are additional examples of specific obstacles to setting and achieving genetic counseling goals:

- Some patients and genetic counselors may lack experience stating problems in positive, goal-oriented terms.
- As we said earlier, some patients have limited familiarity with the nature and scope of genetic counseling and therefore lack an understanding of appropriate goals. You can acknowledge their confusion and invite them to express goals at any point during the session. For example, "Don't feel that you have to come up with something right now. Why don't we begin with…Please let me know if you think of more goals as we go along."
- There are other competing goals (Mann et al. 2013). For example, by avoiding setting a goal of deciding whether to have genetic testing, the patient may believe she can make the issue go away, avoid responsibility for the decision, and/or maintain an illusion that everything will be OK.

Table 6.1 Roadblocks to patient goal attainment

Roadblock	Patient example	Counselor intervention
Lack of knowledge	Patient does not know that there is a risk of passing a gene onto her child	Provide patient with genetic risk information
Lack of skills	Patient does not know how to approach his family members to persuade them to participate in genetic testing	Practice various scenarios for approaching family members
Fear of risk-taking	Patient fears that she could not handle a positive test result	Discuss fears and refer for mental health counseling if appropriate
Lack of social support	Patient has no supportive family members or friends, no religious/spiritual base, etc.	Refer to a support group or to mental health counseling/psychotherapy

- The patient may be trying to set goals that actually belong to someone else (e.g., "My doctor wants me to have this test"; "My parents want me to terminate the pregnancy"; "Can you imagine what my neighbors would say if they knew I wanted to have a baby that has Down syndrome!"). Of course, if a patient is attending genetic counseling primarily to satisfy someone else, or is going through the motions in order to have testing, the goals will be quite limited and not as mutual as you would like. In such situations, you might say, "I know you would rather not be here. However, since you are, I wonder if there's anything that might be beneficial to you. Is there anything you might want to discuss?" It is important to assess the motivation underlying patient goals, that is, whether the goals are for themselves or for doing what others expect of them (Mann et al. 2013).
- Patients may resist goals they perceive as being forced onto them, either by you or by someone else. For instance, McCarthy Veach et al. (1999) found that some former prenatal patients were dissatisfied with their genetic counseling because the genetic counselor insisted on presenting termination as an option after they had explicitly stated it was not an option for them. Clearly, these genetic counselors and patients were at odds over the goal of discussing all available options. Remember, you don't always have to go into detail about every option merely because you think you must *cover all the bases*. It's important to respect your patients' views and feelings.
- Patients may only be considering short-term consequences. For example, a woman with a BRCA1 mutation might not want to share this information with her daughters because she is concerned about causing them to worry. A genetic counselor might help the patient modify her goal of not causing worry to address longer-term consequences (daughters may benefit from testing and appropriate surveillance).
- Cultural worldviews that outcomes are due to chance, fate, God's will, etc. may not be compatible with self-directed goal setting. Patients with such worldviews may have difficulty seeing the value in setting goals. Nevertheless, you might say, "You've made the decision to come for genetic counseling. So, I assume you believe there's something we could do that might be useful for you. How would you like to spend this time together?"
- Cultural variations in explanatory models for illness factors may present obstacles to goal setting. It is important to conceptualize patient concerns in ways that are consistent with the patient's culture. Lewis (2010) suggests a series of questions to assess a patient's explanatory model that can be adapted to genetic counseling:

    1. What do you call your problem? What name does it have?
    2. What do you think has caused the problem?
    3. Why do you think it started?
    4. What do you think the sickness does? How does it work?
    5. How severe is it? Will it have a short or long course?
    6. What kind of treatment do you think the patient should receive? What are the most important results that you hope she receives from this treatment?

7. What are the chief problems that the sickness has caused?
8. What do you fear most about the sickness? (p. 217)

- Cultural differences between the genetic counselor and patient may pose obstacles. As part of the goal-setting process, you may need to explicitly acknowledge ethnic and cultural differences (Cardemil and Battle 2003; La Roche and Maxie 2003).
- Some patients come from cultures that do not have a future time orientation, and therefore goals should be linked less to dates and more to social or natural events (Brown 1997). Also, Western views of change usually are linked to acting upon one's environment and taking control of one's situation, whereas for some patients from other cultures, change is regarded as establishing harmony within the family or tribe and learning to appreciate the ways things are and one's place in this reality (Brown 1997). Patients who hold Eurocentric views will tend to take a goal-oriented, self-expressive approach to dealing with their problems as will many African American and Asian-American patients, while Hispanic-American patients may tend to take a wait-and-see approach, and American Indians may prefer controlled self-expression characterized by thoughtful, rational, carefully controlled responses: "One implication of this value is that different groups may take longer to consider the problem and will have different propensities for action" (Brown 1997, p. 34). Keep in mind, however, that cultural and individual factors interact uniquely for each patient, so you should be careful not to make unfounded assumptions or stereotype patients (Hackney and Bernard 2017)
- Some patients lack an ability to conceptualize the void between where they are currently and where they would like to be (Hackney and Bernard 2017). For example, a patient (following the death of a child with a genetic conditions) says, "We wanted a big family, but now I don't think I will ever want another child." She fails to recognize that she might make a different decision through a series of smaller steps (e.g., gathering information about recurrence risks and available testing; consulting with genetic counselor and family members; seeking out personal counseling). Although these patients recognize where they are currently and where they ideally would like to be, they are unable to visualize what they would need to do to get from here to there. You could ask, "What are some things you need to do in order to make this happen? What will be your first step?" (Cormier and Hackney 2012; Hackney and Bernard 2017).
- Some patients may lack a clear awareness of their values, desires, priorities, etc. (Hackney and Bernard 2017), or they may be in conflict (e.g., wishing to determine if their child has fragile X syndrome, like their brother, but feeling responsible for this condition). You might address patient ambivalence by acknowledging it. For example, "You don't have to come up with a plan right now. Would you like to take a few minutes [or a few days, if feasible] to think about it?" You might try advanced empathy to identify the conflict. For instance, "I wonder if your indecision about fragile X syndrome testing is due to your feeling responsible for your son's condition?"

- When your patients are couples or families, you must simultaneously take into account several individuals' wishes, desires, and needs (Martin 2015; Schoeffel et al. 2018). This can make goal setting difficult, as their interests may be in conflict. Indeed, one of the major challenges experienced by genetic counselors when their patients have genetic concerns involves disagreements among family members about what to do (Abad-Perotín et al. 2012; Alliman et al. 2009; Bower et al. 2002; Gschmeidler and Flatscher-Thoeni 2013; McCarthy Veach et al. 2001). In such situations, you might say, "My goal is to assist you in finding the most satisfying solutions for all of you" (and then ask each individual to express her or his wishes) (Martin 2015; Schoeffel et al. 2018). One possible exception would be situations in which it is a cultural practice for one family member to speak for another (Schoeffel et al. 2018).

6.4 Genetic Counseling Endings

In genetic counseling, there are two types of endings: session endings and relationship endings. In situations where you have only one contact with a patient (e.g., many prenatal genetic counseling cases), these endings occur simultaneously. In other situations, you may have contacts that extend over a period of years (e.g., working in a specialty clinic such as a muscular dystrophy clinic, where patients are seen for ongoing care; patients who return with subsequent pregnancies; BRCA gene families). Ending the relationship in genetic counseling is similar to endings in psychotherapy, where the goal is to "...help clients successfully achieve their agreed-upon treatment goals and then end their work together in a planned and thoughtful manner" (Vasquez et al. 2008, p. 654). In this section, we offer suggestions for effectively managing both types of endings.

6.4.1 Guidelines for Effective Endings

In genetic counseling, you set the stage for successful endings from the outset by describing the nature of the contacts you anticipate having with your patients (number of sessions, session length, follow-up contacts, etc.). We recommend the following strategies:

- *Inform patients.* Explain what genetic counseling is, if they are unfamiliar with the service, and describe the process by which you will work with them. Determine mutually agreed-upon goals (Glasgow et al. 2006; Tryon and Winograd 2011; Vasquez et al. 2008). Include an explanation of how much time you have together so that it doesn't come as a surprise at the end (Kramer 1990).
- *Prepare patients for the end of a session.* Genetic counseling sessions may not adhere to a strict time limit. Nonetheless, you must remain sensitive to the overall

clinic schedule. For example, in prenatal genetic counseling sessions that precede a scheduled ultrasound, it is appropriate to let the patient know your time together is limited or ending (e.g., "I want to make sure that you get to your ultrasound on time, so we only have about 10 min left. I wanted to be sure we had enough time to talk about…"). Be careful, however, not to make patients feel rushed. To the extent that you can, try to maintain some flexibility in your schedule to accommodate the time requirements of an extremely complex and/or difficult case.

- *Summarize the session*. You can do this in different ways. You could provide an overview of the discussion and ask your patient how s/he feels about what you've discussed. Another option is to ask your patient to provide a summary (e.g., "Our time is about up. I'm wondering what stands out for you as far as what we've covered today"). You should fill in missing information and/or correct inaccurate statements; frequently you will need to correct technical/factual information. After the summary of the discussion, you might ask your patients to briefly describe where they are in their decision-making process. For example, "What are your thoughts and feelings about the next thing you will need to do in order to make a decision?" Finally, if appropriate, discuss how test results will be conveyed to them, and possibly walk patients through a discussion of *what if* the results are abnormal.
- *Discuss next steps*. Review what will happen next and what actions they can take. For example, "In about 10 days you will receive a letter summarizing what we discussed today. I will call you in two weeks with the results of your test. If you have not heard from me by then, please call the clinic. Also, if any other questions or concerns come up, please feel free to call me here." Make a specific plan for communicating test results (e.g., What is a good time to call? If you are not in, may I leave a message?)
- *Arrange for follow-up*. If you will interact with the patient again, explain how future contacts can be made. Also, keep the door open, letting patients know they may return at some future time if they need to do so. But do this carefully, as this may be a way to avoid truly ending the relationship. Furthermore, patients may not have health-care coverage for additional sessions.
- *Try to end on a positive note, if appropriate* (e.g., "You seem very comfortable with the decisions you made today"). Be careful not to offer false hope and reassurances. Patients who receive bad news will experience any number of negative feelings (anger, grief, anxiety, shock, despair—see Chap. 9 for a discussion of patient affect). You may be tempted to try to make them feel better. This is probably not possible nor even desirable at this point. Be careful not to offer platitudes such as, "Everything will be fine," "Things will look better after a good night's sleep," "You'll get over this in time," and "It's all for the best." In Chap. 7, we discuss communicating bad news to patients.
- *Reinforce patients*. Express confidence in their decision-making processes and in their ability to get through this difficult time. Be careful to reinforce their process and not their actual choice! For example, "You've done some very careful thinking about your options and seem to know which one is best for you," rather than "You're doing the right thing by pursing this testing."

- *Be sensitive to patient emotional state.* If patients are crying and/or otherwise visibly distraught, allow them a few minutes to compose themselves before leaving the room.
- *Observe social amenities regarding departure.* Hold the door for patients, escort and/or direct your patients to the exit, and shake hands, but *only* at their initiation.
- *Don't counsel outside of the room.* If you have to escort your patients any distance to an exit, some may attempt to continue counseling with you. Try to direct the conversation away from genetic counseling, instead engaging in social conversation about the weather or about where they had to park their car, etc.
- *Respect a patient's autonomy to end early* (Burwell and Chen 2006; Kramer 1990). Some patients may want to end before you believe everything has been adequately covered. There can be several reasons why patients might want to leave prematurely, including patient discomfort with difficult and/or painful information and/or patient denial that anything is wrong; you need to respect your patients' wishes to end early. Remember, however, there is certain information that you must present, such as risk. One option is to send a follow-up letter detailing information that you believe requires additional explanation.

6.4.2 Challenging Genetic Counseling Endings

There are a number of situations in which ending the genetic counseling relationship may be difficult. Generally speaking, the longer you've worked with a patient, or the greater number of contacts you've had with them, the more difficult the endings (Pinkerton and Rockwell 1990; Vasquez et al. 2008). Some patients may feel dependent on you, or they may have really enjoyed working with you (both are more likely when you've had more than one interaction). Research from counseling/psychotherapy also suggests that endings are more difficult when the process and outcome have not gone well; in other words, both the patient and the counselor are dissatisfied (Brady et al. 1996; Quintana 1993). You may have been the bearer of "bad news"; the patient may be angry; you may be a painful reminder of their disappointment; or the patient may not have adequately integrated information from the genetic counseling sessions. Even a skilled genetic counselor may be challenged by an angry, dissatisfied patient (Schema et al. 2015).

In addition to relationship endings, it can be challenging to end individual genetic counseling sessions, especially with highly verbose patients, emotionally distraught patients, patients who are making what you consider to be the wrong decision, patients to whom you've given bad news, and patients with whom you feel a strong connection (e.g., you wonder how things will turn out for them).

Regarding contracting and session endings, in a study of genetic counseling of deaf adults, Baldwin et al. (2012) recommended "Instead of including rapport building at the beginning of a session, the genetic counselor may wish to include rapport building at the end of the session. While in hearing culture, it is common for conversations to terminate quickly, Deaf clients, may find this rude and often prefer a more prolonged good-bye. The genetic counselor may wish to include time at the end of the appointment for rapport building and an extended goodbye session and utilize time at the beginning for contracting and direct statements about the expected content of the genetic counseling session…" (p. 269). Based on their recommendations, we suggest that you spend a little bit of time to establish some rapport at the beginning of the session and save some time at the end of the session for further rapport building.

Perhaps one of the most challenging endings is with terminally ill patients where your good-byes are symbolic of their eventual deaths (e.g., a 17-year-old boy with Duchenne muscular dystrophy). Sometimes counselor difficulties with endings are related to unresolved endings in their own lives. Ending a genetic counseling relationship may represent these unresolved issues (see Chap. 12 transference and countertransference). Clues that you are having trouble with endings include consistently exceeding session time limits and looking for excuses to recontact patients.

Try to anticipate particularly difficult endings whenever possible and carefully plan for them. For example, you could discuss your feelings with your supervisor and brainstorm about how you might best proceed with saying good-bye. You could work on coming to terms with or accepting the limitations of genetic counseling, that is, accepting that it may not be the solution to every patient's problems. We also recommend that you work on being aware of your reactions (see Chap. 12). Try not to let your personal feelings interfere with the ending (e.g., unreasonable fears about what the patient will do, your own feelings of not being helpful, etc.).

6.5 Making Referrals

Some of your genetic counseling patients may benefit from referrals to other sources of information, treatment, guidance, and/or support. In some situations, you might recommend additional medical evaluation (diagnostic or treatment/management). In other situations, you might offer referrals for therapeutic services, such as early intervention services for a child with special needs. You may also identify patients who would potentially benefit from social support services. Genetic counselors frequently provide patients with information about relevant support or advocacy organizations. Finally, you may recognize that your patient might benefit from additional counseling or mental health services. Reasons for this type of referral include patient issues that are beyond your expertise or scope of practice [e.g., patient is suicidal and in need of psychiatric care; intense marital conflict precipitated by the confirmation of a genetic condition (cf. Schoeffel et al. 2018)].

Schema et al. (2015) interviewed genetic counselors about their experiences of patient anger directed at them. Among the counselors' recommended strategies, they suggested "Appropriate referral to other specialists including licensed psychologists is warranted when the psychosocial needs of the patient cannot be met by genetic counseling alone" (p. 728). Wool and Dudek (2013) assessed genetic counselor comfort with referral of prenatal patients to perinatal hospice and found they varied in their comfort. This variation was partly due to level of familiarity with perinatal hospice services. They stressed, "…it is imperative that genetic counselors are aware of palliative care options in their organizations and communities" (p. 539). They identified several options, including written information and referral to support groups, accessing other parents who have experienced similar losses, and online resources that can help families through the decision-making process.

Sagaser et al. (2016) surveyed genetic counselors about their use of religious/spiritual language in sessions and their views about the importance of religion and spirituality. Based on the findings, the authors concluded that, "Just as recognizing traditional coping styles such as distancing, planning, or avoidance is useful in genetic counseling, recognizing a patient's utilization of positive or negative religious coping can be helpful for a genetic counselor, as he or she can either support the patient's use of positive religious coping or consider making a referral for chaplaincy or pastoral services… [Moreover] these data suggest that persons who are experiencing high levels of spiritual struggle are more likely to be receptive to religious actions and would especially benefit from a referral to receive pastoral services" (pp. 929–930).

Murphy et al. (2016) surveyed pediatric genetic counselors regarding their experiences with parents who ask them to provide sex education to their children affected with intellectual disabilities (ID). Based on their findings, they concluded that it is within the genetic counselor's role to "…assess individual sex education needs for patients with ID and provide suitable resources and referrals to those competent in sex education instruction" (p. 559).

Making an effective referral requires careful planning on your part. It is your responsibility to first assess whether your patients might benefit from referral to other sources of help and, if so, to explain how the referral is intended to be in their best interests (e.g., explain why you are suggesting additional support/help and what they might gain from using additional resources). We recommend the following referral guidelines:

6.5.1 Building a Referral Base

- Familiarize yourself with referral sources. You should build and continually update a referral file that contains the names, addresses, telephone numbers, and procedures for contacting various referral sources. Build a file by asking colleagues for recommendations, by checking with patients for sources that have been helpful to them, and by learning about local social services. You should update your file periodically (e.g., checking on which referral sources are currently accepting new clientele).
- In choosing referral sources for your file, select sources that are sensitive to and aware of cross-cultural issues, gender issues, and sexual orientation issues, and sources that are affordable and located a reasonable distance from patients (Owen et al. 2007; VandenLangenberg et al. 2012).

6.5.2 Points to Consider When Making Referrals

- Consider your patient's resources before making a referral. For example, be aware of expense, distance to the source, and whether the patient has insurance or some other means of paying for the referral source (Owen et al. 2007).
- Referrals do not always have to be made immediately. For instance, services may not be available, or the patient may not be emotionally ready. Let your patient know your referral sources are available in the future.
- Offer the referral tactfully so patients realize that it is to provide them with maximum assistance and not that their problems are so severe they need extra help. Start by focusing on the importance of their problems or needs and the desirability of resolving the problem.
- Prepare your patient. Provide details about the referral source (e.g., name, location, fees) to lessen anxieties about this new relationship. Describe the competencies and characteristics of the referral person(s) and how to contact the referral source. You are trying to enhance this person's credibility and expertise.
- Don't be too prescriptive with respect to the type of service or treatment the patient will receive from the referral source. For instance, do not suggest that your patient would receive a certain type of intervention or test.
- Check out patient feelings about the referral. Even patients who seem to readily accept a referral may be apprehensive. Normalize any fear. For instance, "Most people would feel hesitant to bring this issue to their minister." You could point out how the patient took the risk to come to see you and build on this to get the patient to take the referral (Cheston 1991). In some situations, you may decide to call and make the appointment, with the patient's permission.
- Anxious patients may ask a lot of questions about the referral source, and you should patiently answer their questions. In any case, ask them what they feel about the referral, and then what they think about it (Cheston 1991).
- Include the referral in a follow-up letter in order to remind patients.
- For some patients (e.g., a child referred to a special education professional), you may wish to follow up to see if the referral was taken and perhaps schedule another session with the patient after she/he has met with the referral source. Alternatively, you might ask the patient to call you in a couple of weeks to let you know how things went.
- Cheston (1991) cautions against leaving patients to their own resources. If your patient asks for additional help, and you are not immediately aware of any, tell your patient you will look into possibilities after the session and get back to her or him with whatever you find. Then follow through on your promise.

The following list displays the types of referral sources that might be appropriate for genetic counseling patients.

Common Referral Sources

Support groups (genetic condition)
Bereavement groups
Agencies (SSI, medical assistance, WIC, social services, respite care)
Services (infant stimulation, schools, The Arc)
Medical (genetics as well as other specialists)
Psychological (short-term therapy, long-term therapy, psychiatric, career/vocational counseling, family therapy)
Financial services
Adoption agencies
Social workers
Online resources
Clergy/spiritual leaders
Parenting classes
Drug/alcohol rehabilitation
Domestic abuse centers
Homeless shelters
Food banks
Developmental specialists
Unemployment center
Parents/individuals who are experienced with a condition and who are willing to talk with recently diagnosed patients/families

6.6 Closing Comments

You have a great deal of responsibility for beginning and ending genetic counseling sessions and relationships and for helping patients establish feasible goals. Advanced preparation, observing common courtesies, carefully listening to your patients, and setting goals and plans for achieving them will assist you in these important genetic counseling activities. As we've mentioned in other chapters, these responsibilities will become less challenging for you over time and with experience. You will gradually develop your style of structuring genetic counseling relationships and sessions.

6.7 Class Activities

Activity 1: Structuring the Session (Think-Pair-Share Dyads or Small Groups)

Students discuss the following:

- What concerns/questions do you think patients have about genetic counseling?
- What patient questions are you unsure about how to address? Afraid to address?

- How much welcoming should you do? Should you engage in chitchat?
- Should you go to the waiting room to get your patient? Will you escort your patient to the exit at the end of the session?
- How much structure should you give your patients about the genetic counseling process? How much detail would you provide? What would you say?
- Should you provide follow-up, and, if so, how?
- Should you engage in social conversation (chitchat) at the end of the session? Why or why not?

Process

The whole group discusses their responses to these questions

Estimated time: 30 min.

Activity 2: Initiating the Session Model

Instructor and a volunteer genetic counseling patient engage in a role-play in which the counselor demonstrates how to initiate the genetic counseling session. Students observe and take notes of counselor initiating behaviors.

Estimated time: 10 min.

Process

Students discuss their examples of counselor initiating behaviors. They also discuss the effect these genetic counselor behaviors appeared to have on the patient.

Estimated time: 10 min.

Activity 3: Initiating the Session (Triad Role-Plays)

Students practice initiating genetic counseling sessions using the three role-plays described below. The patient selects one of the following roles without letting the counselor know about the role in advance. They should spend about 5–10 min doing each role-play and about 10 min after each role-play to provide feedback. Have the patient read the patient role to the triad after discussion of the role-play.

Patient Roles

1. You are here to see a genetic counselor because you are at risk for Huntington disease. You are worried that potential employers will find out you have the gene. You also worry about how *you* will react if you find out you have the gene. You feel, at some level, that suicide might not be out of the question.
2. You were scheduled to see the genetic counselor as part of your work-up for recently diagnosed breast cancer. You have had some very bad experiences with health-care professionals in the past and feel as if you have been railroaded into coming for genetic counseling. You question what the genetic counselor sitting

in front of you will be like. What are her/his credentials? How can you be sure that s/he will be helpful?

3. You are here to see the genetic counselor because of an abnormal ultrasound finding. Your doctor's nurse told you the ultrasound test was "positive for Down syndrome." You are very scared that something could be wrong with your baby. You have been told by members of your cultural group that genetic counselors can give your baby problems. Furthermore, you are afraid that if you go through with the genetic counseling, it will mean you have lost faith in God's ability to handle things. Still, you desperately want to know if your baby is OK.

Estimated time: 60 min.

Process

The whole group discusses: What did you learn from these role-plays? How did the counselors have to modify their approaches with the different patient roles? What interpersonal skills were required?

Estimated time: 15 min.

Instructor Note

- Observers can use Appendix 1, Observer Checklist for Beginning the Genetic Counseling Session.

Activity 4: Ending the Session (Think-Pair-Share Dyads or Small Groups)

Students discuss patient and counselor resistance to ending. What might be some reasons that *patients* would not want to end the genetic counseling session and/or relationship? What are some reasons *you* might not want to end the session and/or relationship? Do you possess any characteristics that would make it difficult for you to observe time limits? To end the session and/or relationship?

Process

The whole group discusses their responses to these questions.

Estimated time: 30 min.

Activity 5: Ending the Session (Triad Role-Plays)

Students practice ending a genetic counseling session using a combination of the genetic counselor and patient roles described below. The counselor and patient should not reveal to each other or to the observers which role they chose to portray until the end of the role-play. They should spend 10 min doing the role-plays and about 10 min after each role-play to provide feedback. Have the counselor and patient identify the roles they chose to portray during discussion of the interaction.

Genetic Counselor Options	Patient Options
Resist ending	Resist ending
Encourage ending	Encourage ending
Uncertain about ending	Uncertain about ending

Estimated time: 60 min.

Process

The whole group discusses: What did you learn from these role-plays? What interpersonal skills were required?

Estimated time: 15 min.

Instructor Note

- Observers can use Appendix 2, Observer Checklist for Ending the Genetic Counseling Session.

Activity 6: Making Referrals (Think-Pair-Share Dyads or Small Groups)

Discuss making referrals. What do you think is particularly difficult about making effective referrals? (Consider both patient and counselor characteristics as well as external factors such as the referral sources themselves.) What strategies might you use to facilitate a referral?

Process

The whole group discusses their responses to these questions.

Estimated time: 15–20 min.

Activity 7: Making a Referral (Triad Role-Plays)

Students engage in 10-min role-plays. The patient is a prenatal genetic counseling patient who the counselor wants to refer to a psychotherapist. The reason for the referral is that the genetic counselor believes she has unresolved grief over prior multiple pregnancy losses. The genetic counselor realizes these issues are too complex to address during the genetic counseling session. In the first role-play, have the patient accept the referral. In the second role-play, have the patient resist the referral. In the third role-play, repeat either of these two patient roles, without the patient disclosing her role until the triad discusses the interaction.

Estimated time: 30–60 min.

Process

The whole group discusses: What did you learn from these role-plays? What interpersonal skills were required?

Estimated time: 10 min.

Instructor Note

- Observers can use Appendix 3, Observer Checklist for Making Referrals.

Activity 8: Goal-Setting (Think-Pair-Share Dyads or Small Groups)

Discuss these questions: What are your reactions to setting goals in genetic counseling? What might be some challenges in setting goals from the patient's perspective? From your perspective? How do you avoid imposing your goals on patients?

Estimated time: 10–15 min.

Activity 9: Unrealistic Genetic Counseling Goals Brainstorming (Dyads or Small Groups)

Students generate a list of unrealistic genetic counseling goals for patients (e.g., I'm only having this test because my doctor wants me to; I want a test so I can be sure I won't get cancer).

Estimated time: 15 min.

Instructor Note

- This activity could be expanded by having dyads or small groups exchange lists and rewrite the goals to make them more realistic.
- Another way to expand this activity is to have dyads or small groups formulate a response to each patient, as if they were actually speaking to the patient, that clarifies and/or modifies each goal.

Activity 10: Goal-Setting Exercise (Dyads or Small Groups)

Dyads or small groups change the following genetic counseling patient problem statements into goal statements:

- A prenatal patient says, "I'm afraid something's wrong with my baby."
- "My son has just been diagnosed with Klinefelter syndrome, and he needs someone to talk to."
- "My mother died of breast cancer, and I'm afraid I'm going to die like that, too."
- "I'm sick of wondering whether I have the gene for Huntington's!"
- "No one can tell me what's wrong with my son."

- "I was hoping there was some research that could help my daughter with this disease."
- "I don't want to have any test that's going to hurt my baby."

Estimated time: 20–30 min.

Instructor Note
- This activity could be done individually as a written exercise.

Activity 11: Goal-Setting Model

The instructor and a volunteer genetic counseling patient engage in a genetic counseling role-play in which the instructor demonstrates how to establish goals with the patient. Students observe and make notes about counselor behaviors.
Estimated time: 15 min.

Process
Students discuss their examples of counselor goal-setting behaviors. They also discuss what goals were established and share their impressions of the impact of the goal-setting process on the patient.
Estimated time: 10 min.

Activity 12: Goal-Setting (Triad Role-Plays)

Students use the following patient roles to engage in 15-min role-plays in which they attempt to establish genetic counseling goals with their patients. Follow each role-play with 10 min of feedback.

Patient Roles
1. Patient referred for genetic evaluation of her positive family history of breast cancer.
2. Twenty-five-year-old whose father was recently diagnosed with Huntington disease.
3. A prenatal patient who has a child with cystic fibrosis.

Estimated time: 25 min for each role play and critique.

Process
The whole group discusses: What did you learn from these role-plays? What interpersonal skills were required?
Estimated time: 15 min.

6.8 Written Exercises

Exercise 1: Contracting Role-Play

Engage in a 20-min role-play of a genetic counseling session with a classmate. The role-play can be based on a patient you saw in clinic or it can be a made-up patient situation. During the role-play, focus on contracting and setting session goals. Audio record the role-play. Next transcribe the role-play and critique your work. Use the following method for transcribing the session:

Counselor	Patient	Self-critique	Instructor
Key phrases of dialogue	Key phrases	Comment on your own response	Will provide feedback on your responses

Create a brief summary:

1. Briefly describe patient demographics (e.g., age, gender, ethnicity, socioeconomic status, relationship status) and reason for seeking genetic counseling.
2. Identify *two* things you said/did during the role-play that were effective and *two* things you could have done differently.

Give the recording, transcript/self-critique, and summary to the instructor who will provide feedback.

[*Hint*: This assignment encourages self-reflective practice regarding your clinical performance. The goal is not to do a perfect session. Rather the goal is to assess the extent to which you can accurately assess your psychosocial counseling skills. You will gain more from this exercise if you refrain from scripting what you plan to say as the counselor.]

Exercise 2: Ending and Referral Role-Play

Engage in a 15-min role-play of a genetic counseling session with a classmate. The role-play can be based on a patient you saw in clinic or it can be a made-up patient situation. During the role-play, focus on ending the genetic counseling session and making a referral. Audio record the role-play. Next transcribe the role-play and critique your work. Use the following method for transcribing the session:

Counselor	Patient	Self-Critique	Instructor
Key phrases of dialogue	Key phrases	Comment on your own response	Will provide feedback on your responses

Create a brief summary:

1. Briefly describe patient *demographics* (e.g., age, gender, ethnicity, socioeconomic status, relationship status) and *reason* for seeking genetic counseling.
2. Identify *two* things you said/did during the role-play that were effective and *two* things you could have done differently:

Give the recording, transcript/self-critique, and summary to the instructor who will provide feedback.

[*Hint*: This assignment encourages self-reflective practice regarding your clinical performance. The goal is not to do a perfect session. Rather the goal is to assess the extent to which you can accurately assess your psychosocial counseling skills. You will gain more from this exercise if you refrain from scripting what you plan to say as the counselor.]

Exercise 3: Referral Sources

Develop a referral file using the categories in the Common Referral Sources list in this chapter. Include names, numbers, addresses, types of services provided, and fees.

Instructor Note

- This could be done as a group project.
- Students can be instructed to build a list of national resources as well as local ones. The national resources would be useful to them regardless of where they end up practicing.

Exercise 4: Case Preparation Interview Checklist

Develop an interview checklist that you could actually use in your genetic counseling sessions.

Instructor Note

- This can be done as an in-class activity, where small groups develop a list for different case scenarios such as newborn with achondroplasia, adult whose mother has a recent diagnosis of early-onset familial Alzheimer disease (PSEN1 gene mutation), or other known genetic condition in the family. Allow students to select a topic of interest based on their clinical experience or observations.

Exercise 5: Patient Goals

For each patient scenario below, write possible patient genetic counseling goals:

- A couple is referred for genetic counseling to discuss consanguinity (first cousin union). They are from Italy. They have not told their families about their relationship. They are in their early 20s.
- The patients are a young Hispanic couple who have brought their 2-year-old son to see the medical geneticist because of developmental delay. They are uncertain as to why they need to see the medical geneticist but are doing what their pediatrician recommended.

- The patient is a 31-year-old white, G5, P0040 (5th pregnancy, 4 abortions—not elective) woman who is pregnant for the fifth time. She has had four miscarriages and she has no living children. She has a history of seizures and multiple pregnancy loss. You are seeing her in this pregnancy to discuss the possible teratogenic effects of her seizure medications. (Her seizures have occurred only in the past 1 1/2 years due to a serious car accident.) The patient is distraught that she may lose another baby and is also dealing with an unhappy marriage and home life. To make matters worse, she has terrible short-term memory due to the accident, and you have to repeat most of the information.
- The patient is a 24-year-old white woman with a history of type 1 diabetes. She is planning a pregnancy next year.
- The couple have had 7 years of infertility and have learned they are pregnant with twins. The mother is 39 years old.
- The patient is a 6-year-old boy who is developmentally delayed. The family has been to numerous doctors, and someone suggested that he be tested for Williams syndrome.
- The patient is a 37-year-old, G1, P1001 (second pregnancy, one full-term delivery, one living child), woman pregnant for the second time. She is approximately 12 weeks pregnant. She has had one normal delivery resulting in one normal living child. NIPT testing reveals that the fetus is probably affected with trisomy 18.
- The patient is a 14-month-old boy with severe encephalopathy. The family history is significant for a similarly affected male sibling who died at 18 months of age. All studies (done elsewhere) have been negative; no diagnosis has been provided to the family.
- The patient is a 13-year-old girl who is suspected of having Turner syndrome. The pediatrician who referred her spoke only to her parents about his suspicions. Although the parents have researched Turner syndrome on the Internet, they have told their daughter nothing about their concerns or about the condition itself. The patient seems nervous and somewhat frightened.
- A woman comes to clinic for genetic counseling following a recent diagnosis of DMD in her 6-year-old son. Her sister accompanies her to this appointment.

Exercise 6: Obstacles to Patient Goals[1]

For each of the patient scenarios in Exercise 5, identify possible roadblocks (lack of knowledge, lack of skill, fear of risk-taking, and lack of social support) and generate interventions to address one roadblock from each category (i.e., knowledge, skill, risk-taking, and social support).

[1] Adapted from Danish and D'Augelli (1983).

Appendix 6.1: Observer Checklist for Beginning the Genetic Counseling Session

	Yes	No
Initial greeting		
Chairs at comfortable distance		
Faces patient		
Introduces self		
Asks how to address patient		
Makes some small talk, if appropriate		
Orientation		
Presents credentials		
Discusses taping/supervision		
Describes genetic counseling		
Contracting and goal setting		
Asks about patient's reasons for seeking genetic counseling		
Attempts to establish goals		
Seeks patient's agreement to work on goals		
Miscellaneous		
Is sensitive to patient's questions/concerns		
Discusses follow-up to the session		
Additional comments		

Appendix 6.2: Observer Checklist for Ending the Genetic Counseling Session

	Yes	No	N/A
Anticipate conclusion of session			
Summarizes major points			
Reaches consensus on what to do next			
Agrees on time, date, and place of future contact			
Is aware of time constraints (e.g., clinic schedule)			
Gives cues to signal the end			
Determines why patient does not want to leave			
Makes special arrangements for additional time			
Observes courtesies of departure			
Ends on positive note, if appropriate			
Structures end of relationship			
Assesses extent to which goals were accomplished			
Asks patient to summarize decision-making progress			
Summarizes patient decision-making progress			
Plans follow-up			
Makes referral to other sources			
Additional comments			

Appendix 6.3: Observer Checklist for Making Referrals

	Yes	No
Describes patients' issue/problem for which the referral is made		
Selects referral sources appropriate for the patients and their situation		
If possible, provides more than one name for referral		
Informs patients about referral source name, address, phone number, and how to contact		
Contacts the referral source directly		
Presents referral source credentials to enhance credibility		
Makes positive statements about the usefulness of the source for helping the patients		
Secures patients' written permission to send a report of the genetic counseling to this source		
Follows up with patients to inquire about their experience with the referral source		

References

Abad-Perotín R, Asúnsolo-Del Barco Á, Silva-Mato A. A survey of ethical and professional challenges experienced by Spanish health-care professionals that provide genetic counseling services. J Genet Couns. 2012;21:85–100.

Accreditation Council for Genetic Counseling. Practice based competencies for genetic counselors. 2015. http://gceducation.org/Documents/ACGC%20Core%20Competencies%20Brochure_15_Web.pdf. Accessed 18 Aug 2017.

Alliman S, Veach PM, Bartels DM, Lian F, James C, LeRoy BS. A comparative analysis of ethical and professional challenges experienced by Australian and US genetic counselors. J Genet Couns. 2009;18:379–94.

Andrighetti H, Semaka A, Stewart SE, Shuman C, Hayeems R, Austin J. Obsessive-compulsive disorder: the process of parental adaptation and implications for genetic counseling. J Genet Couns. 2016;25:912–22.

Anonymous. A genetic counselor's journey from provider to patient: A mother's story. J Genet Couns. 2008;17:412–18.

Baldwin EE, Boudreault P, Fox M, Sinsheimer JS, Palmer CG. Effect of pre-test genetic counseling for deaf adults on knowledge of genetic testing. J Genet Couns. 2012;21:256–72.

Berger KS. The developing person through the life span. 6th ed. London: Macmillan; 2005.

Bernhardt BA, Biesecker BB, Mastromarino CL. Goals, benefits, and outcomes of genetic counseling: Client and genetic counselor assessment. Am J Med Genet. 2000; 94:189–97.

Bower MA, Veach PM, Bartels DM, LeRoy BS. A survey of genetic counselors' strategies for addressing ethical and professional challenges in practice. J Genet Couns. 2002;11:163–86.

Brady JL, Guy JD, Poelstra PL, Brown CK. Difficult good-byes: a national survey of therapists' hindrances to successful terminations. Psychother Priv Pract. 1996;14:65–76.

Brown D. Implications of cultural values for cross-cultural consultation with families. J Couns Dev. 1997;76:29–35.

Burwell R, Chen CP. Applying the principles and techniques of solution-focused therapy to career counselling. Couns Psychol Q. 2006;19:189–203.

Cardemil EV, Battle CL. Guess who's coming to therapy? Getting comfortable with conversations about race and ethnicity in psychotherapy. Prof Psychol. 2003;34:278–86.

Case AP, Ramadhani TA, Canfield MA, Wicklund CA. Awareness and attitudes regarding prenatal testing among Texas women of childbearing age. J Genet Couns. 2007;16:655–61.

Cavanagh M, Levitov JE. The counseling experience a theoretical and practical approach. 2nd ed. Prospect Heights, IL: Waveland Press; 2002.
Cheston SE. Making effective referrals: the therapeutic process. New York: Gardner Press; 1991.
Cormier S, Hackney HL. Counseling strategies and interventions. 8th ed. Boston: Allyn & Bacon; 2012.
Danish SJ, D'Augelli AR. Helping skills: II: life development intervention: trainee's workbook. New York: Human Sciences Press; 1983.
Fine SF, Glasser PH. The first helping interview. Thousand Oaks, CA: Sage; 1996.
Glasgow RE, Emont S, Miller DC. Assessing delivery of the five 'as' for patient-centered counseling. Health Promot Int. 2006;21:245–55.
Greenberg RP, Constantino MJ, Bruce N. Are patient expectations still relevant for psychotherapy process and outcome? Clin Psychol Rev. 2006;26:657–78.
Griswold CM, Ashley SS, Dixon SD, Scott JL. Genetic counselors' experiences with adolescent patients in prenatal genetic counseling. J Genet Couns. 2011;20:178–91.
Gschmeidler B, Flatscher-Thoeni M. Ethical and professional challenges of genetic counseling–the case of Austria. J Genet Couns. 2013;22:741–52.
Hackney HL, Bernard JM. Professional counseling: a process guide to helping. 8th ed. London: Pearson; 2017.
Hartmann JE, McCarthy Veach P, MacFarlane IM, LeRoy BS. Genetic counselor perceptions of genetic counseling session goals: a validation study of the Reciprocal-Engagement Model. J Genet Couns. 2015;24:225–37.
Ishiyama FI. Culturally dislocated clients: self-validation and cultural conflict issues and counselling implications. Can J Couns. 1995;29:262–75.
Kramer SA. Positive endings in psychotherapy: bringing meaningful closure to therapeutic relationships. San Francisco: Jossey-Bass; 1990.
La Roche MJ, Maxie A. Ten considerations in addressing cultural differences in psychotherapy. Prof Psychol. 2003;34:180–6.
Lafans RS, Veach PM, LeRoy BS. Genetic counselors' experiences with paternal involvement in prenatal genetic counseling sessions: an exploratory investigation. J Genet Couns. 2003;12:219–42.
Latham GP. Goal setting: a five-step approach to behavior change. Organ Dyn. 2003;32:309–18.
Levack WM, Dean SG, Siegert RJ, McPherson KM. Navigating patient-centered goal setting in inpatient stroke rehabilitation: how clinicians control the process to meet perceived professional responsibilities. Patient Educ Couns. 2011;85:206–13.
Lewis L. Honoring diversity: cultural competence in genetic counseling. In: LeRoy BS, McCarthy Veach P, Bartels DM, editors. Genetic counseling practice. Hoboken: Wiley-Blackwell; 2010. p. 201–34.
Mann T, De Ridder D, Fujita K. Self-regulation of health behavior: social psychological approaches to goal setting and goal striving. Health Psychol. 2013;32:487–98.
Martin DG. Counseling and therapy skills. 4th ed. Long Grove, IL: Waveland Press; 2015.
McCarthy Veach P, Truesdell SE, LeRoy BS, Bartels DM. Client perceptions of the impact of genetic counseling: an exploratory study. J Genet Couns. 1999;8:191–216.
McCarthy Veach P, Bartels DM, LeRoy BS. Ethical and professional challenges posed by patients with genetic concerns: a report of focus group discussions with genetic counselors, physicians, and nurses. J Genet Couns. 2001;10:97–119.
McCarthy Veach P, Bartels DM, LeRoy BS. Coming full circle: a Reciprocal-Engagement Model of genetic counseling practice. J Genet Couns. 2007;16:713–28.
Michie S, Weinman J, Marteau TM. Genetic counselors' judgments of patient concerns: concordance and consequences. J Genet Couns. 1998;7:219–31.
Murphy C, Lincoln S, Meredith S, Cross EM, Rintell D. Sex education and intellectual disability: practices and insight from pediatric genetic counselors. J Genet Couns. 2016;25:552–60.
Oosterwal G. Multicultural counseling. In: Uhlmann WR, Schuette JL, Yashar B, editors. A guide to genetic counseling. 2nd ed. New York: Wiley; 2009. p. 331–61.

Owen J, Devdas L, Rodolfa E. University counseling center off-campus referrals: an exploratory investigation. J Coll Stud Psychother. 2007;22:13–29.
Pieterse A, van Dulmen S, Ausems M, Schoemaker A, Beemer F, Bensing J. QUOTE-geneca: development of a counselee-centered instrument to measure needs and preferences in genetic counseling for hereditary cancer. Psychooncology. 2005;14:361–75.
Pinkerton RS, Rockwell WK. Termination in brief psychotherapy: the case for an eclectic approach. Psychotherapy. 1990;27:362–5.
Quintana SM. Toward an expanded and updated conceptualization of termination: implications for short-term, individual psychotherapy. Prof Psychol. 1993;24:426–32.
Resta R, Biesecker BB, Bennett RL, Blum S, Hahn SE, Strecker MN, et al. A new definition of genetic counseling: National Society of Genetic Counselors' task force report. J Genet Couns. 2006;15:77–83.
Sagaser KG, Hashmi SS, Carter RD, Lemons J, Mendez-Figueroa H, Nassef S, et al. Spiritual exploration in the prenatal genetic counseling session. J Genet Couns. 2016;25:923–35.
Schema L, McLaughlin M, Veach PM, LeRoy BS. Clearing the air: a qualitative investigation of genetic counselors' experiences of counselor-focused patient anger. J Genet Couns. 2015;24:717–31.
Schoeffel K, McCarthy Veach P, Rubin K, LeRoy BS. Managing couple conflict during prenatal counseling sessions: an investigation of genetic counselor experiences and perceptions. J Genet Couns. 2018. https://doi.org/10.1007/s10897-018-0252-6.
Spitzer Kim K. Interviewing: beginning to see each other. In: Uhlmann WR, Schuette JL, Yashar B, editors. A guide to genetic counseling. 2nd ed. New York: Wiley; 2009. p. 71–91.
Stone HW. Brief pastoral counseling. J Pastoral Care Counsel. 1994;48:33–43.
Sue DW, Sue D. Counseling the culturally diverse: theory and practice. 6th ed. New York: Wiley; 2012.
Tryon GS, Winograd G. Goal consensus and collaboration. Psychotherapy. 2011;48:50–7.
Uhlmann WR. Thinking it all through: case preparation and case management. In: Uhlmann WR, Schuette JL, Yashar B, editors. A guide to genetic counseling. 2nd ed. New York: Wiley; 2009. p. 93–132.
VandenLangenberg E, Veach PM, LeRoy BS, Glessner HD. Gay, lesbian, and bisexual patients' recommendations for genetic counselors: a qualitative investigation. J Genet Couns. 2012;21:741–7.
Vasquez MJ, Bingham RP, Barnett JE. Psychotherapy termination: clinical and ethical responsibilities. J Clin Psychol. 2008;64:653–65.
Wool C, Dudek M. Exploring the perceptions and the role of genetic counselors in the emerging field of perinatal palliative care. J Genet Couns. 2013;22:533–43.

Chapter 7
Collaborating with Patients: Providing Information and Facilitating Patient Decision-Making

Learning Objectives
1. Describe skills and strategies needed to effectively provide information and communicate risk.
2. Identify factors that impact risk perception.
3. Identify some of the major factors affecting patient decision-making.
4. Develop skills for facilitating patient decision-making through self-reflection, practice, and feedback.

Providing information and facilitating patient decision-making are two genetic counseling competencies that incorporate a set of skills that are fundamental to genetic counseling practice. The principal focus of genetic counseling sessions will vary depending upon the needs of the patient and family. For instance, parents of a newborn with a neural tube defect may mostly need support and resources. Other sessions involve patients who are facing one or more decisions or are just starting to deal with a complicated diagnosis; providing information and facilitating decision-making are essential interventions in such sessions.

Two tenets of the Reciprocal-Engagement Model of genetic counseling practice are particularly relevant to providing information and facilitating patient decisions. The first is "genetic information is key," with these related goals: (1) the counselor knows what information to impart; (2) the counselor presents genetic information; (3) the patient is informed; and (4) the patient gains new perspective. The second relevant tenet is "patient autonomy must be supported" with one major related goal being that the genetic counselor facilitates collaborative decisions (McCarthy Veach et al. 2007). In addition, genetic counselors affirm their ethical responsibilities with regard to providing information and facilitating patient decisions in their Code of Ethics (COE) (The National Society of Genetic Counselors 2017). Specifically, the National Society of Genetic Counselors (NSGC) COE states that genetic counselors strive to "Seek out and acquire balanced, accurate and relevant information required

P. McCarthy Veach et al., *Facilitating the Genetic Counseling Process*,
https://doi.org/10.1007/978-3-319-74799-6_7

for a given situation" (Section I:1) and "Enable their clients to make informed decisions, free of coercion, by providing or illuminating the necessary facts, and clarifying the alternatives and anticipated consequences" (Section II:4).

This chapter focuses on skills associated with these key competencies. It is important to recognize that while the *information* (*content*) of any genetic counseling interaction will vary depending on the indication or focus of the session and may change over time, the *skills* genetic counselors employ in providing information and facilitating decisions are transferrable across all situations and specialty practice areas and remain constant over time.

7.1 Communicating Information

Information giving involves the genetic counselor providing data, facts, and details in an attempt to help patients be as fully informed as possible about their genetic diagnosis and/or risks, including the psychosocial and related medical implications and recommendations, testing options, and potential outcomes. This can be a daunting task. In many situations, you will have to provide complicated and/or ambiguous information about topics such as uncertain risks, sensitivity and specificity of tests, and variable phenotypes (Austin 2010; Facio et al. 2014; O'Doherty and Suthers 2007).

To emphasize that the *skills* employed in providing information are transferable and do not change over time, we note the following statement by Yager (2014). Citing Kessler's (1997) seminal work on teaching versus counseling models of genetic counseling, Yager says the information genetic counselors provide "…needs to be accurate, current, and expressed in a way that is understandable to patients who may have no medical or scientific background. The information-giving (teaching) part of genetic counseling is a complex and difficult task in that it not only requires a depth of knowledge but also a high level of interpersonal skill (e.g., reading a patient's nonverbal confusion after an attempted explanation or recognizing that sometimes a carefully placed question may reveal what the patient is not understanding)" (p. 935).

The types of information you present during genetic counseling sessions can be broadly categorized as: (1) information that sets the agenda and describes what to expect during the session; (2) information pertinent to patients' reasons for seeking genetic counseling (e.g., genetic risk, testing options, testing results, disease information, support services); (3) information that facilitates patients' decision-making processes (e.g., options, outcomes); and (4) follow-up information about what will happen after the session (e.g., support resources, medical recommendations, referrals).

Although patients vary in their information needs, they generally desire relevant medical and genetic information communicated in a way that conveys care, concern, and empathy as well as support in communicating this information to others. Yet, individual differences (e.g., gender, education, age, known or unknown mutation in family, affected or not affected) and cultural differences will influence the type, timing, and amount of information desired by a given patient (Roshanai et al. 2012).

As with other aspects of genetic counseling, you can increase your effectiveness in providing information by employing your skill set, specifically, contracting (Chap. 6), attending behaviors (Chap. 3), effective use of questions (Chap. 5), and empathy (Chaps. 4 and 8).

Through the process of contracting, a genetic counselor can assess a patient's information needs (what the patient *wants* to know, what questions the patient has) and collaborate with a patient to set an agenda that combines the counselor's agenda (critical information the patient *needs* to know) with the patient's needs and agenda. The genetic counselor can use attending behaviors and questions to assess a patient's prior knowledge as well as other factors that may impact her or his ability to hear and assimilate information, such as health literacy. In order to understand a patient's emotional response to the referral and to the information provided during a genetic counseling encounter, the counselor can use empathy. Questions will help a counselor assess a patient's understanding of and response to the information ("Was that what you were expecting to hear?" "What questions do you have?" "How are you feeling about this information?"). As you gain experience, you will be able to use these skills to tailor information to meet the needs of each individual patient. One size does not fit all in providing information in genetic counseling.

Importantly, in most genetic counseling situations, there is *critical* information that a genetic counselor must communicate about topics such as risks, testing options, testing results, and medical management recommendations, regardless of patient preference for discussing them. Presenting critical information in a way that each patient can hear and use it is itself a skill. Every patient is different, and meeting individual needs is the art of genetic counseling.

7.1.1 Providing Information vs. Giving Advice

Providing information, when done effectively, gives patients knowledge they can use to choose their own course of action. Providing information differs from giving advice, in that advice is an attempt to suggest what a patient should do. As discussed in Chap. 10, because genetic counseling is a medically based practice, there will be times where giving advice is not only appropriate but the standard of care. There are many circumstances when a genetic counselor would not hesitate to provide advice. For example:

- Advising a patient with a BRCA mutation to have increased screening for breast cancer
- Advising a pregnant woman against consuming alcohol during the pregnancy
- Recommending that a patient share genetic risk information with at-risk relatives
- Encouraging the parents of a child with a genetic metabolic condition to follow the recommended diet

- Advising a patient with a genetic cardiovascular disorder to follow up with a cardiovascular specialist
- Recommending psychological counseling for a patient with obvious signs of mental health issues (e.g., clinical depression)

7.1.2 Strategies for Communicating Information

Skillful provision of information requires practice and self-reflection. Below are some strategies for effectively providing information:

- *Be organized.* Prepare your information in advance. Gather relevant information and arrange it in a clear order. Think about what might happen in the session that would impact your plans for providing information (e.g., the patient becomes extremely emotional; the patient brings family or friends to the appointment; the patient is physically ill due to treatment).
- *Have a good understanding of the information yourself.* Before meeting with your patient, be sure you comprehend complicated medical details, risk for disease and symptoms, cost of testing, etc., and have thought through how you will explain this information. Practice saying the information and record yourself while doing so. Play back the recording and listen as if you were the patient. Modify accordingly.
- *Do not follow a "cookbook" approach.* In Chap. 6 we discussed the value of preparing a "checklist" of topics you want to be sure to cover in a session. You should, however, avoid writing out a detailed script that you follow more or less verbatim with every patient. The same recipe will not work for all individuals. Instead, tailor how you present the information to each patient and her or his situation. Over time and with supervised experience, you will find yourself gradually working more extemporaneously as you assess how a given patient is responding to your presentation of information.
- *Use terminology patients will understand.* Present information in a language your patients can understand, and remember that this will not be the same for everyone. Some patients will have more science literacy and will understand technical terminology, but most will not. Use analogies that are familiar to patients to convey complicated information (e.g., genes as blueprints, chromosomes as books).
- *Give an appropriate amount of information.* Initially, you may feel comfortable using elaborate drawings and providing extensive information. Although visual aids can be very effective (Garcia-Retamerol and Cokely 2013), they may diminish your ability to attend to patients' nonverbals, may confuse patients whose primary mode of learning is not visual, and may make your presentation seem overly "scripted." Trepanier (2012) describes a case in which she focused a bit

too heavily on information provision at the expense of considering the couple's psychosocial circumstances. As she reflects, "It is not always (ever?) enough to just give people genetic information. It is so very important to consider the context in which patients receive the information" (p. 233). As you become more comfortable and gain experience, you will be better able to discern what is most relevant for each patient.

- *Be selective about the information you provide in a follow-up letter or medical record.* If you write patient letters, keep them relatively short and uncomplicated. Roggenbuck et al. (2015) found that "a short letter [about 1.5-2 pages in length] highlighting the basic facts related to the genetic condition may be more useful to parents of diverse educational backgrounds and may support a positive emotional adaptation at the time of a new diagnosis" (p. 645). The shorter letters contained less technical jargon and simpler sentences. As medicine moves toward electronic medical records, be aware that some written information (e.g., clinic notes) can/will be accessed by patients.
- *Be strategic about deciding whether to give patients information they don't want.* As discussed earlier in this chapter, some information is critical and must be shared with a patient. There are situations, however, where it may be appropriate to consider patient preferences. Researchers have found that a major ethical and professional challenge is deciding whether or not to withhold information when patients don't want to hear it (Abad-Perotín et al. 2012; Alliman et al. 2009; Bower et al. 2002; Gschmeidler and Flatscher-Thoeni 2013; McCarthy Veach et al. 2001). For instance, some patients may resent being given a detailed description of abortion when they have explicitly stated abortion is not an option for them. We suggest you acknowledge a patient's feelings about an option such as abortion and then adjust the amount of information you provide. For example, "I understand that you consider abortion to be an unacceptable option. I respect your feelings about that. I just wanted to make sure you are aware that it's an option. Let's talk about the options that will work for you."
- *Regulate the rate at which you provide information.* Refrain from lengthy statements, especially when they contain threatening information. For example, saying the following, "Your results are back and you do have the BRCA gene, but there are a lot of things you can do to protect your health; you can have regular mammograms, consider having prophylactic surgery, and continue to maintain a good diet and exercise plan," does not allow the patient room to process the test result emotionally and cognitively. You need to give the patient time and space to "catch up." Proceed slowly so your patients can let the information sink in and experience some of their initial feelings and thoughts before moving to the next step.
- *Check patient comprehension.* Periodically assess your patient's understanding of the information. For example, you might ask "What's your understanding of what we've just discussed?"

- *Use questions strategically.* Closed-ended questions like, "Do you understand?" or "Do you have any questions?" are not usually helpful. Most patients will say they understand, and many will deny having any questions. Instead, try open-ended statements: "What questions do you have?" and "Of the information we've discussed so far, what stands out for you?" Their responses to these questions will give you an opportunity to correct any inaccuracies and/or reinforce key points they identify.
- *Refrain from getting into a lecturing mode.* Lecturing tends to lull the patient into passivity. Try engaging your patients by periodically giving them an opportunity to ask questions or react to the information. Try pausing occasionally during your presentation so your patient can digest what you've said. Pauses will also allow you to psychologically attend to their nonverbal reactions.
- *Remember that cognitive content is always emotionally charged.* Your patients may have strong emotional reactions to certain factual information. Consequently, it will take them some time to comprehend and digest the facts. It's generally a good idea to repeat important information.
- *Pay attention to patients' defenses and conscious and unconscious motivations.* You should try to recognize, for example, when patients are intellectualizing their situation and are making decisions without really understanding the long-range emotional impact these decisions will have (Klitzman 2010).
- *Accommodate patient cultural differences.* Patients vary in their cultural interpretations of the causes and significance of genetic conditions (Lewis 2010; Steinberg Warren n.d.). Try to determine their cultural beliefs and values, and then frame your information within their cultural context. For example, Gammon et al. (2011) studied Latina and non-Latina White women at increased risk for hereditary breast and ovarian cancer. They found that both groups wished to discuss family issues, they desired advice, and they wanted more specific information about testing. Latina women, however, were less aware of the availability of testing. The researchers also found that "Women with a personal history of cancer most often mentioned wanting to discuss family issues, followed by personal advice, and specific information about the test, while women without a cancer diagnosis most often mentioned personal advice, followed by information about the test, and discussing family issues" (p. 625). They concluded that it is important to consider both "cultural factors (e.g., ethnic background) and individual differences (e.g., history of cancer) in determining the type of information to focus on during genetic counseling" (p. 625).
- *Remember that you do not have to know every answer.* Don't be afraid to say, "I don't know." Then find out and get back to your patient via phone and/or letter or refer your patient to another professional, if necessary. It may be that no one knows the answer to the patient's question, but this is also important information to convey.

7.1.3 Communicating Test Results

One aspect of providing information is communicating test results. As a genetic counselor, one of the most difficult responsibilities you will have is informing patients their test results are positive (not normal), indicating that they or their unborn child or family member has, or is at increased risk for, a genetic condition. This news has a tremendous impact on patients, and they may respond in a number of ways (crying, "shutting down," getting angry at you, etc.). Patients who test positive may feel an additional burden of worry and guilt about passing the condition to their children (Bottorff et al. 1998). Further complicating matters, learning they are gene positive may affect patients differently, both immediately and in the long term. For example, Hagberg et al. (2011) found that knowing one was gene positive for Huntington disease had both positive and negative effects. The most prevalent positive effects were "greater appreciation for life" and "drawing family members closer," while the most common negative effects were "decisional regret" and decreased "psychological well-being" (p. 70); decreased well-being included distress, anxiety, and loss of hope. The researchers concluded that knowing one's positive gene status "can either be a motivator or an obstacle to invest in one's self" (p. 78).

It may be helpful to prepare people to receive results prior to testing by discussing all possible test outcomes (Semaka et al. 2013) and by carefully exploring patients' "best guesses" of how positive results, negative results, and variants of uncertain significance may affect different short-term and long-term aspects of their life. Specific questions about major domains of functioning may help them to more concretely consider the impact of testing. For example, you might ask how test results could potentially impact future living arrangements, retirement plans, reproductive actions, job or career choices, and decisions about a spouse/life partner.

Positive test results may also have intense emotional effects on the genetic counselor. For example, your empathy for patients makes you, to some extent, feel what they are feeling. You like your patients and don't want bad things to happen to them. You may feel responsible for the positive test result. You may feel guilty for being relieved that it's happening to them and not to you. You have to allow yourself to experience these unpleasant emotions to a certain extent. Communicating positive results should never become routine. Your effectiveness as a genetic counselor depends in part on your ability to remain connected to your patients. At the same time, you need to balance this connection with a healthy distance from their situations (see Chap. 12—countertransference and compassion fatigue).

7.1.4 Strategies for Communicating Positive Test Results

Prepare in Advance

- Make a plan with the patient about how you will provide the testing results. Check to see what phone number to use, with whom you can communicate, and whether it is acceptable to leave a message. If results are only given in person, when is the follow-up visit, and what will happen at that visit? Will you communicate with the patient's primary care provider? Having a plan will help you maintain the patient's privacy in a way that is of their choosing, and it will alleviate some of the anxiety that is natural while waiting for test results.
- Practice giving positive results with a colleague so you know what you want to say and how you want to say it. Be genuine when providing results, and be prepared for strong emotions in the patient. Remember that you might react to those emotions as well.
- For a given patient, visualize the meeting in which you present the results. Try to imagine in detail what each of you will say, feel, and do.
- When you are unfamiliar with the cultural values and practices of your patient, research how positive test results are best communicated. You could, for instance, consult with experienced medical interpreters and review relevant literature. Cultural variables can affect the way in which genetic counselors provide information. For example, Jecker et al. (1995) described a case in which possible bad outcomes were communicated to a Navajo patient by referring to a hypothetical third party; this was done to reduce the patient's likelihood of thinking he was "being witched." For some patients from Middle Eastern cultures, the family is a paramount resource for coping during times of crisis such as illness, and efforts may be made to shield vulnerable family members from unwelcome news (Awwad et al. 2008; Lipson and Meleis 1983). Therefore, a male family member (father or grandfather) may take the lead in the genetic counseling session.
- Help the patient to prepare in advance by using anticipatory guidance. You could ask patients to engage in scenarios prior to undergoing testing. As we mentioned earlier, it may be helpful to prepare people to receive results prior to testing by discussing all possible test outcomes (Semaka et al. 2013). Ask them to imagine and describe what they will feel, think, and do if the results are positive, negative, or a variant of uncertain significance (VUS). In addition to helping patients anticipate their reaction, this strategy gives you some idea of how they may react when you present them with the test results.

Deliver the News

- Proceed slowly and calmly. Patients need time to absorb this type of news, and they will be more likely to express their feelings if you take a low-key approach.

- Sometimes the news is best delivered in stages. For example, you might call a patient with a positive test result, offer to answer her or his immediate questions, and schedule a follow-up appointment as soon as possible. As long as you leave the door open for the patient to contact you with questions before the scheduled appointment, this approach can be helpful.
- Allow patients to react the way they wish. Don't step in with false reassurances, encourage them to stop crying, or go on at length with detailed information they will not be able to hear. Information given too soon tends to block patients from expressing their feelings of disbelief, anger, grief, etc. (Faulkner et al. 1995). Sit quietly while they absorb the news, offer tissues after a few moments, and give them time to pull themselves together. You may want to move your chair closer.
- Be genuine when communicating positive test results. Sometimes you will feel particularly connected to a patient and will find yourself becoming tearful. It's OK to show some of your distress as long as it does not become the focus of the interaction. (Having tears in your eyes and feeling choked-up are probably OK; breaking down and sobbing are not).
- Try saying, "I'm sorry." This simple phrase can communicate the depth of your feeling for your patients and their situations. This is an example of what Kessler (1999) describes as *providing consolation*: "A simple, sincere word or two or even a touch may have an enormous impact on persons who have been devastated by calamity" (p. 339). We suggest you not rush to express your feelings. Rather, wait to say this until after the patient reacts initially to the test result.
- If patients start to cry, do not leave them alone. Stay psychologically and physically present while allowing them to express their feelings. You do not have to say anything. Being there conveys support.
- As appropriate, reassure your patients that mixed feelings are a natural response, and try to draw out their emotions by asking them to tell you what they are feeling.
- Point out that their emotions may fluctuate and/or change over time, and tell them you'll be available to talk to and meet with them in the future when and if new concerns or questions arise.
- Talk with your supervisor or colleague to debrief after delivering positive test results. This will help you to relieve some of your emotion.

Follow-up

- Once patients have regained some composure, assess their understanding and gently inquire about the next steps, that is, what they need. This is a time when an open-ended question such as "How can I be helpful to you right now?" may be particularly effective for drawing out what a patient is feeling and thinking.
- If relevant literature is available, you could give it to patients at the end of the session. This will allow them to take in the information at their own pace, time, and location. This may not be appropriate for all patients and situations, however. For some patients, it's better to provide details during a follow-up visit.

- Follow up with your patients at a later time. Check in to see how they are feeling, what they are thinking, and how much information they have retained. You might need to fill in some gaps. Do not leave it to patients to call you if they have questions. It is unlikely they will do so.
- Referral to counseling/psychotherapy may be appropriate if a patient has an extreme emotional reaction and/or appears to have limited coping skills.

7.1.5 Strategies for Communicating Negative or Inconclusive Test Results

What if the test results are negative (normal)? When reflecting about communicating negative test results, your first thought might be that it's a simple and happy task. On closer consideration, however, you'll find it can be quite challenging. Some patients may not fully understand the meaning of a negative test result (cf. Semaka et al. 2013). So, it is important to talk carefully and repeatedly about the limitations of a test. For example, you might say, "Your prenatal tests are all normal. This means that your baby does not have any of the conditions we were able to look for, but remember we talked about some of the limitations of the test. As you know, the test cannot find all conditions"; or, "You didn't inherit the change in the gene responsible for breast cancer that your mother has. But you still need to have regular checkups because you are at the same risk for breast cancer as any other woman in the general population."

You may need to review complex implications of negative test results. For example, Semaka et al. (2013) found that patients with negative results for HD but with an intermediate allele (IA) did not understand there was a risk of their descendants developing the condition. They noted, "Many participants had difficulty 'grasping the grey,' (i.e., understanding and interpreting their IA results) and their family experience, beliefs, expectations, and genetic counseling influenced the degree of this struggle" (p. 200). Also, you must be sensitive to patients' frustration that a diagnosis is not evident from testing.

Many, but not all, patients will feel relieved and happy about a negative test result. They may also have complex, mixed emotional responses that emerge over a period of time. For instance, a patient whose test for Huntington disease is negative may feel guilty about her siblings who carry the gene, fear rejection by the affected family members, believe she's lost the reason for having a close relationship with her siblings (i.e., the risk for HD), and be depressed about waiting as long as she did to have the testing done. She may also feel overwhelmed by the realization that she will be the primary caregiver for affected family members.

Gray et al. (2000) describe how one of the authors lived for years with the possibility of having the gene for Huntington disease (HD). Once she finally pursued testing, which yielded negative results, her reactions were as follows: "I did not have Huntington's, but for the last 34 years I had lived in the shadow of the disease, and it took a long time to sink in that I was 'normal'—I had the same chance as anyone else to live to be an alert, old person. I also grieved the time I spent not knowing and the choices I had made based on wondering if I had HD. I began to see the ways in which living with the threat of HD had limited my life choices and had narrowed my view of available options. More importantly, I felt that now I could have a life. The implications of this fact and my options were staggering! For a time, I was overwhelmed by the fact that I was HD-free and could live my life anyway I wanted, just like everyone else" (p. 9).

We suggest you try to minimize any preconceived notions about how patients will react and pay close attention to observing their actual reactions. Try to avoid value-laden introductions of test results like "I have good news for you!" Unless you're certain something like a normal prenatal test result is, in fact, good news, consider that some consequences of a normal result might be difficult for the patient/family.

What if the test results are not conclusive? This is one of the major challenges in communicating complicated information. Variants of uncertain significance (VUS) are a type of inconclusive test result that further complicate information provision to patients. Many patients pursue genetic testing because they wish to reduce uncertainty about the future (Semaka et al. 2013). Writing about VUS test results for women at high risk for breast cancer, Frost et al. (2004) noted, "Genetic counselors understand that results may be equivocal and [they] can convey the implications to patients, even if…[patients do not recall] this likelihood from the pre-test counseling session. Results of uncertain significance can be frustrating to hear and must be presented in terms of what the patient needs to understand in her own life as well as the needs of the extended family. When results are of uncertain significance, the family history becomes key to the risk assessment, especially with respect of medical management options for extended family members" (p. 233). They recommended that counselors provide information about the possibility of all three types of results (i.e., positive, negative, and VUS) during the pretesting session and their potential implications for the patient and family members. Speaking about results for a gene test for HD that reveals the patient has an intermediate allele, Semaka et al. (2013) recommended that "genetic counselors explore patients' feelings about receiving a 'grey' result that does not provide the certainty they may desire" (p. 213), correct misunderstandings, and provide additional information and support.

Kiedrowski et al. (2016) interviewed parents whose child had a VUS from a chromosome microarray study (CMA). These parents "…demonstrated a range of recall and personal interpretation regarding whether test results provided a causal explanation for their children's health issues. Participants maintained contradictory interpretations, describing results as answers while maintaining that little clarification of their child's condition had been provided…[and they] described adaptation/coping processes similar to those occurring after positive test results. Recall of terminology, including 'VUS' and precise CMA abnormalities, was poor. However, most demonstrated conceptual understanding of scientific uncertainty" (p. 101). The researchers concluded that "…receiving a VUS result may have an impact similar to that of receiving a definitive diagnosis; it was often viewed as an 'answer,' albeit a more complicated one. Parents described emotional responses ranging from strong feelings of guilt, sadness, and a sense of loss. Others described an evolution in their responses to that of comfort and relief. Some parents reported positive coping through engagement with support groups or advocacy activities. Others discussed that the test results empowered them to seek out medical, educational, therapeutic, and financial services" (p. 108).

Kiedrowski et al. (2016) also stressed the importance of remembering that "Uncertainty itself can have emotional consequences; [e.g.,] parental anxiety, depression, and/or helplessness [and lead to] negative coping such as pessimism, hopelessness, and feelings of failure" (p. 109). They speculated that "in many ways, parental reactions to receiving a VUS are even more complex and have the potential to be more emotionally charged with feelings of loss of control" (p. 109). The authors suggested that when a VUS result occurs "…genetics professionals emphasize the importance of a follow-up genetics evaluation to allow for a review of available databases, the literature, and a re-evaluation of the patient. Otherwise, families may be lost to follow-up and miss updated information that could impact their child's health care" (p. 110).

In summary, communicating test results can be challenging. We described several strategies a genetic counselor can use when communicating test results. As with other aspects of genetic counseling, skills such as careful attending, empathy, and strategic use of questions are critical to effective communication.

7.1.6 *Communicating Risk Information*

> "It is clear that individuals do not act on the basis of the 'actual' risk presented to them but act on the basis of their perception of the risk…." (O'Doherty and Suthers 2007, p. 410).

Risk information is one of the most complicated types of information you can present during genetic counseling. The term "risk" is defined differently by different individuals, and people vary markedly in their perceptions of the relevance and meaning of risk data for themselves and others. The perception of risk "involves more than subjective numeric probability alone…and [it] is an important contributor to, but not the sole contributor to decision-making" (Austin 2010, p. 232).

Relatedly, patients "…find risk difficult to accurately quantify, with a tendency to overestimate. Rather than being a stand-alone concept, risk is something lived and experienced and the process of constructing risk is complex and influenced by many factors" (Sivell et al. 2008, p. 30). "The process by which individuals construct their risk is complex, influenced by many factors including environmental factors, occupation, diet, stress and worry, physical resemblance to an affected relative, as well as genetic or family history factors. Individuals use their framework for understanding risk to aid coping with a risk, which is something that they live with and experience as opposed to being a detached concept" (Sivell et al. 2008, p. 56).

Bylund et al. (2012) noted that "Although counseling sessions do significantly impact individuals' general knowledge of genetics, influencing their personal risk perception or accuracy is more complicated and not always successful and is likely further complicated by diversity in individuals' health and social experiences" (p. 299). Patients often have inaccurate perceptions of their genetic risk, and these misperceptions often are not changed by genetic counseling. "For example, the client may speak of undergoing a genetic test to 'get some certainty' despite the test providing only an indication of risk (uncertainty) of developing cancer by a certain age" (O'Doherty and Suthers 2007, p. 410).

So how can you best present risk information? As percentages? Numbers? With verbal descriptors? Does your patient have a 1 in 100 chance of having a genetic condition or a 99 in 100 chance of not having it? There is no simple answer that fits every patient and situation.

Hallowell et al. (1997) found a majority of their sample of genetic counseling patients who received risk information concerning breast and ovarian cancer preferred quantitative data because these types of data provide clearer and more concrete information. The researchers found little difference in patient preference for percentages, proportions, or population comparisons.

Although the basis of most risk communication in genetic counseling is quantitative data, some patients prefer qualitative descriptions (e.g., the risk is high or low or likely or unlikely). Thus, it can be helpful to include both quantitative and qualitative descriptions. But know that different people in different situations will attach different meaning to risk information. For example, a couple may view a recurrence risk of 1 in 4 or 25% as being low because they came in thinking their chance of recurrence was 100%. Similarly, a relatively low numeric risk (like 3%) may be perceived as insurmountable due to a devastating experience or perceived high burden. You generally should avoid providing only qualitative data since they can be misinterpreted by the patient and/or reflect your biases (Austin 2010; Melas et al. 2012; O'Doherty and Suthers 2007; Sagi et al. 1998).

Typically, in genetic counseling there are five types of quantitative formats for providing risk information (Hallowell et al. 1997):

- Proportions (5 in 100 or 1 in 20)
- Percentages (5%)
- Ratios (1:20)
- Odds against (19 to 1)
- Comparisons with population risks (e.g., risk for breast cancer in women who are carriers of BRCA mutation as compared to the population risk for breast cancer).

Austin (2010) suggests framing risk as a combination of "numeric probability, context, and nature of the potential outcome" (p. 229). She defines *context* as "factors such as the client's perceptions of illness etiology, family history, population prevalence of the condition"; *the nature of potential outcome* as "the perceived severity (e.g. physical, emotional, financial impact) of illness for which numeric probability is being provided"; and *numeric probability* as "the pre-existing subjective numeric probability figure perceived by the client [that] may be modified by the objective numeric probability provided by the counselor" (p. 229). She recommends (p. 231):

- Use risk descriptors cautiously (such as high chance, low chance, etc.). When using risk descriptors, include qualifiers regarding your "own perceptions of context and severity, and acknowledgement that this may be markedly different from that of [the] client," and always provide numeric probability as well.
- Resist conflation of concepts—Be aware that "when we are providing numbers in the context of risk communication…we are providing information only about the numeric probability of an event—not about the broader concept of 'risk,' which would include severity, context, and potentially other factors too…we have a responsibility to make the conceptual distinction...between risk and probability explicit for both ourselves and our clients, by being careful about the language we use relating to the numbers (i.e. not referring to them as risks, but probabilities or chances)…."
- Know that risk perception is not just about the numbers. Help patients make emotionally inclusive decisions—risk perception involves more than rational and logical processing of numeric probabilities. "Perhaps, rather than encouraging clients to make logical decisions based on accurate estimation of numeric probability, we should be ensuring that our clients make the best possible— emotionally inclusive—decisions that they can, based on thorough, conscious awareness of their perceptions of context and nature of outcome."

Patient Factors That May Impact Risk Perception

A number of patient factors may affect how patients and family members perceive their risk.

- Cognitive functioning: for example, the extent to which the patient thinks abstractly and mathematically, abilities that are related to intelligence and education.
- Emotional impact: Etchegary and Perrier (2007) cite evidence that "…people do not always process information, particularly threatening health information, in a deliberate, systematic way. For example, we are frequently motivated to process threatening health information in a self serving manner that allows us to downplay or deny our risk of disease…[One reason is that] messages that contain threatening health information appear to evoke defensive cognitive processing. We may respond by downgrading the seriousness of the illness or the validity of the diagnostic test…scrutinize more carefully the threatening information or generate counterarguments and alternative explanations to discredit it…we may also selectively generate information about ourselves and others in ways that allow us to believe we are at low relative risk for illness…" (pp. 420–421).
- Temperament and personality: for example, pessimists may inflate risk figures, while optimists underestimate their risks; achievement-oriented individuals may believe they can beat the odds, while failure-threatened individuals believe there is little to no chance of winning.

- Attributions/worldview: for example, individuals may have an external locus of control such that they attribute outcomes to chance or fate (Bottorff et al. 1998).
- Personal experience with a condition: individuals with a family history of a condition do not view risk estimates hypothetically (Bottorff et al. 1998).
- Perceived burden: Patients' beliefs about the consequences of being affected by a condition influence their perceptions of risk. Livneh and Antonak (2005) describe seven characteristics of disorders that may influence perceived burden: "(1) degree of functional limitations; (2) extent to which the disorder interferes with one's ability to perform daily tasks and life roles; (3) uncertainty of prognosis; (4) need for prolonged medical, psychological, and/or rehabilitation treatments; (5) degree of psychological stress associated with the condition (e.g., mental illness stigma); (6) impact on family, friends, and other support persons; and 7) financial losses due to unemployment, under-employment, and health care costs" (p. 7). Relatedly, "…the observation that some people tend to overestimate numeric probability even after having been provided with objective assessment is directly in accordance with the expectations based on the concept of 'asymmetric loss functions'. This concept posits that overestimation occurs because the more undesirable the potential outcome, the more costly are underestimates of the probability of that outcome…" (Austin 2010, p. 231).
- Different perceptions by family members of risk, burden, and/or desire for more children: Simonoff (1998) offers this example about how the meaning of risk may vary: "Thus the family who believed all offspring would be affected may receive a 50% risk as good news. Similarly, and more relevant to autism, families burdened by a very disabled child may view a recurrence risk of 5% as unacceptably high" (p. 448).
- Coping styles: for example, information seekers, avoidant style, dependent decision-makers, minimizers, blunters, and monitors (Wakefield et al. 2007) (see Chap. 9).
- Gender: males and females may perceive the implications of the same information differently (Bottorff et al. 1998).
- Temporal factors: for example, time changes how people view their situation (Bottorff et al. 1998).
- Cultural or ethnic identity: for example, in a study of Hmong refugees' English proficiency, Ostergren (1991) had to modify a rating scale of 0% to 100%, changing it to 1–3, because percentage was an unfamiliar concept.
- Religiosity: one's values, philosophy, or meaning of life affect perceptions (Siani and Assaraf 2016). For example, Palestinians and Somali immigrants are likely to believe that disability is determined by God (Awwad et al. 2008; Greeson et al. 2001). Individuals who use religious coping may have a spiritual locus of control which fosters beliefs that "God empowers the faithful to prevent disease, or God can be consulted to actively interfere with a disease process…" (Quillin et al. 2006, p. 456).
- Difficulties grasping the concept of probability and genetics and unresolved issues (Klitzman 2010; Simonoff 1998): patients might not accept the diagnosis in the proband or believe another factor is causative, for example, fall-

ing during a pregnancy caused a child to have Down syndrome. Klitzman (2010) found individuals who were at risk for or had Huntington disease, breast cancer, or alpha-1 antitrypsin deficiency had "Misunderstandings about statistics and genetics [that] often fueled each other, and reflected denial, and desires for hope and control...emotional needs can thus outweigh understandings of genetics and statistics, and providers' input. [Furthermore,] individuals often maintained non-scientific beliefs, though embarrassed by these..." (p. 430).

General Guidelines for Presenting Risk Information

- First and foremost, remember that genetic counseling is a communication process. Thus, risk communication is a conversation with a patient, not a lecture.
- Assess patient risk perceptions. Ask them a question like: "Is this what you were expecting to hear? How does this sound to you – high/low? What is your reaction to hearing this information?" Listen to how patients frame the information you give them "...whether they talk about the 'chance of developing cancer' or the 'chance of not developing cancer' as clues to how they perceive their risk" (O'Doherty and Suthers 2007).
- Present risk information in an unbiased way. Present both sides of a risk (i.e., use positive and negative framing), "There is a 1% chance of ____ occurring, and there is a 99% chance of it not occurring." Terms such as, "the risk is only..." and "as high as..." suggest your own views of risk information; you should present risk information in a few different ways in order to present it more neutrally (Simonoff 1998). When using qualitative descriptors such as likely or unlikely, it is important to also provide numeric information as "people perceive the word likely to imply probabilities anywhere between .5 and .99..." (Austin 2010, p. 231). Point out that an "increased risk" is not always the same as a high risk. Be mindful that certain words may convey a stigma or negative connotation for some patients (Melas et al. 2012; O'Doherty and Suthers 2007, p. 416).
- Be flexible in your approach. You will probably have personal preferences for the way in which you present risk information. Indeed, Hallowell et al. (1997) found this to be the case for their sample of experienced genetic counselors. Just remember that you may need to supplement your personal preference with another way in order to accommodate patient preferences, abilities, situations, etc. In other words, you need to be flexible in how you communicate risk information.
- Remind yourself that your patient's perceptions of risk may be quite different from yours (Bottorff et al. 1998; Hallowell et al. 1997) and that many patients interpret risk as binary or categorical (e.g., either I have the gene or I don't have it) no matter how you present the data (Austin 2010).

- Understand that how you provide risk information has a significant impact on patient interpretations of its meaning. "Informing an individual that he or she has a chance of a particular occurrence of 1.3 in 10,000 compared to the general population's chance of 1 in 10,000 is not particularly impressive to most people. However, if the format was such that the individual was informed that his or her risk is 30% greater than that of the average individual, the situation is likely to be seen as 'riskier,' although the two situations are equivalent" (Bottorff et al. 1998, p. 70). Point out that while population frequencies contribute to estimating their personal risk, they are not the "whole story" for the patient (O'Doherty and Suthers 2007).
- Emphasize that risks are probabilities, not guarantees (O'Doherty and Suthers 2007). Try to help patients understand the uncertainties involved.
- Be aware, as we've stressed in this chapter, that it is very difficult to communicate objective risk to patients (Sivell et al. 2008). Bottorff et al. (1998) offer an illuminating example: "Providing risk information about cancer to individuals who may perceive themselves to be healthy, and who may or may not have directly observed a close relative with the disease, requires these individuals to engage in sophisticated abstract thinking. This issue becomes more pronounced in situations where there is not effective therapy available or the information is only relevant in considerations of possible future outcomes" (p. 69).
- Assess patient reaction to risk information. Austin (2010) and Sagi et al. (1998) point out that risk perception is not equivalent to probability. As mentioned earlier, risk perception actually involves both probability and adversity (or burden of an outcome). So, one of your challenges is to assess how adverse a particular outcome would be for your patient and to associate that adversity with the probability of the outcome occurring. Try working with your patient to identify all short-term and long-range consequences of a particular outcome (medical, psychosocial, financial, lifestyle, etc.) and its relative importance or likely impact (O'Doherty and Suthers 2007).
- Ask patients to summarize their understanding of their risk after you have given them the information (e.g., "What is your understanding of the risk we've just discussed?"). This will allow you to correct any inaccuracies and will provide insight into their subjective perceptions of risk.
- Explore patient feelings about their personal risk. Emotions may include fear, anger, guilt, grief, shame, embarrassment, and lowered self-esteem (Bottorff et al. 1998) and may include "difficulties confronting perceived lack of control and seemingly irrevocable fate, desires to frame genetic information positively in order to avoid despair and helplessness and seek hope, and efforts to reduce anxiety by finding order in the face of fate and seeming randomness" (Klitzman 2010, p. 445). Try an empathy response in which you reflect your patient's feelings. For example, "You've gotten very quiet since I gave you the information about your risk. Are you feeling scared right now?" Be tentative with your empathy as Klitzman (2010) noted, "Given that emotional conflicts may not be fully conscious, providers should proceed very carefully in addressing them" (p. 445).

7.2 Decision-Making: Overview

Genetic counseling patients are often confronted with a number of decisions (e.g., whether to undergo testing, whether to continue or terminate a pregnancy when testing reveals a genetic condition, whether to have further/any children, who to tell and what to tell them, whether and when to undergo predictive testing, and whether to participate in related research). "Facilitating patient decision-making is a critical component of the genetic counseling process. Many decisions are complex, multitiered, time constrained, and emotionally demanding. They may have lifelong consequences and affect people beyond the immediate patient(s)" (Zanko and Fox 2010, p. 31).

Thus far in this chapter, we have discussed two key activities that facilitate decision-making: providing information and risk communication. When patients are presented with options for managing this information and risk, genetic counselors use their skills to support patients by facilitating their decision-making. Two specific competencies related to facilitating patient decision-making are included in the Accreditation Council for Genetic Counseling (ACGC) Practice-Based Competencies: "Use a range of genetic counseling skills and models to facilitate informed decision-making and adaptation to genetic risks or conditions" and "Promote client-centered, informed, noncoercive and value-based decision-making" (ACGC 2015, p. 4; Appendix A).

"Decision-making is a complex process, especially in a domain like genetic testing, which must take numerous considerations into account" (Siani and Assaraf 2016, p. 1093). Often patients must make multiple short-term and long-term decisions. For instance, women with BRCA mutations "...identified multiple decisions to be made when living with and acting upon hereditary breast and ovarian cancer risk. These decisions were more than just having surgery or surveillance and included complex factors related to the person, family, procedure, and healthcare system. Emotional, physical, and social consequences of these decisions, both actual and potential, were important to the decision-making process and require ongoing, long-term support by health care professionals" (Underhill and Crotser 2014, p. 359). You can promote good decision-making when you provide relevant information, recognize factors that are pertinent to patient decision-making processes and outcomes, and "introduce different perspectives as appropriate, and thoroughly explore clients' values and choices with them" (White 1997, p. 305).

Medical Recommendations: Shared Decision-Making

As mentioned previously, and discussed further in Chap. 10, because genetic counseling is a medically based practice, in some situations a genetic counselor will be involved in facilitating patient decision-making about management/treatment options (e.g., mastectomy as a risk reduction strategy for a patient with a BRCA mutation). In these circumstances, a genetic counselor may engage in a type of "shared decision-making" (SDM). The term "shared decision-making" (SDM) describes a process by which a health-care provider collaborates with a patient to make clinical decisions (Barry and Edgman-Levitan 2012; Elwyn et al. 2000, 2012; Makoul and Clayman 2006). Based on a review of literature, Makoul and Clayman (2006) proposed the following as essential elements of SDM: patient and provider define/explain the problem that needs to be addressed; provider reviews options and patient raises additional options of which they are aware; provider and patient discuss the pros/cons of options as they may have different perspectives about the relative importance of benefits, risks and cost; patient and provider discuss patient values and preferences including ideas, concerns, and outcome expectations as well as provider knowledge and recommendations; and patient and provider discuss patient ability/self-efficacy to follow through with a plan. Throughout the process, patients and providers should both periodically check understanding of facts and perspectives and provide clarification as needed (pp. 305–306).

Elwyn et al. (2000) summarized the relevance of SDM to genetic counseling as follows: "The respect for client autonomy that underlies professional enthusiasm for SDM in primary health care is also well developed in GC [genetic counseling], making SDM a natural approach to the negotiation of management decisions in clinical genetics. SDM may also be applicable to negotiations about diagnostic pathways; when investigations are being planned to establish a diagnosis then the likely benefits to emerge may be weighed jointly by clinician and patient along with the inconvenience, anxiety, pain, and other consequences of the diagnostic process" (p. 137).

7.2.1 Facilitated Decision-Making

In contrast to decisions genetic counseling patients face based on medical/clinical recommendations discussed in the previous section, many other decisions in the context of genetic counseling require autonomous decision-making. These include but are not limited to reproductive decisions (e.g., whether to have children, preconception, and/or prenatal screening or diagnostic testing decisions, whether to continue a pregnancy following abnormal prenatal diagnosis, etc.), susceptibility or presymptomatic testing for late-onset conditions (e.g., Huntington disease, early-onset Alzheimer disease), and carrier testing (population screening or targeted carrier testing based on family history). The genetic counselor's role in these types of decisions is to facilitate the patient's decision-making *process*. The remainder of this chapter focuses on factors that may impact patient decision-making processes.

7.2.2 Factors that May Influence Patient Decision-Making

Based on an extensive review of literature, Siani and Assaraf (2016) noted several types of factors that may influence a patient's decision-making about genetic testing and genetic counseling. These include genetic knowledge (e.g., of the condition), attitudes and perceptions (e.g., of the relevance of the services to one's self/family), religion and ethnicity (e.g., level of one's religiosity), personal factors (e.g., patient needs and expectations), practical issues (e.g., cost, access), socioeconomic status, privacy concerns, and emotional factors (e.g., fear of stigma). We discuss several factors in greater detail in this section. Each of these factors may either facilitate or hinder decision-making.

Patient Decision-Making Styles

A number of individual and cultural differences play a role in patients' decision-making. Scott and Bruce (1995) developed and validated an instrument that assesses five different types of decision-making styles:

- *Rational*: characterized by a thorough search for and logical evaluation of alternatives
- *Intuitive*: characterized by reliance on hunches and feelings
- *Dependent*: characterized by a search for advice and direction from others
- *Avoidant*: characterized by attempts to evade decision-making
- *Spontaneous*: characterized by a sense of immediacy and desire to get through the decision-making process as soon as possible.

The author's note that "decision-making styles are not mutually exclusive" and "individuals use a combination of decision-making styles in making important decisions" (p. 829).

Internal and External Factors

- *Medical constraints*: limits regarding information about the disorder, availability of medical options, patient health, and actual or perceived failure rates of tests and procedures (Pivetti and Melotti 2013), availability of diagnosis (Frets et al. 1992), and availability of relevant predictive genetic test(s) (Manuel and Brunger 2014).
- *Financial constraints*: limited financial means, uncertainty about future financial status, and insurance coverage (Pivetti and Melotti 2013).
- *Psychosocial impact*: patient concerns about the emotional and psychological implications of a positive test result (Pivetti and Melotti 2013).

- *Family values*: the nature of family members' values and the ways in which they express them can either be a support or a stress (Cura 2015); sense of relational responsibility or moral obligation to other family members (Manuel and Brunger 2014).
- *Patient motivation*: factors affecting patient desire and ability to make a decision such as intelligence, education level, stress levels, willingness to participate in genetic counseling, and need for scientific information (Pivetti and Melotti 2013).
- *Patient values*: personal attitudes and values about one's options (e.g., contraception, having a normal child, etc.) as well as about taking personal responsibility for the decision, attitudes about medical personnel and concern for others' feelings (Cura 2015), attitudes toward genetic testing and pregnancy termination (Pivetti and Melotti 2013; Siani and Assaraf 2016), and attitudes toward childbearing (Chan et al. 2017). Awwad et al. (2008) recommended "When faced with a decision regarding an affected pregnancy, assess the patient's personal, religious, and cultural beliefs regarding pregnancy termination. Is termination ever permissible? For what reasons? Within what time frame?" (p. 114).
- *Patient emotions*: for instance, regarding reproductive decisions, couples may encounter "difficulties during the decision-making process…[experience] doubts about the decision they made…[feel unable] to make a decision…[and experience] guilt, especially those couples who had an affected sibling" (Frets et al. 1992, p. 25).
- *Ambiguity/uncertainty*: about, for instance, what a particular diagnosis would mean for the health and functioning of an affected child (e.g., What is it like to care for a child with muscular dystrophy?).
- *Burden*: associated with the need to make a decision (e.g., a patient might feel pressured to make a decision about testing to benefit another family member).
- *Patient personality*: affects how the patient approaches decision-making, for example, compulsively, fearfully, dependently, etc.
- *Counselor constraints*: what the counselor is able and willing to provide, legal considerations, rules, and policies, and counselor training and values (e.g., offering predictive testing to minors).
- *Reproductive decisions*: factors may include recurrence risk, desire to have a child, availability of prenatal diagnosis, coping skills, impact of the disorder, family factors (e.g., finances, other resources), diagnosis, norms and values, and reproductive alternatives (Van Spijker 1992).

Multiple studies in genetic counseling have identified additional factors that impact patient decision-making. Dean and Rauscher (2017) explored how women with BRCA mutations but who have not been diagnosed with cancer (previvors) make decisions. They found BRCA mutation previvors used both logical and emotional decision-making styles when making decisions about preventative surgery and when to have children. "Logical decision-making prioritized decreasing their personal risk of HBOC and thus undergoing preventative surgery over having any (or more) children, while emotional decision-making prioritized having children by extending their preventative surgery timeline and in [doing] so gambling with their personal HBOC risk" (p. 1309).

Chan et al. (2017) explored reproductive decision-making in women with BRCA1/2 mutations. They found that knowledge of BRCA carrier status had an impact on patients' decisions regarding relationships and childbearing. "Unpartnered women reported that knowledge of a BRCA mutation influenced their decisions regarding marriage. Almost 40% had a greater desire to get married and 50% felt more pressure to get married after test disclosure" (p. 598). Knowledge of BRCA carrier status also had an impact on patients' attitudes toward childbearing and fertility treatment (e.g., having children earlier, interest in pursuing adoption, deciding not to have children because of risk of transmission of mutation or concern that pregnancy might increase personal risk for cancer, being more likely to consider fertility treatments to become pregnant more quickly, interest in in vitro fertilization and preimplantation genetic diagnosis).

Cassidy and Bove (1998) identified four themes related to parents' decisions about whether to seek or reject presymptomatic testing for their children who are at risk for adult-onset genetic conditions that are treatable: (1) personal experience with the severity of the genetic condition, (2) receipt of accurate information from credible sources, (3) availability of treatment, and (4) risk perceptions.

Reed and Berrier (2017) identified ten distinct factors that may influence decision-making following a prenatal diagnosis of Down syndrome (DS): "rationale for testing, role of information, support, quality of life, effects on family, parenting abilities and goals, personal values, pregnancy experience, age, and experience with disability" (p. 818). The authors further noted "our results indicate that one reason decision-making varies between patients following a DS prenatal diagnosis is that patients assign different meanings to DS—meanings that are influenced by a patients' [sic] lived experience and values, his or her interpretation of information, and the context in which a diagnosis is delivered" (p. 824).

McCarthy Veach et al. (2001) interviewed genetic counselors, physicians, and nurses who identified three factors that pose professional challenges specific to facilitating patient decision-making in genetic counseling:

- Lack of informed consent: patients don't know, don't want to know, and/or don't understand all the pertinent information.
- Facing uncertainty: lack of test specificity and sensitivity and the reality that no one can know all the short- and long-term outcomes.
- Disagreements: with family members, cultural groups, health-care providers, and society about what to do. There is seldom an obvious choice.

7.3 A Rational Decision-Making Model for Genetic Counseling Patients

Because some patients will feel "blocked" in their decision-making process, it may be helpful if you offer them an opportunity to think through their situation (Kessler 1997). Baty (2009) summarized several models of decision-making relevant to genetic counseling (pp. 228–232), and we encourage you to review these models for use in facilitating patient decision-making.

Danish and D'Augelli (1983) created a rational decision-making model based on three major assumptions: (1) it is useful to break decisions down into relevant factors and to weigh each factor according to each alternative (option); (2) a systematic model helps to decrease anxiety about a decision and helps to put the factors involved in a decision into greater perspective; and (3) a rational model includes emotions as a relevant factor, which helps patients deal with the vagueness that feelings often bring to decision-making situations. Their model includes the following steps (which can be written down as they are discussed with a patient):

- Patient briefly describes her or his situation and decision(s) to be made.
- Patient and counselor brainstorm or consider all possible alternatives (options).
- Brainstorm all possible relevant factors (e.g., medical, familial, cultural, psychosocial, financial, ethical, values, etc.). Try to be as comprehensive as possible, including short- and long-term factors, and break global factors into specific ones (e.g., feelings could be broken down into relief, guilt, anger, depression, etc.). Try to bring to the surface irrational factors that patients may be reluctant to acknowledge (e.g., "Having an affected child might mean that I'm a failure as a parent").
- Evaluate each alternative. Does it either satisfy or prevent each factor?
- Patient indicates the most important of the identified factors.
- Patient determines the most desirable and best alternatives. The desirable alternative is the one that attracts the patient the most; the best alternative is the one that is in the patient's best interest in the long run, although it may not be desirable at first glance.
- Clarify and review the decision and revise it as new factors arise.

The following example illustrates the Danish and D'Augelli decision-making model.

Patient Situation

Your patient is a 31-year-old woman whose mother and maternal grandfather were affected with early-onset familial Alzheimer disease (EOFAD). The patient's mother developed symptoms in her late 50s and recently died at age 62. Prior to her death, genetic testing confirmed a mutation in the PSEN1 gene. Your patient is married and has one child, age 2. She and her husband would like to plan additional pregnancies. The patient's primary care physician suggested she seek genetic counseling and testing prior to becoming pregnant. You have explained the autosomal dominant inheritance of the EOFAD in the patient's family and discussed options for predictive testing. The testing would be straightforward as the disease-causing mutation in this family is known. Together you identify the alternatives (her options) and the relevant factors that might be influential in her testing decision, as shown in Table 7.1.

Table 7.1 Example of Danish and D'Augelli (1983) rational decision-making model

Relevant factors	Alternative A Have test	Alternative B No test
Medical		
Address risk, specifically, confirmation of PSEN1 mutation status	X	–
There are no treatments available	–	X
Psychosocial		
Desire to have more children	–	X
Not wanting to pass gene mutation on to future children	X	–
Anxiety about "not knowing"	X	–
Relief of knowing for sure	X	–
Possible impact of test results on marriage and other relationships	–	X
Financial		
Ability to plan for future if test results positive	X	–
Concern about employment/insurance discrimination	–	X
Implications of positive results		
Concern about ability to handle "positive" test result	–	X
Husband may not be willing to have another child	–	X
Fear about possibility of having passed gene on to her daughter	–	X

Decision

Proceed with genetic testing (alternative A) or do not have genetic testing (alternative B).

First List and Then Evaluate Each Factor

As shown in Table 7.1, the patient and counselor identified each relevant factor and then indicated which factors would lead to alternative A or B by placing an X in the column of the alternative most likely to satisfy or prevent each factor.

Choose the Most Important Factors

Upon further discussion, the patient identified the factors that are most important to her decision: Relief of knowing for sure and not wanting to pass gene mutation on to future children.

Determine the Most Desirable and the Best Alternatives

The patient stated that alternative B is the most desirable option, but alternative A is the best alternative because it addresses the factors that she has identified as being most important. To help the patient move forward in her decision-making process, you could work with her to minimize some of the factors such as suggesting she talk things over with her husband before making a decision. You could also point out that she does not need to make the decision quickly.

When using the Danish and D'Augelli model, you should watch for these potential pitfalls:

- Some decisions will have more than two alternatives. Many patients, however, will limit their thinking about alternatives (e.g., having a test vs. not having a test). Deferring testing until a later time might be another option, for example.
- While brainstorming factors, patients may jump prematurely to evaluating alternatives for the factors. Try to stop them from doing this as it usually prevents patients from identifying all relevant factors.
- Patients may be reluctant to admit to irrational factors. You may need to tentatively suggest some, such as choosing an option that others want the patient to choose (having genetic test because your doctor suggested this); worrying about the impact on one's self-esteem (guilt or shame about possibility of passing on a genetic mutation); and superstitious beliefs (e.g., testing for a genetic condition will bring on the disease).
- Sometimes more than one alternative will satisfy a given factor, and this may contribute to the complexity of making a decision. And probably no alternative will satisfy every important factor. If it did, then the decision would be clear. When all alternatives present seriously negative consequences, you might talk with your patient about which option is least risky, as perceived by the patient. Another strategy is to talk through how your patient could eliminate or reduce the negative consequences for different factors. This may allow an alternative to become more desirable. In the above example, discussions with a financial planner may help alleviate some of the patient's concerns about financial impact of the condition if she tests positive (e.g., purchasing long-term care insurance prior to testing); discussions about protections against insurance/employment discriminations based on genetic information are also appropriate.

7.4 Some Suggestions for Assisting Patients in Their Decision-Making

Regardless of the decision-making model you use with patients, the following strategies can help you assist them in their process:

- Reassure patients that they have the ability to make the best decision for themselves.

- Convey understanding and acceptance of your patients no matter what decision they make. Patients tend to approach genetic counseling decisions the way they typically have approached big decisions in their past. So, it may be useful to ask your patients to briefly describe their typical decision-making style (e.g., "Think about an important decision you made in the past. How did you go about making the decision?" or "How does the way you're going about making this decision compare with the way you've made other big decisions in your life?").
- If patients are going about making a decision in an atypical way (e.g., rational deciders who suddenly become very dependent and want you to tell them what to do), this can be evidence that they feel overwhelmed or that some important factor is in the way and needs to be discussed. Consider pointing out this discrepancy and talking about how they are feeling.
- Reassure patients that they do not have to make a final decision on the spot. Even in prenatal counseling, where there may be a greater time pressure, usually a patient or couple can go home and sleep on it. When feasible, offer patients the option to take time to make decisions and encourage them to make one decision at a time (Underhill and Crotser 2014).
- Keep in mind that you have not failed as a genetic counselor if your patient doesn't make a decision. Remember, not deciding *is* a decision. It's a decision not to decide. This strategy allows time and/or a change in circumstances that may help them choose an option or eliminate certain options (e.g., putting off a decision regarding presymptomatic testing means the patient may develop symptoms of a late-onset disorder; similarly, deferring a decision to have carrier testing prior to conception to allow for consideration of PGD may lead to a situation where the patient has an unplanned pregnancy and no longer has this option). It is important that you point out these consequences to indecisive patients.
- Explore with patients their reasons for making the decision. "Questions of a reflective nature are crucial so as to ensure that the clients have gone through an informed process of reaching a decision—the counselor thus focuses on the process of the decision-making rather than the decision reached (Shiloh 1996)" (cited in Sarangi et al. 2004, p. 138). For example, "What will choosing this option mean for you?"; "What do you see as the pros? The cons?"; "Sometimes patients choose this option because it will… Is it possible this is part of what's motivating you to make this choice?" Encourage patients to be honest about their motivation and to consider whether this is the motivation they wish to have driving their decision (e.g., a patient who is rushing into a decision before all the pertinent information is available because she dislikes how anxious she feels).
- Gently "question or challenge clients' views that [may be] poorly reasoned, misguided, or perhaps ethically questionable" (White 1997, p. 305). For instance, a patient says, "I'm not going to share this information with my sister because we don't get along." You may be able to engage a patient in a discussion

that helps her recognize her moral responsibility to a sibling, even if the relationship is poor.

- Explore differences in opinions and attitudes when your patient is a couple or family (Schoeffel et al. 2018; Van Spijker 1992). Go around the group, and ask each individual to express what she/he thinks and feels about each option.
- Recognize and incorporate cultural variables in the decision-making process. For instance, for some Korean and Arab families, it is important to involve the fathers as they are the decision-makers (Awwad et al. 2008; Brown 1997). Cura (2015) states that "…the Philippine society focuses more on collectivistic rules. In addition to personal freedom and rights, social harmony, interpersonal concerns and sanctity are equally emphasized…" (p. 216). He recommends that with Filipino patients you should "assess other key persons in decision-making by noting who accompanies a patient during the clinic visit [and]…questions such as 'Who should we talk to? 'or 'Who can help in making decisions about your treatment (or decisions) in the future?' can yield valuable information…[about] key persons in the family, and whose opinions would influence the other individuals' decisions, especially for patients who are considered as 'dependents' in a family…[as well as help the counselor] to clearly identify with whom information should also be shared…" (p. 216).
- Explore patients' experiences of living with affected family members.
- Let patients know that sometimes the most emotionally painful decisions are the right ones for them. The best decision is not necessarily the easiest to make (cf. Anonymous 2008).
- Suggest that patients listen to their instincts. Often our subconscious is a source of good advice. This may be particularly helpful for patients who are intellectualizing their situation, that is, spending all their time thinking things through without acknowledging how they feel about different options.
- Encourage patients to seek support and guidance from significant others (e.g., family members, friends, community leaders).
- Consider using decision aids or tools to facilitate patient decision-making [for examples, see Birch et al. (2016) and Wakefield et al. (2007)].
- Engage in anticipatory guidance:

  – Use scenarios to help patients evaluate options. As noted by Myring et al. (2011) in their work with couples at risk for having a child with CF, "…decision-making often involved scenario-based thinking. This was reported by participants of both sexes but described more vividly by the women in this study. This process typically began during the adaptation phase and eventually formed a base for decision-making. Women described how they thought through all possible scenarios, including raising a child with CF and the potential impact on the family unit. Personal experience with CF was also central to this process. For individuals with a child with CF, the potential effect of their decisions on their affected child was extremely important in their considerations" (p. 409).

  - Huys et al. (1992) and Van Spijker (1992) also suggest the use of scenarios. This can be particularly helpful when patients are unfamiliar with a disorder and/or have no family history with the condition. For reproductive decisions, after presenting the scenario, Van Spijker suggests that you ask three questions [from the study by Lippman-Hand and Fraser (1979b)]: (1) How likely am I to have an affected child? (2) What will it be like if it happens? (3) How will others react to my choice?
  - Frets et al. (1992) describe scenarios as constructing a plausible story in which the decision-maker is an active participant. Scenarios describe what could happen or could be done under various conditions (e.g., knowing one is at risk for a late-onset disorder vs. living with uncertainty). They point out that you will gain valuable clinical information about how patients represent and reason through information based on the scenarios they construct. In their research, Huys et al. (1992) found people typically construct between three and eight scenarios and that the contents of scenarios are quite divergent, indicating they are highly personalized. These findings suggest patients won't try to come up with every possible outcome but instead will focus on a few outcomes that are particularly important to them.
  - Bottorff et al. (1998) recommend using predisclosure role-plays. These are exercises that invite patients to consider the effect of test results on themselves and their family members. For example, you could ask, "What do you think it will mean for you if the results are positive? How do you think you will feel? What will you do?" Then ask your patient to answer the same questions, but for specific family members (spouse, children, etc.). Finally, ask these same questions, but with your patient imagining the results are negative and, if appropriate, a VUS.
  - Kessler (1997) suggests having patients role-play or pretend they are coping with a specific situation or person. This allows them to try out different strategies and options. For example, role reversal might be helpful for a couple who is disagreeing about a reproductive decision, allowing them to see things from each other's perspective.

- Consider referring undecided patients to psychologists or to others who are familiar with the specific difficulties they are having in the decision-making process (Frets et al. 1992).
- Provide support to assist patients in their adjustment to the outcomes of their decisions. For instance, Underhill and Crotser (2014) identified several support needs of healthy women with a BRCA1 or BRCA2 mutation: "Support for obtaining, interpreting, and applying medical information; Clarification of options and risk; Support while living with anticipated and actual consequences; Recognizing personal values and evaluating over time; Accessing support; Choosing type of medical decision based on personal factors; Seeking information and choosing when to act; Living with impact or consequences" (p. 359).

- Ask yourself, what is a good decision? McCarthy Veach et al. (2001) found that most of the genetic counselors they interviewed felt comfortable when their patients made decisions that would not cause them harm, were consistent with their cultural backgrounds, and seemed to work for those particular patients. The hardest decisions were those perceived by the genetic counselors to be cavalier (e.g., terminating a multiple pregnancy after years of infertility because the couple wanted only one child). One major ethical/professional challenge you likely will face is refraining from talking patients out of decisions with which you disagree.

7.5 Closing Comments

In this chapter, we suggested several strategies to help you walk with your patients through the difficult genetic counseling process. First, you will provide relevant information to help them be informed, recognizing that some of your information (e.g., about risk) may not be fully understood, believed, or have the same meaning for the patient as it has for you. Then, for many patients, you will help them use the information you provide and other relevant information to come to a decision that is best for them. Decisions are complex. Patients select certain options for numerous reasons, some clear, some not so clear. And they often choose options that are different from what you think they should choose. Remember that what seems to be an irrational decision to you may be the best choice for your patient. It is also important to remember that you can't fix situations that aren't repairable—some patients' decisions come down to trying to do the best they can in an impossible situation.

7.6 Class Activities

Activity 1: Stigmatizing Words (Dyads or Small Group Discussion)

First, students brainstorm words that could communicate a negative message or stigmatize the patient when presenting risk information (e.g., mutant).

Process

The whole group generates a list that the instructor writes on the board.

Next, the students identify alternative words/brief phrases for each word they identified as negative or stigmatizing.

Process

The whole group generates a list that the instructor writes on the board.

Estimated time: 45 min.

Activity 2: Medical Recommendations (Group Discussion and Dyad or Triad Role Plays)

First, students work in small groups to come up with a list of patient recommendations specific to genetic counseling such as those from ACOG, ACMG, NSGC, and ASCO for one of the following:

- HBOC
- Hereditary colon cancer
- Communicating a prenatal testing result for Down syndrome
- Communicating a postnatal diagnosis of Down syndrome
- Childhood testing for adult-onset conditions
- Sharing risk information with relatives
- Prenatal carrier screening

Process

Each small group shares the results of their research to identify medical recommendations relevant to genetic counseling.

Estimated time: 45 min.

Next, students select three key information points to be included in the genetic counseling session. Students write out what they will say and where it fits best into the session.

In dyads or triads, students role-play sessions that include the three key information points for the recommendations they found in their research.

Estimated time: 60 min.

Instructor Note

- Students or instructor may select other topics of interest.

Activity 3: Communicating Positive Test Results (Dyads or Small Group Discussion)

Students discuss how they will feel when communicating positive test results to patients. What is difficult about it? What is scary about it? What is the worst thing that could possibly happen?

Process

The whole group discusses their responses.

Estimated time: 20–25 min.

Activity 4: Communicating Risk Data (Dyads or Small Group Discussion)

Using the risk data for the following genetic conditions, students write out how they would communicate this information to a patient using Hallowell et al.'s (1997) five quantitative formats:

- Sickle cell anemia: Pregnant woman is a carrier. Partner has not been tested. Carrier risk is 1/10 for African American population. Explain partner's risk for being a carrier, and then explain risk for having an affected child.
- Neural tube defects: Couple's first child has an open neural tube defect. They want to know the chance of having another affected child. Empiric recurrence risk is 3–5%.
- Abnormal first trimester screen: 32-year-old pregnant patient has an abnormal screening test. Lab report indicates a 1 in 50 risk for Down syndrome.
- Newborn diagnosed with PKU: Parents are Caucasian and this is their first pregnancy. Incidence of PKU in USA Caucasian population is 1/10,000. Explain incidence and recurrence risk.
- Fetal abnormality: A couple is seen for genetic counseling because their first child had a hypoplastic left heart diagnosed on prenatal ultrasound. Parents are concerned about the recurrence risk. General population incidence: 1/4300. Risk for recurrence if one affected child: 2% to 25%.
- Cystic fibrosis (CF): A Caucasian couple with no family history of CF requests testing. Explain their chance of having a child with CF prior to testing. [Population carrier risk (Caucasian) is 1/25.]
- Same couple as in previous example: Wife is tested and is found to be a carrier of the F508 CF gene mutation. Explain how this changes this couple's chance of having a child with CF.

Process

The whole group discusses their responses.

Estimated time: 50–60 min.

Instructor Note

- After writing down their responses, students could role-play actually giving the information to patients.

Activity 5: Anticipating Patient Information Needs (Dyads or Small Group Discussion)

Students brainstorm all of the informational questions patients might have when they seek cancer genetic counseling.

Process

Students discuss their responses in the small or large group.

Estimated time: 45 min.

Instructor Note
- Students can compare their questions to the content in Table 4 of Roshanai et al. (2012, p. 518) which lists patient informational needs.
- Students could be asked to develop a list of questions for a prenatal condition and a list for a pediatric condition. An option would be to provide them with the categories from Roshanai et al.'s (2012) Tables 5 and 6 to stimulate their thinking and to help them organize their questions.

Source Roshanai et al. (2012).

Activity 6: Decision-Making Challenges (Dyads or Small Group Discussion)

Students brainstorm the reasons why it is hard to make decisions.

Process
The whole group discusses the reasons they generated.
Estimated time: 20 min.

Activity 7: Decision-Making Styles (Dyads or Small Group Discussion)

Students think about a major decision they made in their lives (e.g., choice of graduate program). How did they go about making this decision? Next the students try to match their process to one of Scott and Bruce's (1995) five decision-making styles. Then they discuss the advantages and drawbacks to using their own decision-making styles when working with patients.
Estimated time: 20 min.

Activity 8: Decision-Making Styles (Small Group Role-Plays)

Each student takes a turn playing a genetic counselor and patient. The patient selects one of Scott and Bruce's (1995) five decider types and demonstrates that style for a decision about whether to have genetic testing for familial Parkinson disease (assume that the patient is at 50% risk for an AD early-onset form of the condition). The patient should not let the group know in advance which style she/he chooses. Each role-play should last for about 10–15 min.

Process
The students discuss how it feels to deal with different types of deciders.
Estimated time: 90 min.

Activity 9: Rational Decision-Making (Small Group Discussion)

Using one of the following patient scenarios, first go through the Danish and D'Augelli (1983) decision-making steps, and then discuss how to minimize constraining factors.

The patient is coming for genetic counseling because of a family history of individuals with intellectual deficits. Her maternal uncle and some other maternally related males are affected. She is terrified of having a baby who is similarly affected and is adamant that she does not want to be in that situation. She definitely wants every possible test done on her pregnancy.

OR

A 15-year-old female is 12 1/2 weeks into her first pregnancy (g1P0) and has just been told that her fetus has gastroschisis. No other anomalies were found on ultrasound. The father of the pregnancy is not involved. Her mother has accompanied her to the clinic. The mother is adamant that the pregnancy must be terminated.

OR

A 32-year-old woman has two sons; both have fragile X syndrome (one mildly affected, one more severely affected). She wants another child. Her husband is supportive and involved but doesn't want any more children.

Process

If there is more than one small group, each group can present its decision model to the other groups. Then the whole group discusses any questions/difficulties they are having with the model.

Estimated time: 75 min.

Activity 10: Communicating Risk Information (Triads or Small Group Role-Plays)

Role-play presenting risk information to:

- A 24-year-old prenatal patient with neurofibromatosis who has limited cognitive skills. She is concerned about her baby.
- A 39-year-old prenatal patient with a family history of CF who says, "I don't want to hear anything about risks because it scares me. Just tell me what to do."
- A Muslim refugee from Africa in a consanguineous relationship who states that, "How children turn out is God's will, and there is no way to predict or prevent birth defects."
- A 25-year-old woman with a positive family history of breast cancer. Her mother and maternal grandmother both had breast cancer, diagnosed in their 30s; both

are deceased, and no genetic testing was performed. BRCA testing reveals a variant of unknown significance.

Estimated time: 60–90 min.

Activity 11: Risk Information, Positive Test Results, and Decision-Making Model

The instructor role-plays with a volunteer from class. The instructor demonstrates how to (1) present risk information, (2) present positive test results, and (3) assist patient with decision-making.

Process

After the role-play, students discuss their observations of the counselor's behaviors and their impact on the patient.

Estimated time: 45 min.

Activity 12: Decision-Making (Small Group Role-Plays)

The students form small groups (four to five students). In each small group, either the instructor or a student pretends to be a genetic counseling patient. The patient role-plays one of the following scenarios that involve patient decisions:

- The prenatal patient states that she does not want to consider abortion as an option before the genetic counselor has said anything about it.
- The patient wants the genetic counselor to tell him what to do regarding whether to have presymptomatic testing for Huntington disease.
- The patient minimizes the increased risk for cancer when she carries the *BRCA1* gene mutation.
- The patient misunderstands the risk information given to her (she thinks having a 25% chance of having a child affected with cystic fibrosis means that only one of four of her children would be affected).
- The 55-year-old patient with breast cancer with a negative family history greatly overestimates her risk for having a gene mutation (90% when her risk is actually 5–10%).
- The patient has a fetus with anencephaly. She is afraid of what her family will think if she decides to terminate the pregnancy.

The role-plays can last 15–20 min. The counselor or instructor can stop a role-play if the counselor gets stuck and discuss with the group how to proceed.

Estimated time: 90 min.

Activity 13: Correcting Misinformation (Dyads)

Pairs of students practice writing responses to correct some common patient misperceptions listed below:

1. Since there is only one affected person in the family, the condition cannot be genetic.
2. If there is more than one affected person, it must be genetic.
3. The mother did something during her pregnancy that caused the condition in the child.
4. A patient will inherit a family condition because she/he looks like an affected family member.
5. If all affected people in the family are of one gender, the other gender cannot be affected; the condition must be sex linked.
6. Diseases skip generations.
7. Birth order affects the risk.

Process
In a large group, members can discuss and give and receive feedback about their responses.

Estimated time: 60 min.

7.7 Written Exercises

Exercise 1: Risk Communication

The following scenarios provide information about particular patients and their genetic risks. For each scenario identify risks that need to be communicated and what factors might impact their risk. How would you approach risk communication in each case?

1. The patient is a 43-year-old woman, 11 weeks pregnant. This is her first pregnancy; she has a history of infertility for 7–8 years. She works as an elementary school teacher. Her husband is a foreman for a plumbing company. He is of Italian descent; she is of Irish/English descent. She was referred by her obstetrician for discussion of prenatal screening and testing options.
2. The patient has a family history of pancreatic and breast cancer. Her mother had breast cancer in her 40s, was successfully treated, and is currently 54 years old. The patient's maternal aunt and a maternal first cousin both died of pancreatic cancer. The patient, in her early 30s, wants to know her risks.
3. A young couple comes for prenatal counseling. The man's sister has a son with Lesch-Nyhan syndrome. He wants to know if his children are at risk of having the disorder.

4. The same young man in scenario 3 refers his sister (the one with the affected son) for counseling. She has just moved to the USA and has not previously had access to genetic counseling. She wants to know if her other children will develop Lesch-Nyhan syndrome and also what are the risks to future pregnancies.
5. The patient is coming for genetic counseling regarding a history of two sons who had multiple congenital anomalies and died shortly after birth. No genetic evaluation or testing was completed on either baby. She is now married to a different partner and seeks information about her chance of having another child with similar problems.
6. A 32-year-old man was referred to clinic because his father and paternal grandmother both died of a "heart attack" in their early 40s. His brother just had a heart attack at age 41.

Instructor Note
- Students may need to research one or more conditions in order to complete this exercise.
- One variation is to have students select one or more of the patient scenarios and write these patients a letter of summary.
- These scenarios could be role-played in class, with the student verbally presenting risk information to the patient.

Exercise 2: Applying a Decision-Making Model

Observe an actual genetic counseling session, and afterward use the Danish and D'Augelli decision-making model to describe the patient's decision-making process.

Exercise 3: Risk Communication and Cultural Factors

Talk with an individual who is a recognized cultural leader for a specific population (e.g., Hmong, Native American, Latino/Latina, etc.). Discuss how members of her or his community typically understand the concept of risk for health problems and how risk can best be communicated.

Exercise 4: Role Play

Engage in a 30-min role-play of a genetic counseling session with a classmate. The role-play can be based on a patient you saw in clinic or it can be a made-up patient situation. During the role-play, focus on providing risk information and assisting the patient with decision-making. Audio-record the role-play. Next transcribe the role-play and critique your work. Use the following method for transcribing the session:

Counselor	Patient	Self-critique	Instructor
Key phrases of dialogue	Key phrases	Comment on your own response	Will provide feedback on your responses

Create a brief summary:

1. Briefly describe patient *demographics* (e.g., age, gender, ethnicity, socioeconomic status, relationship status) and *reason* for seeking genetic counseling.
2. Identify *two* things you said/did during the role-play that were effective and *two* things you could have done differently.

Give the recording, transcript/self-critique, and summary to the instructor who will provide feedback.

[*Hint*: This assignment encourages self-reflective practice regarding your clinical performance. The goal is not to do a perfect session. Rather the goal is to assess the extent to which you can accurately assess your psychosocial counseling skills. You will gain more from this exercise if you refrain from scripting what you plan to say as the counselor.]

Exercise 5: Preparing Information for a Genetic Counseling Session

Simonoff (1998) lists several types of questions that patients may have when they seek genetic counseling after their first child is diagnosed with autism. These questions, which are generally relevant for reproductive genetic counseling, are listed below. Assign students a genetic condition and have them research the condition, using Simonoff's list of questions for prepping the case:

- What are the recurrence risks?
- Is there increased risk for other conditions?
- Was the diagnosis accurate?
- Would other family members have the same type and level of impairment as the proband?
- What types of prenatal diagnosis are available?
- Are any precautions during pregnancy necessary?
- Is the condition more common in males or females?
- What is the impact of another affected child on the first child??
- What is the impact of a nonaffected child on the first child?
- How early can the condition be detected?
- Would risks differ if either partner were to have children with a different person?

Instructor Note

- Students could then role-play these cases in class using the material they prepared in response to the patient questions.

References

Abad-Perotín R, Asúnsolo-Del Barco Á, Silva-Mato A. A survey of ethical and professional challenges experienced by Spanish health-care professionals that provide genetic counseling services. J Genet Couns. 2012;21:85–100.

Accreditation Council for Genetic Counseling. Practice based competencies for genetic counselors. 2015. http://gceducation.org/Documents/ACGC%20Core%20Competencies%20Brochure_15_Web.pdf. Accessed 18 Aug 2017.

Alliman S, Veach PM, Bartels DM, Lian F, James C, LeRoy BS. A comparative analysis of ethical and professional challenges experienced by Australian and US genetic counselors. J Genet Couns. 2009;18:379–94.

Anonymous. A genetic counselor's journey from provider to patient: A mother's story. J Genet Couns. 2008;17:412–18.

Austin JC. Re-conceptualizing risk in genetic counseling: implications for clinical practice. J Genet Couns. 2010;19:228–34.

Awwad R, Veach PM, Bartels DM, LeRoy BS. Culture and acculturation influences on Palestinian perceptions of prenatal genetic counseling. J Genet Couns. 2008;17:101–16.

Barry MJ, Edgman-Levitan S. Shared decision making—the pinnacle of patient-centered care. New England Journal of Medicine. 2012;366,780-81.

Baty BJ. Risk communication and decision making. In: Uhlmann WR, Schuette JL, Yashar B, editors, A guide to genetic counseling. New York: John Wiley & Sons. 2009; p.207-50.

Bottorff JL, Ratner PA, Johnson JL, Lovato CY, Joab SA. Communicating cancer risk information: the challenges of uncertainty. Patient Educ Couns. 1998;33:67–81.

Birch P, Adam S, Bansback N., Coe RR, Hicklin J, Lehman A, Li KC, Friedman JM. DECIDE: a decision support tool to facilitate parents' choices regarding genome-wide sequencing. J Genet Couns. 2016;25:1298-1308.

Bower MA, Veach PM, Bartels DM, LeRoy BS. A survey of genetic counselors' strategies for addressing ethical and professional challenges in practice. J Genet Couns. 2002;11:163–86.

Brown D. Implications of cultural values for cross-cultural consultation with families. J Couns Dev. 1997;76:29–35.

Bylund CL, Fisher CL, Brashers D, Edgerson S, Glogowski EA, Boyar SR, et al. Sources of uncertainty about daughters' breast cancer risk that emerge during genetic counseling consultations. J Genet Couns. 2012;21:292–304.

Cassidy DA, Bove CM. Factors perceived to influence parental decision-making regarding presymptomatic testing of children at risk for treatable adult-onset genetic disorders. Issues in Comprehensive Pediatric Nursing. 1998;21:19-34.

Chan JL, Johnson LNC, Sammel MD, DiGiovanni L, Vong C, Domchek SM, Gracia CR. Reproductive decision-making in women with BRCA 1/2 mutations. J Genet Couns. 2017;26:594–603.

Cura JD. (2015) Respecting autonomous decision making among Filipinos: A re-emphasis in genetic counseling. J Genetic Couns. 2015;24:213-24.

Danish SJ, D'Augelli AR. Helping skills: II: Life development intervention: Trainee's workbook. New York: Human Sciences Press; 1983.

Dean M, Rauscher EA. "It was and emotional baby": previvors' family planning decision-making styles about hereditary breast and ovarian cancer risk. J Genet Couns. 2017;26:1301–13.

Duane Brown D. (1997) Implications of cultural values for cross-cultural consultation with families. J Couns Dev. 1997;76:29–35.

Elwyn G, Gray J, Clarke A. Shared decision making and non-directiveness in genetic counselling. J Med Genet. 2000;37:135–8.

Elwyn G, Frosch D, Thomson R, Joseph-Williams N, Lloyd A, Kinnersley P, Cording E, Tomson D, Dodd C, Rollnick S, Edwards, A. Shared decision making: a model for clinical practice. J General Internal Medicine. 2012;27:1361–7.

Etchegary H, Perrier C. Information processing in the context of genetic risk: implications for genetic-risk communication. J Genet Couns. 2007;16:419–32.

Facio FM, Lee K, O'Daniel J. A genetic counselor's guide to using next-generation sequencing in clinical practice. J Genet Couns. 2014;23:455–62.
Faulkner A, Argent F, Jones A, O'Keefe C. Improving the skills of doctors in giving distressing information. Med Educ. 1995;29:303–7.
Frets PG, Duivenvoorden H., Verhage F, Niermeijer MF. The reproductive decision-making process after genetic counseling: psychosocial aspects. Birth Defects: Original Article Series. 1992;28, 21–8.
Frost CJ, Venne V, Cunningham D, Gerritsen-McKane R. Decision making with uncertain information: learning from women in a high risk breast cancer clinic. J Genet Couns. 2004;13:221–36.
Gammon AD, Rothwell E, Simmons R, Lowery JT, Ballinger L, Hill DA, et al. Awareness and preferences regarding BRCA1/2 genetic counseling and ting among Latinas and Non-Latina White women at increased risk for hereditary breast and ovarian cancer. J Genet Couns. 2011;20:625–38.
Garcia-Retamerol RG, Cokely ET. Communicating health risks with visual aids. Curr Dir Psychol Sci. 2013;22:392–9.
Gray CA., McCarthy Veach P., Jones KR., Goreczny A, Hoss M. Addressing genetic issues: the interface of psychotherapy and genetic counseling. Minnesota Psychologist. 2000;8–10.
Greeson CJ, Veach PM, LeRoy BS. A qualitative investigation of Somali immigrant perceptions of disability: implications for genetic counseling. J Genet Couns. 2001;10:359–78.
Gschmeidler B, Flatscher-Thoeni M. Ethical and professional challenges of genetic counseling–the case of Austria. J Genet Couns. 2013;22:741–52.
Hagberg A, Bui T, Winnberg E. More appreciation of life or regretting the test? Experiences of living as a mutation carrier of Huntington's Disease. J Genet Couns. 2011;20:70–9.
Hallowell N, Statham H, Murton F, Green J, Richards M. Talking about chance: the presentation of risk information during genetic counseling for breast and ovarian cancer. J Genet Couns. 1997;6:269–86.
Huys J, Evers-Kiebooms G, d'Ydewalle G. Decision making in the context of genetic risk: the use of scenarios. Birth Defects: Original Article Series. 1992;28:17-20.
Jecker NS, Carrese JA, Pearlman RA. Caring for patients in cross-cultural settings. Hast Cent Rep. 1995;25:6–14.
Kessler S. Psychological aspects of genetic counseling. IX. Teaching and counseling. J Genet Couns. 1997;6:287–94.
Kessler S. Psychological aspects of genetic counseling: XIII. Empathy and decency. J Genet Couns. 1999;8:333–43.
Kiedrowski LA, Owens KM, Yashar BM, Schuette JL. Parents' perspectives on variants of uncertain significance from chromosome microarray analysis. J Genet Couns. 2016;25:101–11.
Klitzman RL. Misunderstandings concerning genetics among patients confronting genetic disease. J Genet Couns. 2010;19:430–46.
Lewis L. Honoring diversity: cultural competence in genetic counseling. In: LeRoy BS, McCarthy Veach P, Bartels DM, editors. Genetic counseling practice. Hoboken: Wiley-Blackwell; 2010. p. 201–34.
Lipson JG, Meleis AI. Issues in health care of Middle Eastern patients. West J Med. 1983;139:854–61.
Livneh H, Antonek RF. Psychosocial adaptation to chronic illness and disability: a primer for counselors. J Couns Dev. 2005;83:12–20.
Makoul G, Clayman ML. (2006) An integrative model of shared decision making in medical encounters. Patient Education and Couns. 2006;60:301-312.
Manuel A, Brunger F. Making the decision to participate in predictive genetic testing for arrhythmogenic right ventricular cardiomyopathy. J Genet Couns. 2014;23:1045-55.
McCarthy Veach P, Bartels DM, LeRoy BS. Ethical and professional challenges posed by patients with genetic concerns: a report of focus group discussions with genetic counselors, physicians, and nurses. J Genet Couns. 2001;10:97–119.
McCarthy Veach P, Bartels DM, LeRoy BS. Coming full circle: a Reciprocal-Engagement Model of genetic counseling practice. J Genet Couns. 2007;16:713–28.

Melas PA, Georgsson Öhman S, Juth N, Bui T-H. Information related to prenatal genetic counseling: interpretation by adolescents, effects on risk perception and ethical implications. J Genet Couns. 2012;21:536–46.
Myring J, Beckett W, Jassi R, Roberts T, Sayers R, Scotcher D, McAllister M. Shock, adjust, decide: reproductive decision-making in cystic fibrosis (CF) carrier couples—a qualitative study. J Genet Couns. 2011;20:404–17.
National Society of Genetic Counselors. National society of genetic counselors code of ethics. J Genet Couns. 2017. doi: https://doi.org/10.1007/s10897-017-0166-8 [Epub ahead of print].
O'Doherty K, Suthers GK. Risky communication: pitfalls in counseling about risk, and how to avoid them. J Genet Couns. 2007;16:409–17.
Ostergren JC. Relationships among English performance, self-efficacy, anxiety, and depression for Hmong refugees. Unpublished doctoral dissertation, University of Minnesota, Minneapolis, MN; 1991.
Pivetti M, Melotti G. Prenatal genetic testing: An investigation of determining factors affecting the decision-making process. J Genet Couns. 2013;22:76-89.
Quillin JM, McClish DK, Jones RM, Burruss K, Bodurtha JN. Spiritual coping, family history, and perceived risk for breast cancer—can we make sense of it? J Genet Couns. 2006;15:449–60.
Reed AR, Berrier KL. A qualitative study of factors influencing decision-making after prenatal diagnosis of down syndrome. J Genet Couns. 2017;26:814–28.
Roggenbuck J, Temme R, Pond D, Baker J, Jarvis K, Liu M, et al. The long and short of genetic counseling summary letters: a case –control study. J Genet Couns. 2015;24:645–53.
Roshanai AH, Lampic C, Ingvoldstad C, Askmalm MS, Bjorvatn C, Rosenquist R, et al. What information do cancer genetic counselees prioritize? J Genet Couns. 2012;21:510–26.
Sagi M, Kaduri L, Zlotogora J, Petetz T. The effect of genetic counseling on knowledge and perceptions regarding risks for breast cancer. J Genet Couns. 1998;7:417–34.
Sarangi S, Bennert K, Howell L, Clarke A, Harper P, Gray J. Initiation of reflective frames in counseling for Huntingtons Disease predictive testing. J Genet Couns. 2004;13:135-55.
Schoeffel K, McCarthy Veach P, Rubin K, LeRoy BS. Managing couple conflict during prenatal counseling sessions: An investigation of genetic counselor experiences and perceptions. J Genet Couns. 2018. https://doi.org/10.1007/s10897-018-0252-6.
Scott SG, Bruce RA. Decision-making style: the development and assessment of a new measure. Educ Psychol Meas. 1995;55:818–31.
Semaka A, Balneaves LG, Hayden MR. "Grasping the grey": patient understanding and interpretation of an intermediate allele predictive test result for Huntington disease. J Genet Couns. 2013;22:200–17.
Shiloh S. Decision-making in the context of genetic risk. In: Marteau T, Richards M, editors, The troubled helix: Social and psychological implications of the new human genetics. Cambridge, UK: Cambridge University Press. 1996; p. 82-103.
Siani M, Assaraf OB. Should I perform genetic testing? A qualitative look into the decision making considerations of religious Israeli undergraduate students. J Genet Couns. 2016;25:1093–115.
Simonoff E. Genetic counseling in autism and pervasive developmental disorders. J Autism Dev Disord. 1998;28:447–56.
Sivell S, Elwyn G, Gaff CL, Clarke AJ, Iredale R, Shaw C, et al. How risk is perceived, constructed and interpreted by clients in clinical genetics, and the effects on decision making: systematic review. J Genet Couns. 2008;17:30–63.
Steinberg Warren N. A genetic counseling cultural competence toolkit. n.d.. www.geneticcounselingculturaltoolkit.com/. Accessed 15 Aug 2017.
Trepanier A. Losing sight. J Genet Couns. 2012;21:232–4.
Underhill ML, Crotser CB. Seeking balance: decision support needs of women without cancer and a deleterious BRCA1 or BRCA2 mutation. J Genet Couns. 2014;23:350–62.
Van Spijker HG. Support in decision making processes in the post-counseling period. Birth Defects: Original Article Series. 1992;28:29-35.

Wakefield CE, Homewood J, Mahmut M, Taylor A, Meiser B. Usefulness of the Threatening Medical Situations Inventory in individuals considering genetic testing for cancer risk. Patient Educ Couns. 2007;69:29–38.

White MT. “Respect for autonomy” in genetic counseling: An analysis and a proposal. J Genet Couns. 1997;6:297-313.

Yager GG. Commentary on “conceptualizing genetic counseling as psychotherapy in the era of genomic medicine”. J Genet Couns. 2014;23:935–7.

Zanko A, Fox M. Actively engaging with patients in decision-making. In: LeRoy BS, McCarthyVeach P, Bartels DM, editors. Genetic counseling practice. Hoboken: Wiley-Blackwell; 2010. p. 31–64.

Chapter 8
Responding to Patient Cues: Advanced Empathy and Confrontation Skills

Learning Objectives

1. Define advanced empathy and confrontation.
2. Differentiate advanced empathy and confrontation from primary empathy.
3. Determine guidelines for effectively communicating advanced empathy and confrontation.
4. Identify examples of patient themes appropriate for advanced empathy and confrontation.
5. Develop advanced empathy and confrontation skills through self-reflection, practice, and feedback.

This chapter discusses two fairly advanced helping skills: advanced empathy and confrontation. Typically, genetic counselors use these two types of skills less frequently than other skills such as attending, primary empathy, and questioning. Advanced empathy and confrontation can be very powerful responses when used strategically and sparingly.

8.1 Advanced Empathy Skills

> "…Advanced empathy is necessary. Empathy is a really complicated concept. And it's not a set of behaviors that you can [fully] specify. It's like trying to put your hands on light or something." (Master genetic counselor clinician; Miranda et al. 2016, pp. 771–772).

P. McCarthy Veach et al., *Facilitating the Genetic Counseling Process*,
https://doi.org/10.1007/978-3-319-74799-6_8

8.1.1 *Definition and Functions of Advanced Empathy*

Advanced empathy, variously known as additive empathy, reframing (Kessler 1997), and interpretation, is a helping skill that consists of two components: (1) the genetic counselor's understanding of the underlying, implicit aspects of patient experience and (2) the response or reply the counselor constructs to communicate this understanding. Advanced empathy responses go beyond surface patient expressions by identifying less conscious patient feelings, thoughts, and perceptions (Neukrug et al. 2013). Advanced empathy responses are tentative hypotheses, inference, or hunches about the patient's experience (MacDonald 1996) that reflect "… deeper meanings and/or broader themes" (Bayne et al. 2012, p. 73).

Interpretation about patients and their experiences "requires thinking in a complex way about [their] dynamics and underlying motivations…" (Hill et al. 2014, p. 710). With advanced empathy responses, you "read between the lines," going beyond what the patient has directly expressed by presenting your perspective of her or his experience. You move from patient descriptions of their experiences to offer a deeper and/or new meaning or reason for their feelings, thoughts, and/or behaviors (Kessler 1997; Neukrug et al. 2013). Your intent with advanced empathy expands the ways in which the patient views her or his situation (Hackney and Bernard 2017; Hill et al. 2014; Jackson et al. 2014). With advanced empathy, you become more directive about the discussion, having decided that your patient would benefit from hearing your perspective.

Advanced empathy responses may serve a variety of functions. Psychotherapy research has consistently demonstrated that skillfully used advanced empathy has a positive impact on both processes and outcomes, for example, facilitating patient progress in counseling (Neukrug et al. 2013). When accurate and well timed, advanced empathy responses "…help clients achieve new insights and may facilitate movement towards new ways of thinking about issues…" (Bayne et al. 2012, p. 73). Patients often come to genetic counseling with a vague awareness of their inner thoughts and feelings. Even when they have an idea of what they think and feel, they may hesitate to share this information because they fear judgment, worry that what they have to say is too risky, and/or do not consider such sharing to be culturally appropriate (Hill 2014). When you have reason to believe there is more beneath the surface of your patients' stories, advanced empathy can be helpful because it more directly identifies their inner experience.

In addition to providing patients with greater insight into their thoughts and feelings, advanced empathy can help them clarify their values, thus promoting greater self-understanding. It can also give patients permission to express certain feelings or opinions, which may ultimately help them be more accepting of those feelings and thoughts, thus facilitating their goal setting and decision-making. Advanced empathy can provide patients with an "…explanation [that] can make experiences seem less confusing, haphazard, or inexplicable and give [them] a sense of mastery, security, and self-efficacy" (Jackson et al. 2014, p. 779).

Despite the potential benefits of advanced empathy, there may be risks as "novel information shared and received in the interpretation process may also frighten anger or sadden clients" (Jackson et al. 2014, p. 779). Because advanced empathy addresses hidden or implied content, it can increase patient anxiety (e.g., "Will the genetic counselor judge me now that s/he knows this about me?"; "Do I want to get into this issue with the counselor?"; "Will I completely break down if I say more about how I'm really feeling?"). For these reasons, advanced empathy tends to occur later in the genetic counseling session once you have developed rapport and built trust with a patient.

8.1.2 Distinctions Between Primary and Advanced Empathy

When considering the distinctions between primary empathy and advanced empathy, we like to use the analogy of a dimmer switch on a light fixture. Primary empathy responses are at the lower end of the dimmer feature—they shed some light on a patient's situation. Advanced empathy responses are at a higher level of the dimmer switch—they provide greater illumination, allowing the patient to see even more clearly what is "in the shadows."

Chapter 4 depicted primary empathy on a continuum ranging from minimal encouragers to reflections of content and affect. If we extend that continuum, advanced empathy would be farther to the right.

8.1.3 The Primary and Advanced Empathy Continuum and Distinctions

Minimal encourager	Paraphrase	Summary	Reflect content	Reflect affect	Content and affect reflection	Advanced empathy

Primary and advanced empathy differ in several ways:

Primary empathy	Advanced empathy
• Interchangeable or synonymous with what the patient is saying	Additive—goes beyond what the patient directly states
• Deals with surface content and feelings	Deals with hidden, implied content and feelings
• Reflects patient point of view	Reflects counselor point of view
• Counselor is responsive to discussion	Counselor takes initiative to direct discussion
• Patient is more aware of feelings and thoughts before the counselor reflects them	Patient is less aware of feelings and thoughts until the counselor reflects them

Primary empathy	Advanced empathy
• Reassures patient	Challenges patient
• Lowers patient anxiety	Raises patient anxiety
• Provides clarification and builds trust	Provides insight and promotes change
• May occur throughout session	Usually occurs later in the session
• Used frequently	Used sparingly

Advanced empathy responses are a more leading type of intervention. Clark (2010) describes Welfel and Patterson's (2005) "continuum of lead" that differentiates counselor responses in terms of client awareness and frame of reference. Clark notes that "Particular counselor interventions at one end of the continuum, such as silence and reflection, are minimally leading and are close to perspectives aligned with a client's frame of reference. When a counselor demonstrates empathic understanding in these instances, empathy serves to affirm a client's experiencing. In contrast, other interventions at the other end of the continuum, such as…interpretation, may largely be outside of a client's awareness, and [advanced] empathy provides a means to acknowledge a client's experiencing of new perspectives" (p. 353). According to Clark, the extent of a counselor's leading responses typically increases as the quality of the relationship develops and the counselor more fully understands the client.

8.1.4 Guidelines for Using Advanced Empathy

Skillful advanced empathy requires accurate understanding of and sensitive responding to patients. We recommend the following strategies for formulating and communicating advanced empathy responses:

Generate Hypotheses About Patient Situations, Thoughts, and Feelings

- Do a "psychosocial" case prep. When you have access to patient information prior to the genetic counseling session, review the file. Spend a few minutes formulating tentative hypotheses based on patient demographics (age, gender, culture, etc.), medical data, and reasons for seeking genetic counseling.
- Look for cues when you first meet a patient (e.g., How relaxed or tense is the patient? How eager or reluctant to speak? Whom did the patient bring along to the session?).
- Draw upon past experiences with genetic counseling patients and your knowledge of psychosocial theories to anticipate underlying patient affect and content (see Clark's (2010) objective empathy later in this chapter).

- Use your own professional and personal experiences. In personal essays describing "defining moments" (significant events that comprise a turning point in one's professional development (McCarthy Veach and LeRoy 2012)), many of the genetic counselor authors described enhanced empathy. The impetus for greater empathy included meaningful patient encounters (e.g., Bodurtha 2012; Chin 2012; Knutzen 2012; Lakhani 2012; Oswald 2012) and personal life events involving pain and loss (e.g., Anonymous 2008; Bellcross 2012; Glessner 2012). Peters et al. (2004) similarly found that genetic counselors who had themselves received genetic counseling reported subsequently experiencing increased empathy for their patients (e.g., greater ability to understand patients' decisions), greater connection with certain patients, and a greater emphasis on providing psychosocial support.
- Put yourself in the patient's place, and ask yourself how you might feel if you were this patient. But be careful not to project your feelings onto the patient (see Clark's (2010) subjective empathy later in this chapter).
- Pay attention to patient verbal and nonverbal behaviors.
- Listen for themes and repetitive patterns. Novices often make the mistake of thinking different pieces of information only go together if the patient talks about them at the same time (Mayfield et al. 1999). Patients may provide related information at different points in the session, so you need to fit the pieces together to see the themes. For example, a woman whose mother died of HD comes to clinic for testing. She states that she is concerned about passing HD on to a child. At various points in the session, she mentions her anger with her father who is opposed to her being tested. When the genetic counselor asks the patient to think about why she wants testing, the patient responds, "I cannot imagine watching a child suffer from this condition." The counselor "connects the dots" and uses advanced empathy to help the patient realize this is her father's fear as well. Perhaps that is why he does not want her to be tested, that is, he's likely afraid to find out if she has the condition like his wife.
- Ask yourself, "What is my patient trying to tell me that s/he can't say directly?" (MacDonald 1996). For example, you are seeing a patient with a history of infertility. In reviewing the family history, the patient states that she had an elective abortion when she was a teenager. Later in the session as you discuss the various etiologies for infertility, including both male and female factors, the patient comments, "I'm sure that it's not my husband's fault." You might say, "I wonder if there is something in particular that makes you feel this is *your* fault?" Your interpretation, stated in a tentative (questioning) way, may allow her to say she believes her abortion is the cause of the infertility. If she does not make that connection, and instead says something like, "I don't know, I just know," you might consider tentatively saying, "Some patients think that having an abortion causes infertility." This interpretation opens the door for further discussion of her belief.
- Remember that cultural and individual differences mean no two patients will react to the same experience in the same way. Avoid going overboard with theories that fail to match your patient's experience. Identifying feelings or thoughts incorrectly, referred to as "subtractive empathy," can be worse than saying nothing

(Neukrug et al. 2013). Additionally, it's important to listen for the patient's understanding of illness within her/his cultural context (Lewis 2010). Oosterwal (2009) notes that each ethnocultural group is characterized by its own specific cultural code—"a set of values, assumptions, notions and beliefs that shape the ways that people from diverse cultures act and think, relate and communicate; what they consider right or wrong, good or bad, sacred or profane, important or unimportant. This cultural code shapes the ways that people from diverse cultures interpret disease, death, genetic disorders, and disabilities; perceive of pregnancy and parenting; respond to pain; define family, kinship and ideal marriage partners; share or conceal information; use or refuse certain food and medications; and relate to their counselors and caregivers" (p. 332). Multiculturally competent genetic counselors "...use empathy in all genetic counseling sessions to understand the client's experiences, emotions, and perceptions of the world, and [to] determine how [their] client's behaviors and decisions are influenced" (Steinberg Warren and Wilson 2013, p. 7).

Share Your Hypotheses Through Carefully Formulated Responses

- Be concise, clear, and specific.
- Use responses that are nonjudgmental and nonpresumptive.
- Be tentative. Allow a patient the chance to deny or modify your statement. For example, "Correct me if I'm wrong, but it seems that you're saying..." You can also lead up to advanced empathy response by first asking for the patient's interpretation (Hill 2014). For instance, "What do you think is getting in the way of making this decision?"
- Formulate responses that are moderate in depth. Several psychotherapy studies indicate that interpretations that are of a moderate depth rather than too superficial or too deep have the most positive effect on processes and outcomes (Hill 2014). Refrain from jumping in with dramatic interpretations that will be off-putting to your patients.
- Be sure your response is suitable for a given patient. One way in which genetic counseling patients differ is in their degree of psychological-mindedness. Some patients are more psychologically minded than others and likely will respond well to interpretations about their inner experience; other patients are less interested in the why of their experience, and may be more interested in support, and information (cf. Sarangi et al. 2005). Clearly, you would use fewer advanced empathy responses with the latter type of patients. Another way in which patients differ is in how trusting they are. Some patients are very mistrustful and suspicious; you should stay close to the surface with them, using primary empathy (Martin 2015). Relatedly, in most cases the setting for genetic counseling is a medical clinic. Patients may not be expecting or may be unwilling to share on an emotional level in this setting.

- Give a well-timed response. Usually you will make an advanced empathy statement only after you've built some rapport through other skills such as attending and primary empathy and when you have enough impressions about the patient to be able to trust your hypothesis. Make advanced empathy statements when patients seem to be ready (i.e., have clearly stated their concerns and said there are some things they do not understand and seem eager to understand) (Hill 2014). Also, you should anticipate how your patient will react to your interpretation before giving it (Martin 2015).
- Use advanced empathy sparingly. Psychotherapy research indicates advanced empathy occurs much less frequently than primary empathy (Hill 2014), probably because it is such a powerful response. Patients can usually deal with only a limited number of insights at one time because insights often have a strong emotional impact, such as increased anxiety or sadness.
- Observe the extent to which your patient appears to accept your advanced empathy. Your response has likely missed the mark if your patient rejects what you said, becomes silent and withdrawn, or quickly changes the subject (Martin 2015). Possible patient reactions to advanced empathy include (1) agreeing with your interpretation and exploring its meaning; (2) agreeing, but avoiding, any further exploration; (3) asking for further information about your basis for making the statement; and (4) denying the accuracy of your statement.
- Follow up with primary empathy and questions. Summarize patients' responses by reflecting their emotional reaction to and thoughts about your advanced empathy statement. Then use questions to gather further details about the patient's reactions and their implications. For instance, "What are your thoughts about that….? How is that affecting your decision about….?"

Sources of Advanced Empathy

Clark (2010) proposes a model of empathy that involves "…understanding through three ways of knowing: Subjective empathy, interpersonal empathy, and objective empathy. Clark describes *subjective empathy* as: "…a counselor's awareness of his or her...internal reactions in response to the experiencing of a client. Through a form of personal knowing, a counselor vicariously experiences, for a momentary period of time, what it is like to be the client [by engaging in processes involving] identification, imagination, intuition, and felt-level experiencing..." (p. 349).

Through identification, a counselor engages in a partial and transitory assumption of a client's experiences as if they were his or her own. Use of imagination has the "potential to broaden an empathic understanding of clients in situations or conditions that counselors may personally perceive as culturally distant…[For instance,] the counselor can only imagine the pain that is incurred when one is morbidly obese, chronically disabled, or experiencing a life-threatening illness" (Clark 2010, pp. 349–350). Within genetic counseling, you may need to call on your imagination to understand, for example, the daily physical, cognitive, and emotional challenges a patient experiences as his retinitis pigmentosa progresses. A counselor's intuition

"...enables a counselor to rapidly generate impressions and hunches relating to a client's functioning. Finally, felt-level experiencing refers to a counselor's sensitivity to somatic or physical reactions that arise when empathically listening to a client" (Clark 2010, p. 349). For example, you may find yourself feeling tearful as you listen to a mother describing her child's sudden and unexpected death due to long QT syndrome.

Interpersonal empathy occurs when "...a counselor [is able] to empathically understand a client on an immediate here-and-now basis and also develop a general sense of how the client experiences life from an extended empathic perspective..." (Clark 2010, p. 350). For example, a 25-year-old woman, during a work-up for multiple miscarriages, learns that she carries a balanced chromosome translocation. When she tells her parents about this, they reveal that the translocation was found by amniocentesis when her mother was pregnant with her. She is angry that her parents knew this and didn't tell her. The counselor reflects the patient's immediate feelings of anger and betrayal at what she perceives as her parents' dishonesty and speculates that the patient fears her husband may not be honest with her about his reactions to her diagnosis.

Counselors engage in *objective empathy* when they draw from "...theoretically informed resources to enhance an empathic understanding of a client...." (Clark 2010, p. 351). Examples of resources include multicultural research findings. For example, "familiarity with...a general way that persons experience cultural forces enables a counselor to assess how an individual client responds to influences within his or her particular culture (Ivey et al. 2007; Sciarra 1999)..." (Clark 2010, p. 351).

Clark cautions that the various ways of engaging empathically are vulnerable to bias and distortion. Distortions in subjective and interpersonal empathy may be due to clients' perspectives, and/or the counselor's perspective, and distortions in objective empathy may be due to stereotyping clients based on normative data.

8.1.5 Types of Advanced Empathy Responses

There are several different types of advanced empathy responses that you might use with patients:

- Reflections of feelings and content not directly stated by the patient. For example, you observe the patient's nonverbal behaviors (clenched fists, red face) and comment, "I noticed your fists are clenched pretty tightly...like you might be angry?"
- Reflections of feelings that underlie emotions the patient has expressed. For example, "You say you're angry, but I wonder if you're also scared."
- Clear and direct statements about experiences the patient is guarded or confused about. For example, "You've mentioned a few times that if the test result is positive, you'll have to do something about it. Do you mean terminate the pregnancy?"

- Statements that summarize earlier feelings and content into a meaningful whole. For example, "You've said that since your diagnosis you've lost your appetite, cry a lot, and have trouble concentrating. It sounds like you're feeling depressed."
- Descriptions of patterns or recurring themes. Pay close attention to issues or questions a patient repeatedly raises. For example, to a mother of a newborn with trisomy 13, "You've asked a few times about things you did during your pregnancy, like drinking coffee, eating tuna and having a few drinks before you knew you were pregnant. Are you worried your behaviors may have caused this?"
- Connections between various parts of the patient's problems. For example, "Perhaps some of the difficulty deciding about genetic testing is that, at some level, you're angry with your mother because her cancer put you at risk. Maybe you're worried that if the test comes back positive, your daughter will be angry with you?"
- Logical conclusions to what the patient is saying. For example, "If you decide not to share your test results with your family, then you will not have to deal with their reaction."
- Alternative ways for the patient to view her or his experience. For example, "You said finding out you have the gene would be awful. You've also said it's *pure hell* to be always wondering. Is it possible the test might relieve some of that distress?"

Neukrug et al. (2013, p. 38) describe six types of responses that can express empathy, including responses they characterize as more "creative." Modified slightly for genetic counseling, they are:

1. Reflecting deeper feelings—Of which the patient has little or no awareness. For example, you might say "I hear how frustrated you are that the test results will take a while to come back, yet I also hear how scared you are that you have the gene for spino-cerebellar ataxia."
2. Pointing out conflicts—For example, "I hear that having a child is very important to you, yet I also hear that having an affected child would be too much for you to bear."
3. Visual analogy—A visual image may help patients recognize their nuanced and complex emotions and thoughts. For example, "As I listen to you describe how you will feel if your test is negative for HD, given your sisters' tests were positive, I have an image of you alone on the shore while your family is floating out to sea in a boat."
4. Nonvisual analogy—Not all analogies are visual ones. For instance, with parents who have pursued a diagnostic odyssey, attempting unsuccessfully to obtain a diagnosis for their child, you might say "It's as if you've been trapped in a huge maze, full of twists and turns. And just when you think you've found the way out, you run into another dead end."
5. Metaphors—For example, "When I listen to you talk about your risk for cancer, it sounds like you feel as though you've already been dealt this hand, and you can't do anything about it."
6. Targeted self-disclosure—You might say "You know, as you are speaking, I find my chest tightening, like there is a boulder sitting on it. I wonder if that's what you're feeling – a huge pressure to go through with testing."

8.1.6 Possible Patterns or Themes to Address with Advanced Empathy

With experience, you will begin to recognize patterns or themes that are fairly common to your patients. These generally fall into four broad categories of nonverbal behaviors, affect, attitudes or beliefs, and defenses. In these sections, we briefly cover these themes. Patient emotions, defense mechanisms, and coping are discussed in greater detail in Chap. 9.

Patient Nonverbal Behavior Patterns

- *Patient laughter when discussing painful situations*: Genetic counseling patients may engage in joking and other forms of levity when they in fact are experiencing intense emotions such as grief, anxiety, or fear. Their laughter may create a safe distance between them and you, prevent them from losing their composure, or hide what they regard as unacceptable feelings. You might say, "I notice you're smiling, perhaps because you're afraid you might break down right now?"
- *Omissions*: Listen for omissions of significant information. For instance, a prenatal patient does not mention her partner's thoughts and feelings. You say, "I notice you haven't said anything about your partner's opinion."
- *Other nonverbal behaviors*: Watch for nonverbals that indicate there is more beneath the patient's calm verbal presentation (e.g., sweating, teary-eyed, trembling chin or hands). Counselor: "You say you're OK, but you look like you're ready to cry."
- *Patient word choice*: Certain words or phrases reveal the feelings and relationships among people. For example, does your patient refer to her fetus as a "fetus," "my baby," or "it"? These words can give you clues about the extent to which she is distancing from or bonding with the pregnancy. Do couples refer to each other by first name or as "the wife" or "him"? These words can provide clues about their level of closeness or distance.

Patient Affective Themes

- *Anger*: Anger is frequently the surface expression of sadness and grief. Anger may also be "…coming from a place that's scared, anxious and powerless, and we can bond with patients over those feelings" (Schema et al. 2015, p. 724). Some patients (especially males and patients from some cultural backgrounds) regard certain emotions as evidence of weakness (Schema et al. 2015); anger can be a defense against their perceived weaknesses. You might address their unspoken emotion by saying, "This must be devastating for you."

Schema et al. (2015) investigated genetic counselors' experience of and management of patient anger directed at the counselor. Prevalent counselor strategies for addressing anger included advanced empathy statements about its origins. For instance, "I usually acknowledge their anger and the situation is basically not of their doing, they must feel out of control, and all they want to do is protect the people they love, and…they just can't do that" (p. 724).

- *Depression*: Feelings underlying depression may be anger, sadness, and despair/hopelessness. Depression typically is a reaction to a real or perceived loss of control. You could address underlying feelings by saying, for example, "It must be so discouraging to feel like there's nothing you can do."
- *Shame/guilt*: Patients who pass on genetic conditions to their children often feel guilt and shame, and patients who have a genetic condition may feel shame about being "defective" or "damaged goods" (McAllister et al. 2007). A genetic counselor might say: "It seems like you feel it's your fault your son has Marfan syndrome."

Sheets et al. (2011) recommend that when counseling parents who have received a diagnosis of Down syndrome, you "Assess the emotional reactions of the parents, and validate these feelings. Use active listening and empathic responses to support the parents" (p. 436). They further recommend you "Be empathic and address potential guilt issues" (p. 439).

- *Apprehension/anxiety*: Most individuals experience at least some anxiety in new situations (e.g., genetic counseling), as well as anxiety about what they may learn. Often, they will not tell you that this is how they feel. Counselor: "I wonder if you feel nervous about being here."
- *Despair/fear*: The patient feels there is no solution, no hope, and no way of coping. An example of addressing this feeling is, "Are you afraid you won't be able to deal with the diagnosis?"
- *Feeling threatened*: Of note, feelings of threat (due to the loss of a loved one, physical deterioration, possible rejection by others, etc.) tend to underlie all negative emotions. With advanced empathy, you attempt to reach that deeper level to determine what is threatening for patients and then discuss how that threat may be hindering their ability to hear necessary information, reach a decision, and/or cope with their situation. Counselor: "You keep mentioning how angry your husband gets that you have to spend so much time with your daughter. Are you afraid he might leave?"

Patient Attitude or Belief Patterns

- *Patients who ask you what to do*: Genetic counselors can view these types of questions as "an opportunity to identify and address a key issue that confronts the counselee and/or the genetic counseling process" (Weil 2000, p. 149). Djurdjinovic

(2009) suggests that a "simple and genuine inquiry on the part of the counselor, 'I would like to understand your question better,' sets aside the question and returns the focus on to the counselee" (p. 140).

- *Externalizing beliefs*: Some patients may blame others for their situation. For example, "This wouldn't be so hard if I didn't have to wait this long for an appointment with you!" or "I'd be able to decide about having Huntington's testing if my mother didn't get so hysterical every time I mentioned it." or "My doctor told me I was NOT at risk for cancer, but you are telling me I am!" We suggest you side step these externalizations as they are very difficult to modify and instead steer the conversation toward the patient: "It sounds as if you've been feeling very troubled about your condition"; "Do you feel guilty about burdening your mother with your condition?"; or "I can imagine how difficult it is to talk about these risks."
- *Patient believes fate, destiny, or a higher power brought about the situation*: Such patients may believe they are being punished for some transgression (which they usually cannot articulate). Furthermore, some cultural groups believe strongly in fate or karma. It is important to assess the extent to which this belief underlies the patient's experience. You might say, "I get the impression you think having a child with spina bifida is some sort of punishment" or "I wonder if in your culture, albinism is considered part of your destiny." Later in this chapter, we offer additional suggestions for working within these types of cultural perspectives.
- *Unrealistic expectations*: Some patients believe they should be able to make decisions easily and without any distress, or they may think it is silly or abnormal to feel so distressed. You could point out the unreasonableness of their expectations. For example, "Maybe you're being a little hard on yourself by expecting to have figured everything out already."
- *Feeling too responsible*: Patients may blame themselves for every aspect of their situation. Patient: "I would never have miscarried if I'd quit drinking coffee." Counselor: "It almost seems like you're looking for a reason to blame yourself. Are you feeling responsible?"
- *Forceful family members*: Lafans et al. (2003) interviewed prenatal genetic counselors about how they managed problematic paternal involvement in prenatal sessions. The prenatal counselors used advanced empathy to address overly involved behaviors. For example, "...[I] tried to make him know I'd heard what he was saying...] 'Alright, you're saying if your wife has this amnio and the baby has Down Syndrome, there's no way that you're going to raise a baby with Down Syndrome, and that you'll leave her. Is that what you're saying?'... once he got a chance to talk about his strong feelings... I could turn to her and say 'Ok, I hear what your husband's saying, and he's very clear, but I get the feeling you feel very differently'" (p. 228).
- *Couples or families may want you to take sides*: To be effective, you need to remain as supportive as you can toward each participant (Schoeffel et al. 2018). You might say, "It seems like you want me to agree with you. It's important that you all have a chance to speak and to hear each other." Relatedly, do not let patients speak for each other. At the beginning of the session, state that it is

important to hear from everyone, and then during the session, invite each participant to speak. Exceptions are patients whose cultural practices require that one person do most of the talking. It may also be appropriate for someone to speak on behalf of patients with limited intellectual and/or verbal functioning.
- *Believing their feelings are wrong*: You should validate what patients are feeling when their emotions are appropriate to the situation. For example, "It sounds like you have good reasons for feeling angry."

Patient Defense Patterns

- *Patients who sound as if they are working from a script*: Some patients present with "rehearsed stories" (Fine and Glasser 1996). This may happen if your patient has had to repeat the same information to numerous health-care professionals, family members, and friends. Try breaking into the script. For example, you could say, "You must have felt so angry when your father-in-law said you shouldn't have any more children." This redirects the patient to feelings and away from the rehearsed script.
- *Rationalization*: The patient is trying to justify her or his feelings, beliefs, or choices. You might say, "You keep saying that you're worried about how your wife will feel if you find out you're at increased risk for early onset Alzheimer disease. I wonder if you're worried about how *you* will handle this information."
- *Projection*: Patients may attribute their feelings or attitudes to others. Patient: "Everyone will think I'm selfish if I terminate this pregnancy because the baby has trisomy 18." In fact, it is the patient who feels that she is being selfish. Counselor: "Perhaps you're afraid that *you* are being selfish."
- *Either-or thinking*: For example, in a prenatal genetic counseling session, both partners are carriers for cystic fibrosis (CF). They see two options—risk having an affected child or do not have children—because abortion is not an option for them. The couple has not mentioned any other reproductive options. You could introduce the possibility of other options by saying, "So you see only two options, risk having an affected child, or have no children. I wonder if there are any other options you haven't considered."

8.1.7 Challenges in Using Advanced Empathy

Beginning genetic counselors usually find that advanced empathy is a complex and difficult skill to learn to use effectively. Common advanced empathy mistakes include:

- Going overboard with too many interpretations that overwhelm the patient. For example, some counselors may need to come across as all knowing, or insightful (Hill 2014).

- Making advanced empathy statements before patients are ready for them and/or making your statements too long.
- Inaccurately projecting your own experiences onto your patients (Clark 2010; MacDonald 1996).
- Lacking theoretical and personal frameworks to see the bigger picture and give patients alternative hypotheses (Hill et al. 2014; Jackson et al. 2014).
- Avoiding advanced empathy responses because you're afraid of being wrong about the patient; you are scared of how the patient will react; you are concerned you might damage the genetic counseling relationship; you fear you are being too intrusive (Jackson et al. 2014); or you don't want to hurt or embarrass your patients (Hill 2014).
  "At some level clients are well aware of their own feelings and perceptions of what has happened to them. We do not need to protect them against the pain of their lives. They have their own defenses to deal with that. More often, they need a witness to hear their pain, their concern, their anger—not someone to change or deflect it" (Fontaine and Hammond 1994, p. 223).

8.1.8 Some Cultural Considerations in Using Advanced Empathy

In some cultures, it is important to be less direct in making advanced empathy responses (Hackney and Bernard 2017; Pedersen and Ivey 1993). A less direct approach helps the patient "save face" (This approach can be effective with defensive patients as well). Consider, for example, the following subtle ways to address patient inner experience:

- "In the past when I've had patients in a situation similar to yours, some of them have felt…"
- "Some people might feel [think, do]…if they were in your situation."
- "Some people find it very difficult to…and they choose to…"
- "You say you're fine with this news, but I want you to know it's OK if you're not. I hope you'll talk it over with me or, if you're not comfortable discussing it here, then talk with someone close to you."
- "If I were in your situation, I might be thinking about the following…What do you think?"

Generally speaking, it is not a good idea to challenge a person's cultural perspective (e.g., that a genetic condition is God's will). First, it is very ethnocentric to believe your way of viewing reality is better for patients than their own way. Second, patients are quite unlikely to change their perspective based on one or two genetic counseling sessions. Third, this sort of challenge will probably damage any trust you have established. Try to work with patients within their cultural perspectives. For example, "I understand that you regard your child's metabolic condition as

God's will. You may be wondering how we can be of any help. Our team can certainly help manage your child's condition."

8.2 Confrontation Skills

8.2.1 Definition and Functions of Confrontation

Confrontation involves responses in which you directly challenge patients to view themselves and their situations differently. Confrontations are a type of feedback that is discrepant with or contrary to the patient's self-understanding, and they usually involve behaviors the patient has neither publicly nor privately acknowledged. Confrontation responses can include identification of patient self-defeating behaviors as well as patient strengths. Indeed, Kessler (1997) stresses the importance of genetic counselors' identifying "key areas of client functioning which they use throughout the session to strengthen the latter's sense of competence. This might involve parenting, work, interpersonal, or other issues and requires the professional to say rewarding things to the client" (p. 381). Confrontations ultimately are intended to help patients consider changing their behavior.

Confrontations can challenge discrepancies, contradictions, defenses, or irrational beliefs, encourage individuals to think or feel in new ways (Hackney and Bernard 2017; Hill 2014), and/or challenge patients to recognize and use their strengths or potentials. By helping patients explore hidden feelings, attitudes, and beliefs, confrontation can remove some of the barriers to goal setting and decision-making. Confrontation shares similarities with advanced empathy, as both are counselor-initiated attempts to elicit greater patient self-understanding. An important distinction, however, is that advanced empathy expresses part of the patient's experience she/he is vaguely aware of, whereas confrontation points out experiences that are discrepant with or contradictory to the patient's self-understanding. Returning to our analogy of a dimmer switch, with confrontations, the switch is turned up to its maximum, meaning the brightest amount of light possible. As such, confrontation has the potential to be both a more powerful and a more threatening response. Confrontation should occur infrequently, even less often than advanced empathy. You must be extremely careful when using confrontation in genetic counseling.

8.2.2 Guidelines for Effective Confrontation

When making a confrontation, you should attempt to be *with* rather than *against* your patient (Miller and Rose 2009). We recommend the following strategies when using confrontation:

Formulate a Response

- *Time your response*: Use confrontation when your patient is likely to be open to it. Direct confrontations at the very beginning have been found to be ineffective in consultation relationships (Dougherty et al. 1997). Rapport and trust must be present before patients are likely to hear confrontations. Lafans et al. (2003) found that genetic counselor confrontation was sometimes an ineffective management strategy for problematic paternal involvement and concluded that confrontation should occur only after you have some understanding of the patient's experience and culture and the couple's dynamics. As those researchers reported, "Indeed, several participants noted that some mothers seem to accept their partner's under- or over-involvement, and they tried to read the mother in deciding what to do about the father's involvement" (p. 239).
- *Begin with accurate empathy*: You must understand your patient's experience before you can detect and raise issues of discrepancies or distortions.
- *Moderate the depth*: Decide how big a difference there is between what you want to say and what the patient believes to be true. If the difference is too big, your patient will be more likely to reject your confrontation.
- *Anticipate impact*: Estimate your patient's ability to handle the confrontation before you intervene. If your patient seems to be confused or disorganized, you should wait until she/he is in a more receptive state.
- *Use successive approximations*: Introduce confrontation gradually; begin with small aspects the patient has some likelihood of being able to take into consideration. Describe your patient's behavior and its significance and/or consequences.
- *Choose your vocabulary and syntax carefully*: Confrontation responses can sound accusatory or patronizing. You should speak tentatively ("I wonder if…"; "Perhaps…"; "Maybe…"; etc.) and use a questioning tone that leaves the patient room to disagree.
- *Check your motivation*: Use confrontation to help the patient, not to be right, to release your anger or impatience, to get back at the patient, or to put your patient in her or his place. It is not appropriate to confront a patient because you are bored, anxious, need to feel in control, or want to dominate the interaction.
- *Be sincerely concerned*: Communicate your confrontation in a way that demonstrates you have a sincere interest in your patient's welfare. Confrontation should be grounded in empathic understanding. For example, "You seem very anxious, and I wonder if we could talk about how that may be part of the reason you're so undecided about testing." Furthermore, if your confrontations imply criticism, that is, if patients think you're accusing them or getting into a power struggle, your relationship and the session can quickly deteriorate (Martin 2015).
- *Put your feedback skills to work*: Since confrontation is a type of feedback, it is useful to consider guidelines for delivering feedback effectively. As discussed in Chap. 1, Danish and D'Augelli (1980) suggest a skillful feedback giver:
  - Is focused on behavior rather than on the patient's personal characteristics.
  - Gives only as much information as the patient is ready to handle.

- Makes the confrontation as soon as possible after the behavior has happened.
- Is concise, tentative, and descriptive rather than judgmental and only confronts about behavior that she/he believes the patient can control or change. For instance, it is judgmental and does no good to ask a patient who says they did not want to be pregnant again if they used birth control.
- States the consequences of the behavior for the patient and/or family members (e.g., "You said you resent not knowing you were at such a high risk for cancer, but now that you know, you're finding it difficult to talk to your brother. How do you think he will feel about not knowing his risk?").
- Focuses on both strengths and weaknesses, asks the patient to respond to the confrontation, and is willing to modify it based on the patient's feedback.
- Is definite (i.e., does not give the feedback and then take it back).

Follow Up on a Confrontation Response

- *Monitor the impact of your confrontation*: Sometimes patients perceive your statements differently from the way you intended them (e.g., you may intend to point out a discrepancy in your patient's story, while the patient thinks you're saying she/he is too confusing or stupid). To check out the impact of a confrontation, you could ask, "What do you think about what I just said?" or "How do you feel about what I just said?"
- *Be supportive after a confrontation*: Confrontations can be threatening and painful to hear. You should follow up with supportive empathy statements that acknowledge your patient's experience. For example, "I know this is hard for you. I can see why you try to cut me off when I'm telling you these painful things. Let's try to go more slowly, so you can take this in gradually."
- *Don't expect miracles*: Not all confrontations produce insights that lead to change (Pedersen and Ivey 1993).

8.2.3 Possible Patient Behaviors to Confront

Discrepancies in Information

Confrontation of discrepancies is important for preventing confusion and to verify the accuracy of information. This type of confrontation is common in genetic counseling because you must gather accurate data in order to help patients set goals and make decisions. Three types of information discrepancies might be addressed:

- *Gaps*: an issue usually associated with a particular genetic situation the patient does not raise. Parents of a child with NF who never mention that they also have multiple neurofibromas, even though you asked about this specifically in gathering the family history.

- *Omissions*: the patient fails to include relevant information in her or his personal narrative. Patient is being seen for genetic counseling about a family history of Duchenne muscular dystrophy. She fails to mention that she is currently pregnant.
- *Inconsistencies*: in what the patient says at different times in the session. For example, "Earlier you told me this is your first pregnancy, but now you mentioned several miscarriages."

Discrepancies Between Ideas and Actual Behavior

It's not unusual to think one thing and do another thing. For instance, a prenatal patient's partner says, "I only want what's best for my wife" but argues strongly against testing, even though the wife says this is what she wants. You respond, "You say you only want what's best for her. It sounds like she wants testing, but you don't agree."

Ambivalence

Ambivalence is a common human experience, and patients should be given permission to feel uncertain (Fine and Glasser 1996). For example, "You say you want to have the testing done, but you keep canceling your appointment. I wonder if you have mixed feelings." Or the patient says, "I'm only here because my doctor sent me. But since it took me hours to get here, and since I'm here already, I might as well go ahead and have the test." Counselor: "That's not a good enough reason. Let's consider the reasons you might and might not want this test."

Discrepancies Between What the Patient Says and the Real-World Context

For example, your patient says, "My child is just a little developmentally delayed, but the doctors told me he'll catch up if we just work with him." You might respond, "You say he's going to catch up, but your medical records indicate that he has Prader Willi syndrome, which is known to be associated with intellectual deficits."

In the Lafans et al. (2003) study, some of the prenatal genetic counselor participants confronted under-involved fathers through education. For example, "[I say] 'This is a couple decision...whatever happens with the amnio has ramifications for both of you.' He says, 'Well, she's the one who gets the needle in her belly.' I said, 'Well, that's true, but it's a minimal part of the amnio experience.' "Did he feel he could support her if she chose to have it?..." (p. 255).

Discrepancies Within the Patient's Messages and/or Internal Dialogue

"You've said you could never have an abortion; you've also said you couldn't deal with another child who has cystic fibrosis." Or "You've said you want to know if you have an increased risk for breast cancer, but you've also said you would be devastated by a positive test result."

Discrepancy Between Patient Self-Perceptions and Genetic Counselor Perceptions of the Patient

The patient says, "I'll never be able to make a decision by myself!" You say, "And yet, you made the decision to come here and to have the testing done even though your family was against it, which suggests to me that you can be strong and decisive."

Distortions

"I'm wondering if blaming your child's condition on the way he was delivered keeps you from having to acknowledge your own medical history."

Evasions/Avoidance

"You've told me you've forgotten to ask your siblings to be tested. Is this perhaps because you know it would mean a more definite answer about your own cancer risk?" Or the patient was supposed to request that his medical record be sent to the genetic counselor. Patient: "I really didn't have a chance to call the doctor's office." Counselor: "I'm wondering if you're sure you want to pursue testing."

Lafans et al. (2003) found behaviors that characterized partner under involvement in prenatal genetic counseling sessions included lack of affect and comments such as "It's her body; it's her decision." Counselor confrontations included saying: "You seem withdrawn, uncomfortable, or confused about how to make this decision...to allow him to say either, 'I don't care,' or 'I don't want an amnio, and that's why I'm doing this.'..."; "I don't think you're hearing what she's saying ...paraphrase what she said and ask her... 'Is that what you're saying?'; then to him, 'Is that what you're hearing?'"; and "'What would you do if you were making the decision all by yourself'...that will get just about any male to state an opinion, and then...you can start discussion in coming to a compromise" (p. 230). Some counselors also used humor. For example, "[I] say to them, 'You realize you're talking to a counselor. I'm not going to let you get away with not talking about your feelings'" (p. 255).

Nonverbal Contradictions

The patient says, with tears in her eyes, "I'm OK with these test results." You reply, "You say you are OK, but you look very sad."

Some prenatal counselors in the Lafans et al. (2003) study confronted paternal nonverbals. For example, "…'your wife is crying and you're not really...looking at her. What's going on with you?'[and] ...some just want to read the newspaper; I'll address that—'I'd like you to be part of this'" (p. 255).

Games, Tricks, and Smoke Screens

You say, "I wonder if interrupting me lets you protect yourself from hearing this painful information?" Or, if the patient repeatedly says "Yes, but…," you could respond, "I notice you say 'Yes, but…' every time I suggest a resource for you to learn more about fragile X syndrome. Perhaps you don't feel ready to learn more about the condition?"

Self-Defeating Statements

Patient: "I can't think of anything I could say to my sister to convince her that genetic testing is in both of our best interests."
Counselor: "I think you've raised several persuasive points in talking with me."

Patient: "I'm just not strong enough to face a test result that says I have a gene for breast cancer."
Counselor: "You say you're too weak to handle that sort of news. However, you seem strong and able to reach out to others for support."

Lafans et al. (2003) found that with overly involved fathers (who spoke for the mother and/or otherwise dominated the conversation), some prenatal counselors used confrontation to encourage them to "own" their behavior, separately from their partner's behavior. For example, "...[I] bring it back to the wife and say, 'Do you have strong feelings about that?... How do you think [his feelings] affect your relationship as a couple?'" (p. 228).

8.2.4 Possible Patient Reactions to Counselor Confrontation

Egan (1994) describes six ways patients could respond to a confrontation:

- *Deny the feedback*: Your patient may calmly tell you that your feedback is wrong or angrily refuse to accept what you said.

- *Discredit the source*: A common genetic counseling patient response might be, "You don't understand. After all, you don't have Huntington's disease in your family."
- *Try to change your mind*: Your patient might try to argue you into believing her or his point of view (e.g., "Oh, if you knew me better, you'd realize I really can't handle this type of news!").
- *Devalue the topic*: For example, "I'm only kidding when I say our daughter's genetic condition is my husband's fault. I don't really mean anything by it."
- *Seek support elsewhere*: "Well, all of my family members and friends agree with me!"
- *Your patient may pretend to agree with you*: "You're probably right. Of course, you have more experience than I do with this disease."

Pedersen and Ivey (1993) identify several additional ways patients might respond:

- Patient is willing to admit to part of what you have confronted.
- Patient agrees with the confrontation but refuses to do anything about it.
- The patient chooses to compromise or accommodate the problem.
- The patient hears the confrontation and uses the insight to change the behavior.

It is important to realize that it may take time for patients to respond fully to confrontation. Their full reactions may not be evident in the genetic counseling session.

Prior to using confrontation, it is important that you assess your patient's general demeanor. Research suggests that you should generally avoid confronting patients who are high on reactance (resistant to giving up control in interpersonal interactions) and/or angry patients (Karno and Longabaugh 2005; Schema et al. 2015). Confrontation may intensify their emotions.

8.2.5 Challenges in Using Confrontation

Confrontation is not an easy intervention. If you look up "confrontation" in a thesaurus, you will see terms such as challenge, oppose, antagonize, provoke, meet, threaten, defy, tackle, face, encounter, handle, face up to, deal with, and meet head-on. Some of these terms sound quite negative, suggesting behaviors to avoid doing.

Moreover, when confrontations are about difficult issues, we may want to avoid them because we fear patient's negative reactions, and/or it makes us feel bad or uncomfortable to think we've caused someone else's pain. Moreover, "Beginning counselors tend to avoid confronting…because it deviates from what they have been taught is polite behavior; therefore, they fear that doing so might damage the relationship" (Hackney and Bernard 2017, p. 29).

Similarly, in genetic counseling you may avoid using confrontation with your patients because:

- You want to be liked and are afraid patients won't like you after you confront them.
- You don't want to hurt or embarrass patients (especially likely if you regard patients as fragile and vulnerable). In reality, patients are already experiencing pain and conflict; rather than directly causing their distress, your honesty allows it to come out in the open (Wilbur and Wilbur 1986).
- You have a cultural belief that confrontation is a rude or otherwise inappropriate behavior.
- You might be off base, that is, you're afraid you are biased against or wrong about the patient.
- You might open yourself up to feedback from the patient.
- Your patient might get angry, shut down, or even get up and leave!
- You are unsure how to confront in a way that is supportive while also being direct (Chui et al. 2014).
- Confrontation is not just difficult when it's about painful issues. You may also be afraid of sounding phony if you confront patients about their strengths (e.g., you feel uncomfortable giving compliments) or you think your opinion will not matter to them.

8.2.6 Cultural Considerations in Using Confrontation

You cannot use confrontation in the same ways with patients from all cultural groups. You need to be sensitive to cultural differences and modify your approach depending on a patient's background. For instance, direct challenges with Asian, Latino, and indigenous American patients generally should be avoided (Ivey 1994). Additionally, cultural practices for some Chinese individuals involve being extremely careful not to hurt another person or to make the person "lose face." Another implication of these differences is patients from some cultural groups might feel compelled to agree with your confrontations because they don't want to hurt you. The appropriateness of confrontation also differs between men and women across cultures (e.g., a female genetic counselor communicating with a male from the Middle East should be particularly careful about using this type of intervention).

Pedersen and Ivey (1993) recommend addressing the different rules that various cultures have about confrontation by:

- Being aware of your own cultural assumptions as well as those of your patient's culture.
- Framing confrontations in ways that make it appropriate to your patient's culture. Change the words or the process of communicating the confrontation; translate it into the patient's cultural style, so your confrontation can be understood. For example, the use of the word *problem* might be ineffective for a patient who comes from a culture where it is unacceptable to have a weakness.

- Trying not to be "distracted by behaviors—no matter how discrepant they might seem—until they are understood from the viewpoint of the patient's values and expectations" (Pedersen and Ivey 1993, p. 196). For instance, some African American patients may look away when listening to you.

You will encounter many different types of beliefs and practices that are culturally based. Consider the following example:

> A Middle Eastern couple is counseled regarding prenatal testing. The husband does all the talking but states that it is his wife's decision. The wife keeps her eyes on the floor and says nothing. Counselor: "Mr.—, you've said several times that it's up to your wife to decide about testing this pregnancy, yet she has said very little today. Help me understand how she will make this decision."

In this example, it is important to assess the reason for the woman's silence. For instance, Awwad et al. (2008) interviewed native Palestinians and first-generation, Palestinian Americans and asked them to imagine themselves as patients in hypothetical premarital and prenatal situations. Among their results, they found most interviewees preferred a joint decision-making process with their partner; this process, however, would happen at home, not during a genetic counseling session. Furthermore, if the couple was in strong disagreement, most Palestinian Americans said the decision should be made by the woman, while most native Palestinians preferred the decision either remain a joint one or that the man should decide. These results demonstrate clear differences in culture and acculturation that might be one explanation for the perceived discrepancy in the above example.

Keep in mind that confrontation is unlikely to work when patients hold strong cultural beliefs. In such situations, you need to respect their view and move on. For example, a couple from Pakistan who has a child with Friedreich's ataxia does not believe their consanguinity caused this condition. You could say, "I understand that you do not think your child's condition happened because you and your wife are related. Can we talk about some tests that would tell us if the next baby will have the same thing?" This accomplishes the genetic counseling goal of offering options to patients, without disrespecting their beliefs.

Remain flexible in using confrontation with patients whose cultural backgrounds differ from yours. You generally should strive to make your confrontations gentle, as such feedback is difficult for most individuals to hear. Remember it is always appropriate to ask patients to help you understand their cultural perspective on an issue. It may be sufficient to say, "You and I come from different cultures. Can you help me understand how we can approach this issue together?"

Note that there will be times when you can incorporate your patient's cultural beliefs into the session. For example, Greeson et al. (2001) interviewed Somali women immigrants and found unanimous belief that "…Allah, not inheritance, makes a person disabled" (p. 375). The researchers recommended that instead of confronting this belief, genetic counselors could "mesh science and religion by… [helping] Somali patients consider risk by using the example that Allah decides which gene the child gets, but that there are four choices" (p. 375).

Religious beliefs comprise another cultural variable that may present inconsistencies, and you might think the beliefs are impeding the genetic counseling process. Knapp et al. (2010), speaking about psychologists, recommend that practitioners "…(a) consider carefully how to identify a belief as religious; (b) listen carefully to their clients; (c) recognize that religious beliefs, like other beliefs, may be fluid and changing; and (d) accept that religious beliefs are multifaceted and multi-determined" (p. 406). They further assert that "…situations where it is necessary to directly challenge a client's religious beliefs are exceptional" (p. 409).

8.3 Closing Comments

Advanced empathy and confrontation are less frequent responses than other genetic counseling behaviors such as primary empathy, questioning, and information giving. Nevertheless, when used strategically, they can foster patient insights about themselves and their situations. Often these insights will help patients achieve greater acceptance of their feelings, thoughts, and actions. They may also prompt changes in behaviors that are getting in the way of patient goal-setting and decision-making processes. As a beginning genetic counselor, you may feel anxious about using these powerful responses. With supervised practice, you will gradually become more comfortable incorporating advanced empathy and confrontation skills into your counseling repertoire.

8.4 Class Activities

Activity 1: Empathy and Confrontation Discussion

Students talk about what they think advanced empathy and confrontation are, how the two skills are similar and how they differ, and the functions each serves in genetic counseling. This discussion can be started by having students respond to the questions in dyads.

Estimated time: 10–15 min.

Activity 2: Conceptualizing Patients (Small Group Exercise)

In small groups, each student selects and reads aloud a patient statement (listed below) then discusses what it might be like to be this patient. The student generates as many ideas as she or he can about:

- The patient's surface feelings, thoughts, and issues
- The patient's underlying feelings, thoughts, and issues

Then the student speculates on what issues s/he might need to confront the patient about during genetic counseling.

Students are NOT to give advice or solve the patient's problem. Other group members can add their ideas to the student's speculations.

Patient Statements

- "I'm 39 and this is my first pregnancy. I had prenatal testing and just learned that there is something wrong with my baby. They say there's a chance my child could have a lot of behavior problems in school and may not be able to learn. Oh, and I remember they also said he would be really tall. But they aren't real sure, because hardly any research has been done on people with this condition. What should I do?"
- "I've just found out that my brother is gay. I already know that two of my cousins on my dad's side are gay. I've read that homosexuality may be inherited. Are my wife and I more likely to have a gay child if she ever gets pregnant?"
- "I asked to see you first before my husband comes in because I'm not sure I want to go through with this NIPT test. He knows I was pretty wild in my younger days, and I did a lot of partying, including smoking pot and using other drugs a few times. What if the results come back and there's something wrong with the baby?"
- "I've just tested positive for Huntington's disease. I'm not symptomatic yet, but I want to know exactly what to expect. How do other people deal with this? Have you ever heard of people with Huntington's committing suicide?"
- "My husband and I want to have a baby. I believe my health is good and there are no genetic problems in my family. However, my husband is an active alcoholic. I'm concerned about fetal alcohol syndrome."
- "I came here today for prenatal testing. This is my second pregnancy. My first child has a severe form of autism, which means that he will be completely dependent on my husband and me for the rest of our lives. I'm afraid this might happen again, but I don't believe in having an abortion. If our next child does not have autism, I will feel better that this is not my fault."
- "This is my fourth pregnancy. I have three sons. My husband and I really want a girl this time. We have heard that some prenatal testing could determine the sex of the child. I'd like to get that testing done here."
- "I was diagnosed with breast cancer a few weeks ago. Because my mother died of breast cancer in her 40s, my doctor said I should have genetic testing. I know it will help to have this test. But, I have two teenage daughters. I'm so worried that I might find out that they will get breast cancer, too."

Estimated time: 60–75 min.

Activity 3a: Low-Level Advanced Empathy and Confrontation Skills Model

The instructor and a volunteer genetic counseling patient engage in a role-play in which the counselor demonstrates poor advanced empathy and confrontation behaviors (e.g., overanalyzes patient motives and feelings; confronts the patient in punitive, inaccurate, judgmental ways). Students observe and take notes of examples of poor advanced empathy and confrontation.

Estimated time: 10 min.

Process

Students share their examples of poor advanced empathy and confrontation responses. Then they discuss the impact of the counselor's poor skills on the patient. The patient can offer her or his impressions of the counselor's behaviors after the other students have made their comments. The instructor could divide the group of students and instruct half to focus on counselor behaviors and half to focus on patient behaviors, or half of the class could focus on advanced empathy behaviors, and the other half could focus on confrontation behaviors.

Estimated time: 15 min.

Instructor Note

- Students often have difficulty differentiating advanced empathy from confrontation. The instructor should assist them in categorizing the responses they observe in the role-play.
- One issue that may come up is the counselor's intended response (e.g., advanced empathy) may be perceived differently by the patient or observers (e.g., as a confrontation).
- One option is to continue with a role-play used earlier in the class, so the counselor can more quickly move to advanced empathy and confrontation skills.

Activity 3b: High-Level Advanced Empathy and Confrontation Skills Model

The instructor and the same volunteer repeat the same role-play, only this time the counselor displays good advanced empathy and confrontation skills. Students take notes of examples of good advanced empathy and confrontation behaviors.

Estimated time: 15 min.

Process

Students discuss their examples of good advanced empathy and confrontation responses and the impact of the counselor's behaviors on the patient. They also contrast this role-play to the low-level role-play. The instructor could divide the group of students and have half focus on counselor behaviors and half focus on patient behaviors, or half of the class could focus on advanced empathy behaviors, and the other half could focus on confrontation behaviors.

Estimated time: 15 min.

Instructor Note

- Students could work together in think-pair-share dyads to identify advanced empathy and confrontation examples and their impact on the patient.

Activity 4: Triad Role-Plays

Using the patient statements in Activity 2, three students practice advanced empathy and confrontation skills in 15–min role-plays taking turns as counselor, patient, and observer. Allow another 10 min of feedback after each role-play. The students should focus on using good helping behaviors.

Criteria for Evaluating Counselor Advanced Empathy and Confrontation
Well-timed
Accurate
Tentative
Language is respectful
Specific
Identifies themes, underlying issues, and/or discrepancies
Addresses content and/or feelings
Follow-up with primary empathy
Estimated time: 75 min

Process
In a large group, students discuss what they learned from the role-play.

- How was it to do this exercise?
- What are you learning about advanced empathy and confrontation in general?
- What are you learning about yourself with respect to these two skills?
- What questions do you still have about advanced empathy and confrontation?

Estimated time: 15 min.

Instructor Note
- The observer or counselor may wish to stop the role-play if the counselor is obviously "stuck." The triad (except for the patient) then engages in a brief conversation about the patient's dynamics, issues, etc., with a goal of prompting the counselor. Then the counselor and patient resume the role-play.

Activity 5: Conceptualizing Patients (Small Groups)[1]

Instructor reads aloud the following patient description:

> The patient is a 34-year-old pregnant woman. Her 4-year-old son has Duchenne Muscular Dystrophy (DMD). She had prenatal testing for DMD for her current pregnancy and learned that she is carrying a boy who is also affected with DMD.

[1] Adapted from: McHenry and McHenry (2015).

Next the instructor reads one patient statement at a time. After reading a statement, the students write three responses—one primary empathy response, one advanced empathy response, and one confrontation response.

Students should write the responses as if they were actually speaking to the patient. Tell students they can assume more knowledge about the patient and her situation than is evident in the description when formulating their advanced empathy and confrontation responses.

Have volunteers share their written responses to each patient statement, one type at a time. In other words, ask volunteers to read their primary empathy responses first. Provide feedback to the students on those responses. Next have volunteers read advanced empathy responses and provide feedback. Finally, have volunteers read confrontation responses and provide feedback. Reinforce responses that are skillful. Be corrective about inaccuracies (e.g., a response the student thinks is advanced empathy but is actually primary empathy, a response that "misses the mark" with respect to patient experience/situation) and responses that are too lengthy, too threatening in tone, and too awkward/mechanical. Ask the group to help a student revise a response to make it more effective. Follow this process for each of the five patient statements.

Pt: I was so certain this baby would be just fine. We told everyone right away that we were expecting another baby.

Co:

1. Primary empathy response—
2. Advanced empathy response—
3. Confrontation response—

Pt: I don't understand why God did this to me.

Co:

1. Primary empathy response—
2. Advanced empathy response—
3. Confrontation response—

Pt: This is such a hard decision to make. Do I have an abortion? And if I do, what do I tell people?

Co:

1. Primary empathy response—
2. Advanced empathy response—
3. Confrontation response—

Pt: What do I tell my son? He knows that "Mommy has a baby in her tummy." I can't lie to him.

Co:

1. Primary empathy response—
2. Advanced empathy response—
3. Confrontation response—

Pt: I just can't face the thought of having another baby who is going to get so sick. Does this mean that I don't love my son?

Co:

1. Primary empathy response—
2. Advanced empathy response—
3. Confrontation response—

Estimated time: 60 min.

Instructor Note
- This activity could be done as a written exercise.

8.5 Written Exercises

Exercise 1: Journal Entry

Ask students to write a journal entry or short paper addressing the following:

1. Describe what you consider to be a confrontation.
2. Discuss how confrontations were/are handled in:
   - Your family
   - Your peer group as a child
   - Your current peer group (Do *not* include your classmates in this group)
   - The cultural group with which you identify
3. How might these experiences impact the way you will approach confrontation with your genetic counseling patients?
4. In general, is it easier for you to make confrontations about a person's strengths? Limitations?
5. Are certain types of patients easier for you to confront?

Exercise 2: Primary Empathy, Advanced Empathy, and Confrontation

Read each of the following patient statements, and write one primary empathy response, one advanced empathy response, and one confrontation response for each statement. Write your responses as if you were actually talking to the patient.

[*Hint*: You may have to infer more knowledge about the patient than is written here when formulating your advanced empathy and confrontation responses.]

For example, a 40-year-old man at risk for Huntington disease, says, "I'm sick of worrying about this all the time! Every time I trip over something I think I have it. I think, 'Oh no, you're gonna end up just like your father.' Everyone made fun of him because of his disease. It was so hard being a child when your father acted so goofy. I don't know what I'll do if I find out I have this gene."

Primary empathy: "You seem scared that you have Huntington's, too."

Advanced empathy: "Are you afraid people will be saying the same things about you?"

Confrontation: "This seems to be very distressing for you, and I'm wondering about the fact that you haven't had testing until now."

- 35-year-old prenatal patient: "I'm afraid my husband will not understand my reasons for wanting to continue with this pregnancy. He might try to talk me out of my plan. I'm afraid he won't understand how I feel."
- 25-year-old male patient: "I don't know whether or not to be tested for SCA (spinal cerebellar ataxia, type 6). I'm so frustrated! You'd think after watching my father with this disease that I'd know what to do."
- 50-year-old woman talking about her 25-year-old child: "He knows that he can take advantage of me because of his albinism. If he gets sunburned or begins to talk about how he feels worthless and hopeless, I go crazy. He gets everything he wants out of me, and I know it's my own fault. But I still love him very much."
- 17-year-old male prenatal partner: "My girlfriend is pregnant, and the baby has abnormalities. She says she want to have an abortion. She says it's her problem and she can handle it without me. She never even asked me what I think she should do! I mean, it's my baby, too!"
- 10-year-old boy with Duchenne muscular dystrophy: "My classmates don't like me, and right now I don't like them! Why do they have to be so mean? They make fun of me because I can't walk or play with them. Gee, they don't have to like me, but I wish they'd stop making fun of me."
- 16-year-old with neurofibromatosis (NF) and a lot of visible nodules: "I'm only here because my mother made me come."
- 32-year-old mother and her husband who are from India and have three daughters: The mother says (looking tearful), "We want to have a boy."
- 38-year-old woman with a history of five miscarriages and no living children: "No one really knows how I feel. I know it's just miscarriages, and not like losing a real baby."
- Prenatal patient who has a child with cystic fibrosis (CF): "My husband wants me to have prenatal testing for this pregnancy, but I just don't know. Susan, our daughter, is doing so well, and we love her so much."
- 30-year-old woman: "My family does not talk about how so many people in our family have cancer. I can't talk to my husband about it, either. And I don't know what to think about my two daughters!"
- Consanguineous couple from the Middle East: "I don't think this is a genetic problem. All of my sisters married cousins, and their children are all normal."
- 25-year-old African American woman who has one child with sickle cell anemia, had an elective abortion of her second pregnancy, is pregnant again and considering prenatal testing: "Everyone tells me that this baby will be affected because I ended the last pregnancy."
- 35-year-old Arabic woman whose newborn has Down syndrome: "What will she look like when she is older? Will she look abnormal?"

- 20-year-old Catholic, Hispanic prenatal patient. Prenatal testing revealed anencephaly: "My doctor thinks I should have an abortion, but my priest and my husband are so against it."

Instructor Note

- As an addendum to this exercise, students can be asked to describe a cross-cultural genetic counseling experience they were involved in or observed and to write three responses for that situation (i.e., primary empathy, advanced empathy, and confrontation).

Exercise 3: Role-Play

Engage in a 20–30-min role-play of a genetic counseling session with a classmate. The role-play can be based on a patient you saw in clinic, or it can be a made-up patient situation. During the role-play, focus on all the helping skills you've learned so far. Try to include at least one advanced empathy and one confrontation response. Audio record the role-play. Next transcribe the role-play and critique your work. Use the following method for transcribing the session:

Counselor	Patient	Self-critique	Instructor
Key phrases of dialogue	Key phrases	Comment on your own responses	Will provide feedback on your responses

Create a brief summary:

1. Briefly describe patient *demographics* (e.g., age, gender, ethnicity, socioeconomic status, relationship status) and *reason* for seeking genetic counseling.
2. Identify *two* things you said/did during the role-play that were effective and *two* things you could have done differently.

Give the recording, transcript/self-critique, and summary to the instructor who will provide feedback.

[*Hint*: This assignment encourages self-reflective practice regarding your clinical performance. The goal is not to do a perfect session. Rather the goal is to assess the extent to which you can accurately assess your psychosocial counseling skills. You will gain more from this exercise if you refrain from scripting what you plan to say as the counselor.]

Exercise 4: Advanced Empathy: Letter to Your Genetic Counselor[2]

Imagine that you and your partner have an appointment to see a pediatric genetic counselor because your four-year-old child (your only child to date) has been diagnosed with autism. Several other children in the family (nieces and nephews) have

[2]Adapted from: Slendokova (2005) and from research by Siemińska et al. (2002) involving an intervention to develop sensitivity to healthcare patients.

learning disabilities. Your pediatrician questioned whether autism runs in the family. Write a letter to the genetic counselor in which you describe your *surface* thoughts and feelings, your *deeper* thoughts and feelings, what you *expect* about the genetic counseling appointment, and what you *want* from the counselor. Try to write about things you might *initially be reluctant to share* with the genetic counselor.

Instructor Note

- This exercise could be done as a journal entry, small reflection paper, or with a dyad partner.
- The letters generated could be used for genetic counseling role-plays. The "patient" could either act out the content from her/his own letter or from a classmate's letter.

References

Anonymous. A genetic counselor's journey from provider to patient: a mother's story. J Genet Couns. 2008;17:412–8.

Awwad R, Veach PM, Bartels DM, LeRoy BS. Culture and acculturation influences on Palestinian perceptions of prenatal genetic counseling. J Genet Couns. 2008;17:101–16.

Bayne HB, Pusateri C, Dean-Nganga L. The use of empathy in human services: strategies for diverse professional roles. J Hum Serv. 2012;32:72–88.

Bellcross C. A genetic counselor's story of birth, grief, and survival. J Genet Couns. 2012;21:169–72.

Bodurtha J. 46 chromosomes and me. J Genet Couns. 2012;21:173–4.

Chin SR. It's not always about the "genetics": giving patients what they need. J Genet Couns. 2012;21:181–2.

Chui H, Hill CE, Ain S, Ericson SK, Ganginis Del Pino HV, Hummel AM, et al. Training undergraduate students to use challenges. Couns Psychol. 2014;42:758–77.

Clark AJ. Empathy: an integral model in the counseling process. J Couns Dev. 2010;88:348–56.

Danish SJ, D'Augelli AR, Hauer, AL. Helping skills: a basic training program. New York: Human Sciences Press; 1980.

Djurdjinovic L. Psychosocial counseling. In: Uhlmann WR, Schuette JL, Yashar B, editors. A guide to genetic counseling. 2nd ed. New York: Wiley; 2009. p. 133–75.

Dougherty AM, Henderson BB, Lindsay B. The effectiveness of direct versus indirect confrontation as a function of stage of consultation: results of an exploratory investigation. J Educ Psychol Consult. 1997;8:361–72.

Egan G. The skilled helper. Pacific Grove/Monterey, CA: Brooks/Cole; 1994.

Fine SF, Glasser PH. The first helping interview. Thousand Oaks, CA: Sage; 1996.

Fontaine JH, Hammond NL. Twenty counseling maxims. J Couns Dev. 1994;73:223–6.

Glessner HD. Will my voice be heard? J Genet Couns. 2012;21:189–91.

Greeson CJ, Veach PM, LeRoy BS. A qualitative investigation of Somali immigrant perceptions of disability: implications for genetic counseling. J Genet Couns. 2001;10:359–78.

Hackney HL, Bernard JM. Professional counseling: a process guide to helping. 8th ed. London: Pearson; 2017.

Hill CE. Helping skills: facilitating exploration, insight, and action. 4th ed. Washington, DC: American Psychological Association; 2014.

Hill CE, Spangler PT, Chui H, Jackson JL. Training undergraduate students to use insight skills: overview of the rationale, methods, and analyses for three studies. Couns Psychol. 2014;42:702–28.

Ivey AE. International interviewing and counseling: facilitating client development in a multicultural society. Pacific Grove, CA: Brooks/Cole; 1994.

Ivey AE, D'Andrea M, Ivey MB, Simek-Morgan L. Theories of counseling and psychotherapy: a multicultural perspective. 6th ed. Boston, MA: Allyn & Bacon; 2007.

Jackson JL, Hill CE, Spangler PT, Ericson SK, Merson ES, Liu J, et al. Training undergraduate students to use interpretation. Couns Psychol. 2014;42:778–99.
Karno MP, Longabaugh R. An examination of how therapist directiveness interacts with patient anger and reactance to predict alcohol use. J Stud Alcohol. 2005;66:825–32.
Kessler S. Psychological aspects of genetic counseling. X. Advanced counseling techniques. J Genet Couns. 1997;6:379–92.
Knapp S, Lemoncelli J, VandeCreek L. Ethical responses when patients' religious beliefs appear to harm their well-being. Prof Psychol. 2010;41:405–12.
Knutzen D. Genetic counseling through hope. J Genet Couns. 2012;21:205–6.
Lafans RS, Veach PM, LeRoy BS. Genetic counselors' experiences with paternal involvement in prenatal genetic counseling sessions: an exploratory investigation. J Genet Couns. 2003;12:219–42.
Lakhani SB. It's a small world: fusion of cultures in genetic counseling. J Genet Couns. 2012;21:207–8.
Lewis L. Honoring diversity: cultural competence in genetic counseling. In: LeRoy BS, McCarthy Veach P, Bartels DM, editors. Genetic counseling practice. Hoboken: Wiley-Blackwell; 2010. p. 201–34.
MacDonald G. Inferences in therapy: processes and hazards. Prof Psychol. 1996;27:600–3.
Martin DG. Counseling and therapy skills. 4th ed. Long Grove, IL: Waveland Press, Inc.; 2015.
Mayfield WA, Kardash CM, Kivlighan DM Jr. Differences in experienced and novice counselors' knowledge structures about clients: implications for case conceptualization. J Couns Psychol. 1999;46:504–14.
McAllister M, Davies L, Payne K, Nicholls S, Donnai D, MacLeod R. The emotional effects of genetic diseases: implications for clinical genetics. Am J Med Genet A. 2007;143:2651–61.
McCarthy Veach P, LeRoy BS. Defining moments in genetic counselor professional development: one decade later. J Genet Couns. 2012;21:162–6.
McHenry B, McHenry J. What therapists say and why they say it: effective therapeutic responses and techniques. 2nd ed. New York: Routledge; 2015.
Miller WR, Rose GS. Toward a theory of motivational interviewing. Am Psychol. 2009;64:527–37.
Miranda C, Veach PM, Martyr MA, LeRoy BS. Portrait of the master genetic counselor clinician: a qualitative investigation of expertise in genetic counseling. J Genet Couns. 2016;25: 767–85.
Neukrug E, Bayne H, Dean-Nganga L, Pusateri C. Creative and novel approaches to empathy: a neo-Rogerian perspective. J Ment Health Couns. 2013;35:29–42.
Oosterwal G. Multicultural counseling. In: Uhlmann WR, Schuette JL, Yashar B, editors. A guide to genetic counseling. 2nd ed. New York: Wiley; 2009. p. 331–61.
Oswald GL. Being the genuine me. J Genet Couns. 2012;21:220–1.
Pedersen PB, Ivey AE. Culture-centered counseling and interviewing skills: a practical guide. Westport, CT: Praeger/Greenwood; 1993.
Peters E, Veach PM, Ward EE, LeRoy BS. Does receiving genetic counseling impact genetic counselor practice? J Genet Couns. 2004;13:387–402.
Sarangi S, Bennert K, Howell L, Clarke A, Harper P, Gray J. (Mis) alignments in counseling for Huntington's disease predictive testing: clients' responses to reflective frames. J Genet Couns. 2005;14:29–42.
Schema L, McLaughlin M, Veach PM, LeRoy BS. Clearing the air: a qualitative investigation of genetic counselors' experiences of counselor-focused patient anger. J Genet Couns. 2015;24:717–31.
Schoeffel K, McCarthy Veach P, Rubin K, LeRoy BS. Managing couple conflict during prenatal counseling sessions: An investigation of genetic counselor experiences and perceptions. J Genet Couns. 2018. https://doi.org/10.1007/s10897-018-0252-6.
Sciarra DT. Multiculturalism in counseling. Itasca, IL: FE Peacock; 1999.
Sheets KB, Crissman BG, Feist CD, Sell SL, Johnson LR, Donahue KC, et al. Practice guidelines for communicating a prenatal or postnatal diagnosis of down syndrome: recommendations of the National Society of Genetic Counselors. J Genet Couns. 2011;20:432–41.

Siemińska MJ, Szymańska M, Mausch K. Development of sensitivity to the needs and suffering of a sick person in students of medicine and dentistry. Med Health Care Philos. 2002;5:263–71.

Slendokova B. Genetic counseling students' empathic understanding of a prenatal patient's reactions to the diagnosis of Down Syndrome: a simulation study. Unpublished master's paper, University of Minnesota, Minneapolis, MN; 2005.

Steinberg Warren N, Wilson PL. COUNSELING: a 10-point approach to cultural competence in genetic counseling. Perspect Genet Couns. 2013;Q3:6–7.

Weil J. Psychosocial genetic counseling. New York: Oxford University Press; 2000.

Welfel RE, Patterson EL. The counseling process: a multi theoretical integrative approach. 6th ed. Pacific Grove, CA: Brooks/Cole; 2005.

Wilbur MP, Wilbur JR. Honesty: expanding skills beyond professional roles. J Humanist Educ Dev. 1986;24:130–43.

Chapter 9
Patient Factors: Resistance, Coping, Affect, and Styles

Learning Objectives

1. Define resistance.
2. Identify counseling responses for addressing patient resistance.
3. Differentiate defense mechanisms from other coping behaviors.
4. Describe selected types of patient affect and their impact on the genetic counseling relationship.
5. Describe patient stylistic differences and their effects on the genetic counseling session.
6. Develop skills for addressing patient factors that impact genetic counseling.

This chapter discusses several patient characteristics that impact the processes and outcomes of genetic counseling, including resistance, coping behaviors, emotional reactions, and individual and cultural stylistic differences. Your challenge as a genetic counselor is to recognize and address these factors using the counseling skills presented in this book.

9.1 Patient Resistance

9.1.1 Definitions of Resistance

Within genetic counseling, resistance refers to patient behaviors that contribute to the complexity of genetic counseling practice. Weil (2010) defines resistance as "attitudes, behaviors, emotions, and ways of thinking by which a patient limits full engagement with the process of genetic counseling" (p. 155). Resistance is rather

P. McCarthy Veach et al., *Facilitating the Genetic Counseling Process*,
https://doi.org/10.1007/978-3-319-74799-6_9

common in genetic counseling, and it is a normal reaction, especially when patients perceive an issue as important (Weil 2010). Resistance, often an unconscious process, indicates a patient is not fully committed to the genetic counseling relationship/session. Resistance arises whenever patients oppose any aspect of genetic counseling processes and/or outcomes.

9.1.2 Causes of Resistance

Resistance "serves an important self-protective function…[For instance, it may be prompted by] "…a desire to avoid conflict – internal and/or with others. The resistance may also involve ambivalence, an inability to make a decision in the face of mutually conflicting possibilities, each of which has value to the patient" (Weil 2010, p. 159).

Resistance may occur for many reasons, such as opposition to testing, termination, communicating with family members, the legitimacy of genetics services, and/or the information you aim to provide. Weil (2010) notes several reasons for resistance including inadequate referral in which the purpose and possible outcomes of genetic counseling/testing are unclear, the information and/or diagnosis a patient receives creates anxiety, the patient feels overwhelmed by the amount/complexity of information, the patient has expectations you are unable to meet, and the patient's feelings such as guilt and shame. Resistance also often occurs when patients perceive genetic counseling and testing as contrary to their religious/spiritual beliefs and/or their personal/familial/cultural values (Weil 2010, p. 158).

Below we elaborate on some reasons for patient resistance in genetic counseling. These reasons involve fear, resentment, misunderstanding, and/or disconnection from the counselor.

Fear

Some patients:

- Are afraid to take personal responsibility for their situation and resulting decisions (e.g., patient who always lived as if she had the Huntington disease (HD) gene and did not want to find out she does not have the gene as it would "invalidate" the way she has lived her life).
- Feel demoralized because of the genetic condition and also view their privacy and independence as threatened (e.g., late-onset progressive neurological disorder, such as spinocerebellar ataxia).
- Feel a loss of control and use resistance as a way to hold on to some power and self-esteem. Also, they may be ambivalent about making a decision that has important benefits but also significant restrictions (e.g., having genetic testing for breast cancer to better plan monitoring for the disease, but not wanting to learn they have the gene).

- Have already experienced a great deal of emotional pain (grief, anger, fear, shame, or guilt) from their genetic concerns and are reluctant to discuss these feelings further (e.g., they may be ambivalent, wanting answers to their questions, but scared of what those answers will be).
- Fear the unfamiliar (e.g., they do not know what genetic services involve, feel apprehensive about discussing personal matters with a stranger, etc.).
- Are afraid the genetic counselor will tell other people what they said. For example, some individuals are resistant to preconception genomic carrier screening because of concerns about how and when information would be shared (Schneider et al. 2016).
- Feel threatened (i.e., they fear being unable to cope with a diagnosis of a genetic condition). For example, individuals at risk for cardiomyopathy or long QT syndrome may avoid testing as they do not feel able to handle the continual threat of sudden death (Smart 2010).

Resentment

Some patients:

- Feel coerced (e.g., a patient was told she could only have genetic testing if she first spoke with a genetic counselor).
- Feel angry about being referred by another health-care provider (family doctor, infertility specialist, etc.) and carry this resentment over to the genetic counselor.
- See no reason to speak with a genetic counselor in the first place.
- Have a negative attitude about medical agencies and/or are suspicious of medical personnel (Peters et al. 2011).
- Do not believe in discussing genetic information with family members and resent any suggestion they might do so (Peters et al. 2011).
- Feel offended by options they consider as unacceptable and resist discussing them. For example, some individuals at risk for HD resist discussion of abortion because they believe the quality of life for a gene-positive individual is good prior to becoming symptomatic (Klitzman et al. 2007). As one at-risk individual expressed, "My brother has HD, but is a beautiful human being...a lot of people out there would do anything to have 30 good years. I'm taking care of him. He's not draining society" (Klitzman et al. 2007, p. 356).

Misunderstanding

Some patients:

- Do not know how to participate effectively in genetic counseling and/or testing because they lack understanding of what the services entail. For example, resistance by some individuals to DNA testing and cascade screening for hypertrophic cardiomyopathy and long QT syndrome may be due to a perception that there are no personal health benefits from such testing (Smart 2010).

- Believe genetic counseling is essentially the same thing as psychotherapy, and therefore it may involve extensive probing into their innermost experiences and motivations.
- Have unrealistic expectations about what genetic counseling can offer and become resistant upon realizing their expectations cannot be met (e.g., the counselor cannot guarantee a healthy baby). In a study of informed consent for genomic sequencing, a genetic counselor described this interaction with a patient who had unrealistic expectations of the testing: "I felt like I needed to absolutely pour cold water on her in the sense that no matter what was stated, she overstated it…And she was just so far over the top with her own desires for information and I was having a lot of trouble getting her to hear what was being said and that this was not being promised and that we could not figure all this out" (Tomlinson et al. 2016, p. 66).
- View the genetic counselor's goals as different from their own (e.g., a patient who believes the counselor's agenda is to persuade her to have presymptomatic testing when she does not wish to do so). Kaimal et al. (2007) found that some parents resist pursuing testing for their child's hearing loss because of cultural differences in perceptions of deafness as a disability and because they do not understand the varied purposes of testing. They recommended the following actions to address this resistance: "It is also important [for providers] to differentiate between testing to rule out associated medical issues that can have a significant impact on medical management from genetic (DNA) testing to determine a mode of inheritance. A parent may be quite willing to consent to an EKG on their child to rule out a cardiac conduction defect while at the same time, not see the utility in determining whether a connexin mutation exists as a cause for isolated deafness. Providing parents with testing options also exhibits the health care provider's trust in their decision-making ability and allows parents to maintain a sense of control" (p. 785).
- Do not understand or accept genetic information. For example, Shaw and Hurst (2008) found that some British Pakistani mothers who experienced problems and unexpected infant deaths postnatally "…blamed medical services for not detecting abnormalities early and suspected medical malpractice or negligence. Their complaints can be viewed as expressions of women's covert resistance to being blamed or blaming themselves for their child's problem…and [resistance] to accepting genetic explanations, but also indicate a need for counseling to address patients' understandings of the problem in their pregnancy, infant or child" (p. 380).

Disconnection with the Counselor

Some patients:

- Are testing the genetic counselor's level of support and competence.
- Dislike something about the genetic counselor but do not voice their negative reaction directly.
- Are culturally distant from the counselor with respect to gender, ethnicity, social class, religion, previous experiences with prejudice and discrimination, etc.

9.1.3 Behaviors That May Indicate Resistance

Resistance may occur when patients:

- Do not seem to know what they want from genetic counseling
- Present themselves as not needing any help
- Are only there because of someone else's urging, referral, etc.
- Express resentment about being there
- Talk only about safe or low-priority issues (e.g., focus on the risk numbers and not on the condition itself)
- Are directly or indirectly uncooperative (e.g., refuse to discuss certain issues or *selectively forget* important aspects of their family history)
- Unwarrantedly blame others for their situation
- Show no willingness to establish a working relationship with the genetic counselor
- Are slow to accept responsibility for the decisions they need to make
- Are abrasive or actually hostile toward the genetic counselor
- Seek to get support for a decision they've already made rather than being open to exploring and engaging in a decision-making process
- Fail to complete requested forms, arrive late for the appointment, exhibit a closed body posture, and/or give minimal responses to the counselor (Schema et al. 2015)
- Use one or more defense mechanisms (discussed later in this chapter)

9.1.4 Mimics of Denial as Specific Types of Resistance

In discussing what he defines as "mimics of denial," Lubinsky (1994) described three patient behaviors that Weil (2010 pp. 162–164) classifies as specific types of resistance: disbelief, deferral, and dismissal.

Disbelief involves accurate patient perceptions of the information but a refusal to accept or believe it because it does not make sense to them given prior information and expectations (e.g., "But my daughter is so healthy"). Disbelief also allows patients to remain hopeful, especially early in the adjustment process.

Deferral occurs when patients accept information as correct but the implications as incorrect (e.g., parents accept the diagnosis of Down syndrome in their child but are convinced their child will only be mildly affected because they will be vigilant about seeking developmental interventions for him). Deferral helps prevent the emotional impact of information from overwhelming patients' psychological resources and gives them time to adapt and cope before fully acknowledging the consequences.

Dismissal occurs when the patient denies or attacks the genetic counselor's professional competency or the competency of someone/something else. (For example, patient challenges the genetic counselor who reports abnormal NIPT results because their obstetrician has assured them the pregnancy is normal based on a recent ultrasound. Surely a trained physician knows more about pregnancy than a genetic counselor.) This form of resistance provides relief from a seemingly unbearable situation by dismissing information and expertise and providing a rationale for disengaging.

9.1.5 Responding to Patient Resistance

There are several strategies you might use to address patient resistance:

Strategy: Explore the reasons for their resistance. Keep in mind that patients have no obligation to attend genetic counseling, and part of your job is to determine whether they want counseling.

Examples:

- If a patient seems rushed or in a hurry, acknowledge this: the patient may truly have somewhere else she/he needs to be and will appreciate that you took the time to notice and understand this need. Clarifying that a patient is indeed in a hurry will also alert you to be as efficient as possible in your use of session time.
- Patients may be resistant or afraid because they're worried about having to pay out-of-pocket for yet another service. Find out if financial coverage is a concern.
- A patient was referred for genetic counseling to discuss her risk for having a baby with tuberous sclerosis (TS). The patient was diagnosed with TS 3 years ago during her first pregnancy, when fetal cardiac tumors were identified by ultrasound. The baby and mother were examined upon delivery, and both were given a diagnosis of TS. The patient never returned to the medical geneticist, and a cardiologist had followed only her son. When the counselor was assessing the patient's understanding of why she was referred, the patient said she had no idea. The counselor explored this further with her, and the patient admitted that the cardiologist wanted her to come in to discuss TS and her risk for having another affected child. Further exploration revealed that she did not believe she had TS, rather her findings of TS were familial birthmarks. Because she was in denial about her diagnosis, the genetic counselor focused on her feelings about her diagnosis, why she did not believe it, etc. The patient was able to engage in a dialogue about these issues, feelings of guilt that she passed this on to her son, her fear of passing the condition on to other children, etc.
- A patient came in and sat down with a *huff* and crossed her arms. The counselor said, "You seem uncomfortable. Is there something I can do?" The counselor hoped this response would allow the patient to vent her anger, and the counselor could determine the reasons for her feelings.
- The genetic counselor's role is to briefly consult with the patients in the craniofacial clinic to determine the need for a complete evaluation in pediatric genetics. Some of the patients have multisystem involvement (not just craniofacial abnormalities) and consequently have been seen by multiple specialists. When the

genetic counselor recommends yet another evaluation (medical genetics), she is often met by some amount of resistance. In most cases, it relates to a lack of understanding and/or a view that the counselor's goal of evaluation is different from that of the family's (e.g., the family mistakenly believes it is *to provide a label* rather than to ensure quality care). This can be addressed by discussing the goal of the medical genetics evaluation.

Strategy: View some degree of resistance as natural and normative (usual).
Examples:

- A genetic counseling patient appeared to be hostile right at the start of the session. She was unhappy with the appointment time, felt that staff should be available in the evening as the hospital is open 24 h, and thought the directions to the clinic were confusing and she had to pay for parking. She was also (understandably) unhappy that there was an hour's delay before she was seen. The patient proceeded to instruct the genetic counselor to "fix these problems." The genetic counselor tried to empathize with the patient's frustration about appointment time, etc. "It sounds like getting to clinic has been a very frustrating experience for you, and I apologize that we are behind schedule today. I'm glad you are here now. Let's talk about how I might be able to help you."

Strategy: Understand that sometimes resistance is patients' avoidance of what they consider to be a frightening and/or unhelpful experience. Concretely discuss the potential benefits of genetic counseling. We recommend doing this at the beginning of the session.
Examples:

- The patient was referred for genetic counseling late in the pregnancy (24 weeks). She had an abnormal screening test 2 months ago and did not follow up on the referral for genetic counseling until just recently. The patient expressed frustration at her limited options. The genetic counselor acknowledged that the patient was in a difficult position. The counselor's empathy allowed some alignment and also gave the patient time to express her frustration, which helped her move forward in the session.
- A patient came in for a consult prior to an ultrasound for evaluation of possible intrauterine growth failure and said, "I don't see why I have to have a *consult*. I'm not having any testing." The counselor explained that a consult was being done so the patient could understand the potential outcomes of the ultrasound. The genetic counselor also explained that if problems were identified, she would be available to help review options so the patient could make informed decisions.
- Often families have the impression that a genetic evaluation will always involve genetic testing, which they may perceive (for whatever reason) as a negative experience. When the counselor explains that the process will involve gathering information, obtaining a history, doing a physical exam, and then considering or discussing testing if applicable, their resistance often disappears.

Strategy: Examine the quality of your own responses. Ask yourself if you are doing anything to generate resistance from your patient.

Examples:

- The patient was a young woman with Turner syndrome who was extremely anxious. She had numerous misconceptions about genetic counseling. The counselor realized toward the end of the session that the patient had imagined all sorts of horrible procedures that were going to be done to her. The counselor told her they would not be doing any tests that day, and the patient immediately calmed down and began to listen to the counselor. Picking up on this earlier in the session would have allowed the counselor to address the patient's anxiety and misperceptions even sooner.

Strategy: Accept and work with the patient's resistance. Start with your patient's frame of reference. Let your patient know you understand how she/he might feel. Accept your patient's right to think differently.

Examples:

- A patient referred for genetic evaluation of his family history of colon cancer said, "I don't want to hear any numbers or anything that is scary." The counselor responded, "Genetic counseling can be scary; sometimes we tend to give too many numbers in the hopes of helping patients make informed decisions. What kind of information can I give you that may make you more comfortable with this situation?"

Strategy: Invite patient participation in every step of the process. Share your expectations, and discuss your patients' reactions to being referred for genetic counseling. Give patients as much power as possible; focus first on their reasons for being there (Weil, 2010). Ask them what you can do to help make their situation/decision easier.

Examples:

- Sometimes it's apparent that the patient has a need to be in control of what happens during the session. It's sometimes possible to accommodate this type of patient depending, of course, on the circumstances. For instance, a genetic counselor was counseling the mother of a boy with developmental delay. The mother said she wanted an appointment for fragile X syndrome testing only. She was initially reluctant to agree to a complete evaluation, but once it was made clear that the fragile X test would be done and the other components were necessary for completeness, she became a willing participant. She had also initially refused to consent to follow-up counseling if the results were positive, but at the end of the session, she agreed to it, in part because she felt she had maintained some control.
- A genetic counselor had an emergency session with a woman who had spastic cerebral palsy and was pregnant with her third child. She was in a wheelchair, and although she appeared to have some cognitive impairment, she was actually quite sharp. It was clear from the beginning that she did not want to be there, and

when the counselor asked her why she came, she responded, "My doctor made me come down here because he thinks it would be terrible if I had a child just like me. He thinks I would want an abortion if the chances are high. Well, my mother gave me a chance at life, and I intend to do the same for my child. I'm doing just fine." By the end of the session, it was clear she had come not for the counseling but to make a point. In this situation, the genetic counselor effectively attempted to see the issue from the patient's perspective. She was willing to hear her out, established a working relationship, and allowed the patient to leave with the understanding that genetic counselors are not gatekeepers to abortion but individuals trained to help patients meet the challenges presented by any given scenario/diagnosis.

Strategy: Help patients see how their resistance is impeding the genetic counseling relationship, if it is. Advanced empathy and confrontation (Chap. 8) may be helpful responses.

Example:

- A patient came to learn more about her chance of having a baby with a birth defect. Her sister had a baby that died, and she did not know the cause. She refused to talk to her sister even after the genetic counselor explained that she needed the baby's medical records to determine if there was any familial risk. The patient, however, kept calling the counselor to ask if there was any prenatal test or other kind of test she could have. The genetic counselor tells the patient that she cannot help unless the patient talks to her sister.

Strategy: Search for incentives for moving beyond resistance, but use these sparingly.

Example:

- A 38-year-old woman who was 18 weeks into her first pregnancy came for genetic counseling because her second trimester maternal screening (quad screen) showed her risk for trisomy 18 was 1 in 100. She could not decide whether to have an amnio. She was insistent on having the maternal serum screening test repeated despite the genetic counselor telling her this would not provide her with useful information. The genetic counselor steered the conversation toward a discussion about what the patient would do should she find that her baby had trisomy 18 syndrome. The counselor pointed out that if the patient would consider a termination, then repeating the maternal serum screening would not be a realistic option because of time constraints. The counselor was also able to offer an ultrasound.

Strategy: Do not take patient resistance personally.

Example:

- McCarthy Veach et al. (2001) found that a major challenge for genetic counselors and primary care providers was addressing diversity issues. In their focus group study, they heard accounts of Mexican immigrants who believed that if they discussed the possibility of a genetic condition with a health-care provider, the provider would "give" the condition to them. It was important for the health-care providers to recognize that this resistance was not due to their own competency or personality. Rather, it resulted from a deeply held cultural conviction.

Strategy: Avoid getting into power struggles, which you will almost never win. Plus, this would damage your relationship with your patient, making effective counseling impossible.

Examples:

- A patient states that he does not want to have a genetic counseling student involved in his care. The genetic counseling supervisor honors this request.
- After explaining the genetic counseling process, the patient is adamant that she does not want to proceed. Tell her that is fine, but leave the door open for future contact.
- It can be very frustrating when patients don't listen to what you are saying. You may find yourself becoming visibly agitated. Periodically, tune in to your body language, especially when you feel your "buttons" are being pushed. First, you need to know what your buttons are (see countertransference in Chap. 12) and then practice checking on your reactions during the session. Finally, step back and ask yourself why the patient is not listening before deciding how to respond.

Strategy: Use less threatening terms.

Example:

- If your patient is reactive, use "consultation" or "discussion" rather than "counseling," "we are going to talk about some available options" rather than "testing procedures," "testing options in pregnancy" rather than "prenatal diagnosis," and "changed" or "altered" gene rather than "mutation." Listen to the words your patients use to determine terms that may be acceptable to them.

Additional strategies involve keeping in mind that cultural differences may lead to patient resistance. Shaw and Hurst (2008) recommend: "…when counseling individual patients, regardless of their ethnic background, it may be valuable for genetic counselors to elicit patients' prior understandings of the causality and inheritance of the condition they have come to discuss. This might be done by providing patients with opportunities to describe their own perception of the condition and their understanding of its inheritance or etiology. Genetic counselors would also need to be prepared to challenge mistaken beliefs because mistaken beliefs may influence an individual or couple's reproductive decision-making and risk communication in the family in clinically significant ways" (p. 382).

Weil (2010) recommends considering whether there might be alternative explanations before concluding patient behaviors are a sign of resistance; asking yourself how you are feeling, as resistance can feel like an attack on your competence; and trying to talk about the resistance if the patient seems open to doing so. He further suggests "…whenever possible, affirm the patient's dignity, integrity, and sense of responsibility…support the patient's feelings of control and autonomy…[For example] 'I can see that you have been doing your very best to try and deal with this difficult situation…' [as well as] providing relevant information, promoting informed decision making, and facilitating the patient's role in planning and implementation…" (p. 163).

9.2 Coping Behaviors

Patients will exhibit a variety of coping behaviors and strategies. Some of their strategies are more likely to lead to positive outcomes such as acceptance and adaptation. Others, when used predominantly and/or for too long, may hinder desired outcomes.

Djurdjinovic (2009) identifies eight coping behaviors, which she defines as strategies for solving problems or for modifying the meaning of an experience. Three of these coping styles——seeking social support, plan, and positive reappraisal——have the greatest likelihood of leading to positive outcomes for patients. The other five are more likely to lead to negative outcomes if used exclusively and for very long periods of time:

- Seek social support: talks with others in the hope of learning more (e.g., attending support groups for people with similar genetic conditions).
- Plan: identifies next steps and follows through on them.
- Positive reappraisal: tries to see any possible positive results or outcomes (e.g., "I'm glad I found out that I am BRCA positive, because now I can do something to lower my risks").
- Confrontative: tries to change the opinions of the person who is in charge (e.g., genetic counselor, physician, etc.)
- Distancing: acts as if nothing has happened (e.g., the patient leaves the session after learning that he has a very high risk for having the gene for a form of colon cancer, and therefore his children are at risk and says, "Well, I really didn't learn anything new today").
- Self-controlling: keeps feelings to oneself (e.g., when asked how she is feeling after receiving abnormal test results, the patient says, "I'm fine" and says nothing more).
- Accept responsibility: criticizes or blames one's self (e.g. "My doctor told me a while ago that I should be tested for BRCA, but I didn't follow through. Now I have advanced cancer, and it's my fault for not having testing sooner").
- Escape-avoidance: hopes for a miracle.

9.2.1 Defense Mechanisms

Defense mechanisms are attempts to cope as a way of maintaining some measures of personal control and self-esteem and to reduce painful emotions in the face of a threat (Clark 1991). Defense mechanisms temporarily protect an individual from painful feelings such as anxiety, grief, guilt, shame, remorse, embarrassment, and fear; they allow an individual to continue believing the world is the way she/he thinks it is or wishes it to be (Weil, 2010). Defenses "that function flexibly and in a midrange of intensity are normal and essential to adaptive psychological functioning" (Weil 2000, p. 159). Defense mechanisms are not necessarily conscious behaviors, but they are used to some extent by all individuals, including genetic counselors (Reeder et al. 2017)! Keep in mind that although all defense mechanisms are attempts to cope (coping behaviors), not all coping behaviors are defense mechanisms.

Table 9.1 Patient defense mechanisms

Definition	Patient examples
Denial: Rejecting the possibility that an event happened	"Nobody ever told me I was at risk:" "He'll grow out of it:" "She looks just like my mother, and my mother is ok."
Displacement: Shifting response from the original aim to a vulnerable target	"I won't get any useful information from your incompetent lab."
Identification: Assuming the attitude or behavior of an idealized person or group	"My sister says it's foolish to worry about a few ultrasound *glitches*." "My friend says that if I have an amnio I'll have a miscarriage."
Intellectualization: Avoiding intolerable feelings through abstract, precise thinking with little or no feeling	"So, it is a statistical probability that with this type of translocation a fetus would expire."
Projection: Blaming other people or situations for difficulties the patient experiences	"I know you think I'm a fool to continue this pregnancy." (in reality, the *patient* feels foolish.)
Rationalization: Justifying objectionable information with plausible statements	"Everyone has some *abnormal* genes... I'm probably not any more at risk than anyone else." "But I take my prenatal vitamins every day!"
Regression: Reverting to developmentally less mature behavior	A well-educated and articulate couple, upon hearing abnormal test results, suddenly were unable to process any further information. They kept saying, "what do you mean?"
Repression: Putting intolerable thoughts and feelings out of one's mind	"I don't remember how many miscarriages I had."
Undoing: Canceling out a distressing experience through a reverse action	An obsessive need for prenatal testing after having a child with anencephaly

Adapted from Clark (1991)

There are several different types of defense mechanisms, in addition to those described earlier in this chapter, that we define and illustrate with examples in Table 9.1.

9.2.2 *Examples of Patient Defenses*

In a study of challenging situations involving informed consent for genomic sequencing (Tomlinson et al. 2016), one genetic counselor participant expressed concern that a "…genetically savvy participant who had an advanced degree in molecular genetics was focused on the details and limitations of sequencing rather than the implications of results for herself and her family: 'I think at least on the pre-test side if I had to guess, based on how much she was focusing on that, it was almost like a defense mechanism for her [intellectualization]. You could already see her skepticism with any results that might come back and whether she would actually believe any of them because she was focused so much on the limitations of the technology and our interpretation [displacement]…. So, it was just difficult because I've never been pushed that hard on the technical aspects by a patient before and I was trying to just remember what were my main goals for her to walk away with…'" (p. 165).

Klitzman (2010) found evidence of denial among individuals who had or were at risk for HD, breast cancer, or alpha-1 antitrypsin deficiency: "A therapeutic misconception about testing appeared: that testing would be helpful in and of itself. Many believed they could control genetic disorders (even HD), yet these beliefs were often incorrect, and could impede coping, testing, and treatment. Misunderstandings about statistics and genetics often fueled each other, and reflected denial, and desires for hope and control. Emotional needs can thus outweigh understandings of genetics and statistics, and providers' input. Individuals often maintained non-scientific beliefs, though embarrassed by these…" (p. 430).

Another patient in the Klitzman (2010) study "…did not think that the fact that her grandmother and aunt had breast cancer might increase her own chances of developing the disease. 'One of my siblings said: It's good you're having aggressive treatment because of the history in our family. I was a little startled, because I had never thought of it that way. I didn't think it was related to their cancer. I knew my maternal grandmother died of breast cancer. But I didn't know how it was related genetically. I was in incredible denial, and didn't really want to know too much about it…' Individuals may have little desire to counter such minimization of genetic risk. Yet such avoidance, if challenged by external events, can prove devastating. This woman continued, 'When it did hit me, it hit me like a ton of bricks…I was a wreck—angry, frightened, crazed'" (p. 439).

Alluding to denial, Shiloh (2006) states that "…illness representations have an important role in clients' coping efforts. Cognitive coping strategies are often used by genetic counselees, especially if behavioral acts to control the condition are not available. Therefore, holding on to misconceptions in the face of contradictory information provided by counselors may result from defensive coping functions that these beliefs serve…" (p. 332).

9.2.3 Addressing Patient Defenses

Patients need coping strategies to deal with intense experiences, and some patients may need to engage in a certain amount of defending before they can move on to more positive coping strategies that support effective problem-solving and decision-making. Thus, defense mechanisms are not always negative coping strategies. In a study of couples coping in prodromal HD, Downing et al. (2012) concluded that the defense mechanism of denial "…can be helpful in coping with an illness that is severe and has a poor prognosis (Lazarus 1999). Another way to characterize denial as a positive coping strategy is to view it as normalization (Deatrick et al. 1999), which occurs when people living with chronic illness attempt to construct their lives as normal (Robinson 1993). While this can have a positive effect by allowing people with chronic illnesses to experience life as normal, denial can have negative consequences if people minimize problems to the extent that they fail to take action when it might be beneficial" (p. 668).

If you decide to address patient defenses, you must first establish a trusting relationship. Begin with primary empathy and questions to help you understand your patient's perspective. Then indirectly point out defenses by commenting on patient inconsistencies between verbal and nonverbal behaviors, contradictions, omissions, and misinformation (Clark 1991). (See Chap. 8 on advanced empathy and confrontation for examples of possible counselor statements.) Be careful about confronting defenses *head on* as that may actually increase their intensity and decrease patient trust (Clark 1991). Klitzman (2010) recommended "Misunderstandings might best be reduced by addressing the emotions that may underlie them (e.g., difficulties confronting perceived lack of control and seemingly irrevocable fate, desires to frame genetic information positively in order to avoid despair and helplessness and seek hope, and efforts to reduce anxiety by finding order in the face of fate and seeming randomness). Given that emotional conflicts may not be fully conscious, providers should proceed very carefully in addressing them" (p. 445).

Shiloh (2006) asserts that genetic counselors "…should weigh the costs and benefits of changing misconceptions against the costs and benefits of keeping them for clients' health and well-being, before undertaking to change them. And, when they undertake to change them, they should appreciate how difficult it may be to disabuse someone of an attribution that may serve as a defense mechanism, and try to facilitate adaptation of substitute coping mechanisms" (p. 332).

9.2.4 Promoting Effective Coping

Speaking about HD, but relevant to other life-threatening genetic conditions, Downing et al. (2012) recommended assessing "individuals' coping strategies, which may provide insight about their future coping abilities and whether coping is likely to be adaptive and healthy vs. maladaptive and possibly problematic. This may include understanding of how individuals at risk for HD and their companions use denial as either a positive method of coping through normalization, or as a negative method of avoidance when other coping strategies might be more effective" (p. 669).

Chaplin et al. (2005) interviewed parents with a prenatal diagnosis of spina bifida or hydrocephalus and who decided to continue with their pregnancy. They explored parents' experiences of receiving the diagnosis and their coping throughout the antenatal period. They found many parents were confident about their ability to cope with a child with a disability, drawing "strength from their personal and professional skills, relationships, and financial and practical resources" (p. 157). They also found some parents coped by avoiding contact with support agencies until their child's diagnosis was confirmed. The researchers concluded that genetic counselors must respect individual variation in coping strategies when parents receive unexpected diagnoses. For example, "Professionals need to recognize that both avoidance and active problem solving are valid ways of coping for parents" (p. 159).

Another consideration when you wish to promote coping behaviors is that, in many cases, patients' coping and adaptation do not really begin until they leave your office. They face a lifetime of adaptation to their risk and/or their genetic condition. Having a conversation with them about the changing nature of their needs and possible resources as they go forth in their lives may be warranted (Arnold et al. 2005; Hallowell et al. 2017; Ramdaney et al. 2015; Vos et al. 2013).

9.3 Patient Affect

Patients experience a myriad of emotions. These feelings are central to many genetic conditions/situations, and you should address them in genetic counseling. Direct expression of feelings may provide insight, reduce their intensity for patients, and result in more effective problem-solving and decision-making. To help patients express their feelings, you should be accepting and encouraging and invite them to fully describe what they are experiencing.

Patient Anger

Patient anger is relatively common in genetic counseling. Schema et al. (2015) interviewed genetic counselors about experiences of patient anger directed at them and found, "Nearly every participant expressed that [patient] anger (justifiable or not) functioned as a coping mechanism in one or more ways: a cover-up for other emotions, allowed for expression of a socially-acceptable feeling, a form of catharsis, a way to gain control and/or attention. A few mentioned some people are 'angry by their nature'" (p. 723).

Anger is a complex emotional reaction that may mask deeper feelings such as fear and despair (Baty 2010; Djurdjinovic 2009; Schema et al. 2015). Anger may be an expression of frustration about one's situation (e.g., that a diagnosis has not been possible or encountering one obstacle after another when attempting to obtain appropriate health care), or it may mask feelings of vulnerability (e.g., extreme fear about the implications of a genetic condition). Patients may be more likely to feel anger when a genetic condition is uncommon in their family and respond with statements such as, "Why did this happen to me?" or "What did I do to deserve this?" (Djurdjinovic 2009). The more important or meaningful an issue is for a patient, the more likely the patient is to be angry. Positive aspects of anger include that it gives patients emotional energy to deal with problems and it "clears the air," allowing patients to release pent-up feelings (Schema et al. 2015). Visible clues that a patient may be angry include breathing more rapidly, sweating, clenching muscles (for instance, in the jaw or the hands), becoming flushed, and raising one's voice.

Anger can be a difficult emotion to address, especially for beginning counselors (Schema et al. 2015). Nevertheless, it's important that you do so because unexpressed anger will impede the work of genetic counseling. You must be prepared to be the target of patient anger, and you should respond nondefensively (Schema et al. 2015). First, realize you usually are not the real target (Baty 2010; Schema et al. 2015); the patient may be displacing anger (e.g., about abnormal test results) onto you. You may, however, want to check with the patient to see if you have perhaps done something to elicit anger and then apologize when at fault: "…say, 'You're right, that was a mistake on my part. I'm not going to let it happen again. Thanks for bringing it up, and I'm really sorry'" (Schema et al. 2015, p. 725). Be honest with yourself about how you are feeling and what you're thinking—you may be thinking you'd like to retaliate, but it's essential that you not do so. Use basic primary empathy instead: "I can see you're very angry right now." This type of reflection indicates that you respect the patient's feelings. Finally, you should talk about what's making your patient angry (e.g., "Can you tell me what you're angry about?") (Schema et al. 2015).

Examples of empathy from Schema et al.'s (2015) participants include: "I usually acknowledge their anger and the situation is basically not of their doing, they must feel out of control, and all they want to do is protect the people they love, and…they just can't do that" (p. 724); and "normalizing and validating patient anger and then working towards opening a space to allow the patient to express it: 'You're a human being, why wouldn't you be angry? It's a normal emotion'" (p. 724). Some participants further suggested proactive responses: "'How can we make this better? How can we help you become more comfortable with the situation?'…'I see you are angry. I'm not sure where that's coming from; can you tell me a little more about that?'…; and 'I'm going to do everything I can to help you'…" (p. 725).

Grief

> "As we held our son in the delivery room the day my wife and I became parents, he looked too beautiful and peaceful for us to believe there could be much of a problem. Three hours later, the pediatric cardiologist surprised us with the diagnosis. He discussed "single ventricle," "congestive heart failure," and "palliative surgery," but the words simply floated in and out of our heads without comprehension. There was a vague notion that his life would be different because of his heart, but it didn't register that ours would be as well. In fact, nothing registered. Time stopped, sounds became muffled, and it seemed as if we were always walking sideways and uphill. It wasn't just that we were emotionally numb; our world was suddenly thrown off course and we were totally unprepared. We lost confidence in our thinking and had difficulty making even simple decisions. It became hard to know what to say or do." (Batton 2010, p. 1303)

Gettig (2010) asserts that "the [genetic counseling] profession makes us bereavement specialists. The literal meaning of the word *bereavement* is 'robbed'…Whether it is the physical loss of a family member, the loss of an anticipated child, or experiences in life that are now altered due to genetics, it is a genetic counselor who guides the family through the adjustment to a diagnosis or who guides the mourning of a family member. We assist families who are robbed of future events, memories, or envisioned life experiences. By providing anticipatory guidance as to how the process of grief works, we help individuals and families adjust to the circumstances of their lives that genetics has altered" (p. 96).

Douglas (2014) similarly states that, "Genetic counselors frequently meet with patients who are bereaved. Being diagnosed with cancer, having a relative or child die of a genetic condition, giving birth to a child with a disability, and experiencing infertility, a miscarriage or a stillbirth are all examples of common genetic counseling contexts in which our patients are experiencing grief" (p. 695).

Grief occurs when individuals lose something important to them (e.g., the perfect baby, the loss of one's health) (Djurdjinovic 2009; Gettig 2010). Grief is universal because we all experience losses in our lives, and we all go through a recovery process (Gettig 2010). The grieving process, however, may take several years (Gettig 2010, p. 96) and, in some ways, may never be finished: "Years after the onset of the disability, mothers describe feeling sad and wanting to take away the disability from their children, while at the same time feeling content and happy and loving their child just the way they are. These sorts of findings show us that the traditional idea of 'acceptance' does not apply to parents of children with a disability; instead, their happiness may co-exist with chronic sorrow" (Douglas 2014, p. 697).

Patients may exhibit a variety of behaviors when they are grieving, and their responses are affected by a variety of individual factors (e.g., temperament, personality); personal, family, and cultural beliefs and practices; and religious/philosophical values (Gettig, 2010). Although patients experience and express their grief in highly individualized ways and will vary in the sequence and timing of their grief process, the following aspects of grief are fairly common (Gettig 2010; Ormerod and Huebner 1988):

- Shock, especially when the loss is unanticipated. The patient may have a great deal of difficulty accepting the meaning of a diagnosis (cf. Wool and Dudek 2013).
- Denial that it really happened. "Denial allows a patient or parents to 'take in' *only* what they are capable of handling mentally, emotionally, and physically" (Gettig, 2010 p. 103). As mentioned earlier in this chapter, genetic conditions can be so traumatic that individuals will deny their existence. For example, unless an infant has obvious physical abnormalities, the parents may act as if the child is fine. A possible counselor response in this situation is: "I get the impression you think your baby will be fine. Yet, I also heard you say your doctor thinks your baby has Down syndrome." Your response allows your patient the opportunity to either stay in denial or move forward.
- Making "snap" decisions. Sometimes, people initially deal with their grief by making rushed and/or extreme decisions. Such decisions usually are based almost entirely on their emotions in the moment. For example, shortly after the birth of a child with a genetic condition, a patient tells you she is going to have a tubal

ligation. It's reasonable to suggest that patients put off decisions that seem "rushed" until more time has passed and they are able to weigh all of their options.
- Physical and psychological symptoms (e.g., insomnia, loss of appetite, depression, hopelessness).
- Guilt for passing along a defective gene to one's child.
- "Anger is a recognized aspect of the grieving process, arising from feelings of loss of control, dignity, or well-being, and/or from dormant feelings about past experiences that result in anger towards family members or caregivers…" (Schema et al. 2015; p. 718). Anger may be directed at the medical professionals for not arriving at a diagnosis, or for not arriving at a diagnosis sooner, for not being sympathetic enough, etc. or toward the person they lost——"If she had treated her breast cancer sooner, she might have lived"—or anger at God/higher power, which can be particularly problematic for religious patients who believe it's not OK to be angry with God. In this latter situation, you might explain that anger is a normal part of the grieving process and suggest the patients look for support from their religious community.
- Idealization of the person or thing they have lost (e.g., believing their lives would have been perfect if their baby had lived).
- Realism that the loss is permanent. At this phase, and in the subsequent acceptance process, patients will be more capable of hearing and understanding information, and they will be better able to evaluate the information they receive.
- Acceptance of the loss. Until your patients can accept their situation, you must show patience and support and allow them to be indecisive, confused, angry, etc.
- Readjustment—the "new normal."
- Personal growth.

Strategies for Addressing Grief

Often grieving individuals will cry. During the genetic counseling session, many patients will be on the verge of tears, although some may attempt to hold back their tears (out of embarrassment, fear of appearing weak, etc.). You should give them permission and provide an accepting atmosphere in which to cry. Both verbally and nonverbally show that you will listen with concern: "It's OK to go ahead and cry." Move your chair a bit closer; move a box of tissue within easy reach. These actions suggest you are comfortable with patients who lose their composure. Allow yourself to become tearful if that is what you are feeling. Research has found "When a provider was tearful with the family, several parents indicated that this seemed appropriate" (Gold, 2007, as cited in Sebold and Koil 2009, p. 201). Along with a safe supportive environment in which to discuss their grief, provide relevant resources (Douglas 2014; Helm 2015).

It's also important to reassure patients that what they are feeling is a normal reaction to loss and that grieving takes time (Gettig 2010). Experts estimate the grieving process can take from 6 months to 5 years. To reassure patients and to normalize their experience, you might say, "You've lost so much. I can see how you would feel so much pain." After your patient responds to your statement, you could follow up with a statement such as, "Grief takes a long time, so don't feel you have to get through it quickly."

Allow patients to discuss their grief, even if it's a story they've told before. It may be helpful to let patients repeatedly discuss their loss because grief is a repetitive and ongoing process (Gettig 2010). This may help them experience some acceptance of their loss (Gettig 2010).

It's a mistake to try to falsely reassure grieving patients that everything will be fine or to try to cheer them up. You must let them freely express their feelings, some of which may be quite intense. One problem, however, is that beginning counselors often are uncomfortable with intense patient emotion. If this is the case for you, acknowledge your discomfort internally, and later discuss it with your supervisor or a colleague.

When genetic counseling involves prenatal or perinatal loss, it's important to attend to the partner's grief as well as to the mother's. The literature emphasizes maternal attachment and mourning, which has led to some fathers/partners feeling marginalized, invisible, and as if they are responsible for the mother's well-being (LaFans et al. 2003; Rich 1999).

Attention to cultural variations is also important (Helm 2015): "...every ethnic group and religion has its own grief traditions...Grieving and death rituals vary widely across cultures and are often heavily influenced by religion...These [rituals] include the degree of openness in discussing family history and health problems in a medical setting, the way in which different types of mental and physical disabilities are viewed in terms of their impact on individuals and families, and barriers to receiving services, such as language and health care beliefs at variance with Western medicine... Any counselor who is unsure as to what to do should consult the family or their traditions expert: rabbi, priest, minister, elder family member, anyone who understands the traditions" (Gettig 2010, p. 118).

Work on becoming comfortable with patient expressions of strong emotion, but "...know your own limits; set boundaries; nurture yourself. You will witness great pain but you will also assist families at a critical point in their lives and affirm the resilience of the human spirit" (Gettig 2010, p. 119). Read firsthand accounts such as those describing "...intense reactions to having a baby with a disability: numbness, disappointment, isolation, withdrawal, defensiveness, protest, despair, shock, denial, sadness, anger, self-doubt, humiliation, confusion, disbelief, and guilt" (Douglas 2014, p. 696).

In closing this section on grief, we ask you to consider this description by a cancer genetic counselor who worked with the wife of a young man who died from gastric cancer:

> Listening to her grief about missing her husband, her anxiety regarding her children growing up without a father and being a single parent, financial concerns, and her support systems...has helped me remember that every person who I see may be experiencing the hardest days of their life. Every person has a story, and I must anticipate that some patients will only need me as a knowledgeable resource while others will need much more long-term support. (Flynn 2012, p. 186)

Anxiety

Patients are frequently fearful and anxious about genetic counseling (Kessler 1992a, b; Klitzman 2010; McCarthy Veach et al. 1999; Weil 2010). If their anxiety is too intense, it will disrupt their thoughts and behaviors. For example, they may have difficulty comprehending and retaining genetic and medical information. Patients typically will not express their anxiety directly. Instead they may show it indirectly (e.g., repeating the same question, avoiding sensitive topics by changing the subject, joking, making trivial comments, frequently interrupting you, seeking excessive reassurance from you, behaving dependently). Anxiety is a very contagious emotion. Often you will find yourself beginning to feel uneasy; and this can be a clue that your patient is anxious.

First you must recognize your patient's anxiety. Next you should remain calm (take a couple of deep breaths); your demeanor may have a calming effect on your patient. Finally, you should reflect your patient's anxiety: "You seem to be nervous. Can you tell me what's making you feel that way?" Talking about your patient's anxiety in a relaxed, accepting way may help to diffuse it.

Guilt and Shame

Guilt and shame are common emotions, especially when patients are the parents of children who have genetic conditions (Djurdjinovic 2009; Douglas 2014; Sexton et al. 2008; Weil 2000, 2010). Some patients feel guilty for having negative feelings about a child or family member with a genetic condition. Other patients feel guilty because they believe they've done something wrong and are being punished by God or a higher power (Sheets et al. 2012). It can be very difficult to discuss the scientific basis of genetic situations with patients who view their situation as punishment for their own or their ancestors' transgressions. Until you address some of your patient's guilt, you probably will not be very successful at communicating genetic information.

Consider the following example: The genetic counselor was counseling a Korean couple who shared with her their belief about why their son had muscular dystrophy. They had an ultrasound study early in pregnancy, and their doctor said the fetus was "likely" female. So, the couple had prayed for a boy. They felt this "conversion" from a girl to a boy resulted in the mutation causing the disorder in their son, and thus they felt responsible (guilt) for having caused the disorder. The genetic counselor certainly could not dispel their belief, but she felt the couple's awareness and their willingness to share their belief with her spoke volumes about their progress toward acceptance of this diagnosis.

Shame is a feeling of being flawed and/or unworthy as a person (Cavanagh and Levitov 2002). Shame is a difficult feeling to acknowledge. Patients who feel shameful may engage in repression by keeping awareness of their shame out of conscious experience and by refusing to think about the situation that has led to this feeling (e.g., a diagnosis of a genetic condition). Emotional clues that a patient may feel shame include chronic low levels of depression, uneasiness or anxiety, and guilt.

Behavioral clues include shaming others ("If you had taken better care of yourself you wouldn't have lost this pregnancy!"), being critical or blaming ("This whole process wouldn't be so awful if you had been clearer about how severely affected our child would be"), focusing outside of oneself (talking about everyone else's feelings and reactions except one's own; keep in mind, however, that in some cultures *externalizing* is a typical behavioral pattern), forgetting or lying about critical information, and overcontrolling another person (e.g., the overprotective parent of a child with hemophilia).

As with other emotions discussed in this chapter, unexpressed guilt and shame impede the genetic counseling process. If you have developed rapport with patients, you may be able to invite a discussion of their guilt and shame by using primary empathy and by maintaining an accepting, nonjudgmental attitude. You might also try addressing guilt and shame by using advanced empathy to reframe the issue for patients. This may help them see things from a different perspective (Kessler 1997). For example, parents whose child has Down syndrome were struggling with guilt and shame because they came into the session believing they had caused this to happen. The genetic counselor explained the simple mechanics of meiosis and emphasized that it was no one's fault—no one can make it happen or prevent it from happening. She reinforced this message by saying this is a simple error in the division of the genetic material, which can happen to anyone.

9.4 Patient Styles

No two patients will behave exactly alike. They will have stylistic differences. A *style* suggests a certain degree of consistency in the way a given individual behaves across different situations. For instance, a person who expresses emotions easily and intensely may be very emotional in most situations, including genetic counseling. On the other hand, individuals who typically are controlled would be less likely to express strong emotions during genetic counseling. Patient stylistic differences influence how they respond during genetic counseling sessions. Additionally, counselors have preferred intellectual and emotional styles that affect how they approach their patients. To the extent possible, counselors should vary their approach to effectively work with different types of patient styles.

Cheston (1991) identified patient styles for two major dimensions: emotional and intellectual.

9.4.1 Emotional Styles

- Spontaneous style: These types of patients are active communicators, who respond easily and expressively. Often, they have a good sense of humor which they will use even when they are sad (e.g., joking while crying). They will tend to use both humor and denial as defense mechanisms. You must attend carefully to these patients because they may portray everything as being fine when it is not. Also, you can help them "own" their reactions by gently encouraging them to express their true feelings.

- Nonexpressive style: These types of patients are very articulate but in a highly intellectual way. Although they feel their emotions, they deny their feelings have any importance. They may even express some annoyance or disregard for individuals who do show their emotions. They appear to be confident and in control. You should try to moderate the intensity of your own emotional expression, because these types of patients tend to shut down even further when other people are very emotive.
- Reserved style: These patients express their feelings to a limited extent, but do not allow their full expression. You can usually draw out these patients a bit with primary and advanced empathy reflections of feelings and with questions (e.g., "Please tell me more about what it's like for you to be so sad"). Then, after your patient discloses, you can ask what the patient will do to cope with her or his feelings.
- Explosive style: These patients express everything they are feeling, sometimes in overly intense ways. They can be demanding, histrionic (dramatic), and may lack good interpersonal boundaries. You need to set clear limits (e.g., regarding session length, physical contact, what you will and will not provide, etc.). It is also important that you remain calm if they have outbursts, such as crying uncontrollably.

9.4.2 *Intellectual Styles*

- Inductive reasoners gather a large amount of data and then make generalizations based on these data. Inductive reasoners may display a fair amount of confusion until they can find the patterns in the data (i.e., draw a conclusion from the facts). Then they may have "light bulb" experiences as the data suddenly fall into place for them. Inductive reasoners may also provide you with a great deal of detail. You must not allow yourself to get bogged down in these details. The most effective counseling strategy is to sort through the details to identify common threads and patterns and then share these patterns with your patient.
- Deductive reasoners tend to have a rigid framework from which they view reality. They may disregard important information that does not fit into their framework (e.g., "I can't have this condition, I'm a healthy person!") and only take in information that supports their view. You will need to be tentative with patients who have rigid frameworks, helping them to see that reality is not so clear-cut. Deductive reasoners may be particularly frustrated with the uncertainty that is inherent in genetic counseling (e.g., "What do you mean you can't tell me how severely affected my child will be?").

- Synthesizers can take in information that both confirms and challenges their frameworks. Synthesizers can absorb a great deal of information rather easily and use it to make decisions. They tend to spend most of their information processing time in their heads to the neglect of their feelings. You will need to encourage synthesizers to discuss their emotions.
- Confused reasoners are not less intelligent than other patients, but they have never learned how to prioritize information. They may experience intellectual confusion because they cannot differentiate between important and trivial information. Confused reasoners may spend a great deal of time on a small point while missing the larger issue, for example, the patient who wonders if her unborn child who has Down syndrome will look like her while missing the point that the child will be cognitively impaired, or the patient who wants to know every statistic associated with any report on his disorder and yet is unable to discuss how the disorder has and will affect his life.

Other researchers have investigated individual differences in information processing styles. They have demonstrated that people differ in their information-seeking preferences and preferences for how actively involved they wish to be in decisions about personally threatening situations (Miller 1995). One way individuals cope under situations of threat includes cognitive confrontation ("monitoring") versus cognitive avoidance ("blunting"). Monitors, characterized as information seekers, are motivated to minimize uncertainty and may benefit from receiving as much health-related information as possible (Roussi and Miller 2014; Miller 1987). Blunters are more likely to seek distractions to avoid thinking about the threat due to emotional discomfort or cognitive dissonance (Case et al. 2005). Monitors prefer to receive detailed health-related information and desire a more active role in decision-making about their health (Lindberg 2012; Lobb et al. 2005; Miller 1995; Pieterse et al. 2007; Wakefield et al. 2007; Williams-Piehota et al. 2005). Blunters prefer to avoid threat-relevant information and seek distraction from threat and are more likely to follow medical advice if provided with less complete and mainly less threatening information (Lindberg 2012; Lobb et al. 2005; Miller 1995; Wakefield et al. 2007; Williams-Piehota et al. 2005).

9.5 Religious/Spiritual Dimensions

Religion and spirituality comprise an important aspect of life for a majority of individuals in many countries such as the USA (Sagaser et al. 2016). "Religiosity is primarily understood as one's adherence to a denominational belief system or practice, and can be characterized by a person's obedience to an explicit set of religious rules or parameters…In contrast, spirituality is widely-acknowledged to have a broader definition than religiosity in which both religious and nonreligious perspectives are encompassed, as spirituality is not restricted by the boundaries of any one religious tradition and is frequently a self-defined concept...Spirituality often centers on the search for meaning or purpose in life, and spiritual beliefs and practices aid a person in looking outside of the self for support and/or guidance in crisis situations…" (Sagaser et al. 2016, pp. 923–924).

Several genetic counseling studies demonstrate that patients' spiritual beliefs and practices affect their interpretation of genetic information and subsequent decisions, as well as their coping strategies (Morris et al. 2013). For example, Greeson et al. (2001) interviewed Somali immigrants who were Muslim and found their religious beliefs profoundly influenced their perceptions of the causes and consequences of disability. The authors concluded that these religious views would significantly affect the utility of genetic services. Seth et al. (2011) interviewed Latina women about their religious beliefs and thoughts while considering the option of amniocentesis and found they drew upon their faith in God's will for comfort and validation of their decision-making process. Moreover, "Belief in God's will was not an outright deterrent to testing; rather, it consoled them while either accepting or declining the offer of amniocentesis and provided validation for their ultimate decision" (p. 670).

Hurford et al. (2013) found that the most impactful personal factors on women's decision to continue a pregnancy affected by Down syndrome were religious and spiritual beliefs and feeling attached to the baby. Sheets et al. (2012) found that for Latina mothers of a child with Down syndrome, many at first believed they or their partner was being punished for a wrong doing. Eventually, however, their perspectives shifted to include, in many cases, a genetics/inheritance explanation alongside their religious beliefs; and most mothers developed a belief that their child is a "blessing." The researchers concluded that, "Intertwining religiosity with other beliefs about Down syndrome seemed to play a role in bonding with their child" (p. 587).

Shaw and Hurst (2008) studied British Pakistani families referred to a genetics clinic. Similar to Sheets et al. (2012), they found almost every parent viewed the condition as God's will, despite either believing or denying there was a genetic cause. Furthermore, "Acceptance of the problem as expressing 'God's will' or a test from God was compatible with seeking treatments or cures (ilāj), by medical, spiritual, or other traditional means. As Mr Y put it, 'Allah says there is a cure for every disease, whether the doctor finds it or whether the spiritualist guide finds it. So, you must try all routes'..." (p. 378).

Ahmed et al. (2008) explored Pakistani and European UK women's reasons for and against prenatal testing and termination for various conditions. "The main difference between the two groups was the role of religion in decision-making. [Only] One European white woman spontaneously mentioned religion, compared to most of the Pakistani women who spontaneously mentioned that Islam does not allow termination of pregnancy. This interpretation of Islam's stance on termination of pregnancy is a misconception, which…[may be] due to the difficulty people have in distinguishing between their religious and traditional or cultural beliefs. In fact, a number of Islamic states have ruled that termination of pregnancy for a foetus with a serious disorder is permissible, but before soul-breathing (ensoulment) occurs at 120 days of gestation, and even beyond this point if the pregnancy endangers the mother's life" (pp. 568–569).

Sheppard et al. (2014) interviewed African American women either diagnosed with or at risk for breast cancer. They found that perceptions of women in both groups regarding their genetic status and genetic testing were related to their relationship with God. Their beliefs and religious/spiritual connection served as an "anchor" (p. 318) in these stressful situations.

Quillin et al. (2006) investigated perceived risk for breast cancer and use of spiritual coping mechanisms in a sample of at-risk women. While they found no significant relationship for women with negative family histories, there was an inverse relationship for women with positive family histories. Specifically, use of spiritual coping was related to lower perceived risk of breast cancer for those women. The authors speculated that "Frequent spiritual coping may be a manifestation of one's spiritual locus of control, the belief that God empowers the faithful to prevent disease, or God can be consulted to actively interfere with a disease process, in this case genetic susceptibility for cancer…" (p. 455).

Williams et al. (2017) interviewed genetic counselors and former patients who had maintained a long-term professional relationship after a life-limiting prenatal diagnosis. One effect of the relationship on the counselors was their recognition of the "strength that faith can have in a patient's life" (p. 350).

9.5.1 *Strategies for Addressing Religious/Spiritual Issues in Genetic Counseling*

> "…As a new genetic counselor, I was often unsure how to proceed when families turned the discussion towards religion and spiritual issues. I'm still not sure I'm very accomplished in this realm, but I've learned to be more comfortable with these discussions and I've found that this theme works well for me. I've had the good fortune of having one of our hospital chaplains (who also happens to be the mother of a young boy with Down syndrome) partner with me in discussions with families who were having a difficult time resolving their spiritual beliefs with the birth of their baby with Down syndrome. Your hospital chaplains are an underutilized resource! It is interesting that it is in these discussions with families, where we are talking about how to find meaning in the birth of this child with Down syndrome, where I feel I am making the most difference with my families. This is the heart of genetic counseling to me, not the review of chromosomes and recurrence risks and features, but the relationship between human beings and the discussion of what it means to be human" (Brasington 2007, p. 733, reflecting on her experiences counseling about Down syndrome).

You should consider the possibility that spiritual issues are relevant to some extent for most of your patients even those patients who do not mention them. Research suggests "Unless invited patients may assume these topics are 'off limits' or that care providers are indifferent to their beliefs" (Anderson 2009, p. 52). You do not need to be of the same faith or have the same belief system as your patients in order to consider religious/spiritual issues. It's not necessary to share the same religious faith any more than you need to share the same sex, race, or background. What matters is that you convey openness and nonjudgmentalness and connect empathically with patients' worldviews (Cheston 1991).

Some authors advocate the use of limited spiritual assessment to determine the relevance of religious and spiritual beliefs for genetic counseling patients (D'Souza 2007; Peters et al. 2016; Seth et al. 2011; Sheets et al. 2012; White 2009). D'Souza

(2007) recommends a brief spiritual assessment in which you might ask: "It sounds like your faith (religion, spirituality) is important to you. Have these beliefs been important to you at other times in your life? Have these beliefs helped you reach other important decisions?" (D'Souza 2007, as cited in Seth et al. 2011, p. 670).

We suggest you directly inquire about the importance of religion/spirituality. For example, you could ask patients:

- What religious/spiritual beliefs do you hold, and how do they relate to your concern?
- What values do you hold?
- Would you want your beliefs to be part of your decision-making process?

To use a cardiovascular setting as an example, you might ask: In the past 2 weeks, have you frequently worried about your future due to genetic testing or your cardiac condition? Had concerns about your sense of purpose in life? Felt as if you were getting down on yourself? Had difficulty setting meaningful goals for yourself? (Adapted from Rhodes et al. 2017, p. 228). When a patient endorses these types of items, a referral to mental health professional, chaplain, or spiritual counselor might be in order (Rhodes et al. 2017).

We recommend the following article that describes a tool for assessing patient spirituality and general social functioning: Peters et al. (2006).

9.6 Closing Comments

In the other chapters in this book, you read about and practiced several basic helping skills. Part of the art of being an effective genetic counselor involves timing and choosing, that is, knowing when and how to intervene. "Genetic counselors should remind themselves not to stereotype a given patient on the basis of ethnicity or religion, and to consider the beliefs and preferences of individuals" (Ahmed et al. 2008, p. 569). Different patients require different choices on your part. This chapter described a few of the ways in which patients differ stylistically, discussed some of the patient emotional issues you will encounter, and considered how patients may resist, defend, and cope when they feel threatened. Patients differ in many other ways, more than we could adequately cover in one chapter or even one book. As you gain supervised experience, you will increase your sensitivity to patients' individual and cultural differences and learn to more effectively tailor your counseling approaches, accordingly.

Finally, we wish to stress that even the most skillfully crafted and implemented responses on your part may not have a positive effect. Despite your best efforts at assessing patients and applying the other skills you are learning, you sometimes will feel as if you did not make a difference. You are only one of the individuals in the genetic counseling relationship. The patients play just as critical a role. They must be "ready, willing, and able" to engage in the process. Some patients will lack one or more of those critical elements because of diminished intellectual and/or psychological functioning (e.g., cognitive impairment, mental illness), challenging life events (e.g., divorce, job loss), and/or lack of resources (e.g., poor or no social support, isolation). Be careful not to take too much of the responsibility onto yourself for a "lack of success." Moreover, even when you do not have an obvious and immediate effect, if you behave in a caring and professional manner, you may "plant a seed" for later thought and action by some patients.

9.7 Class Activities

Activity 1: Res (Triad Role-Plays)

Students work in triads, each taking a turn being the genetic counselor, patient, and observer. They should engage in 10-min role-plays in which the patient presents a very specific issue (e.g., sharing relevant genetic risk/testing information with siblings). The patient and counselor should act out this issue using one of the following resistance role-plays:

Role-Play 1
When the genetic counselor provides some information about the patient's options, the patient should respond to all counselor's suggestions with "Yes, but.. ." In other words, the patient should refute, counter, and find fault with all counselor's options.

Role-Play 2
The patient should be silent, giving one- or two-word answers, refusing to answer, and trailing off in her responses. The patient is making it evident that nothing is going to happen until the counselor addresses her resistance (which was caused by the genetic counselor telling the patient that she should share information with her siblings; the patient thinks the counselor does not understand her family situation.).

Role-Play 3
The patient should get angry in response to the first question the genetic counselor asks.

Process
Discuss with the counselor how it felt to be resisted in this way. What did the counselor do to respond to the patient's resistance? Why might patients use these types of resistance?

Estimated time: 60 min.

Instructor Note
To make this activity more challenging, the student playing the patient could select the role-play without telling the individual playing the counselor which role she/he selected.

Activity 2: Defense Mechanisms (Small or Large Group)

Using the list of defense mechanisms in Table 9.1, students generate additional examples of patient statements or behaviors to illustrate each defense mechanism. They can first work in think-pair-share dyads to generate ideas.

Estimated time: 20–30 min.

Instructor Notes

- Following the generation of examples, the instructor could lead a discussion of which defenses each student finds particularly challenging to work with in genetic counseling.
- Students could generate counselor responses to address each patient statement or behavior.

Activity 3: Counseling a Grieving Patient (Triad Role-Plays)

Students work in triads, each taking a turn as counselor, patient, and observer. Using the following patient roles, they should engage in 10–15-min role-plays in which they discuss the patient's feelings.

Patient Role 1

A woman just found out from her routine ultrasound that the fetus died.

Patient Role 2

A 50-year-old woman was told by the neurologist that she has symptoms of Huntington disease.

Patient Role 3

A mother of a 6-year-old boy found out last week that testing showed her son to be affected with Duchenne muscular dystrophy.

Estimated time: 45–60 min.

Process

Students discuss in the large group: What are you learning about patient grief and how do you respond to it? What is difficult about it? What is the genetic counselor's role in addressing patient grief? How did you feel responding to strong patient emotion?

Estimated time: 15–20 min.

Activity 4: Assessing Patient Coping Strategies (Dyad or Small Groups)

Students work in dyads or small groups to develop a set of five to eight questions they could ask to assess the impact of Huntington disease (HD) on a patient's and her/his family's coping strategies. Students should write the questions as if they are actually talking to the patient.

Estimated time: 15 min.

Process
Dyads or small groups share their questions with the large group.
Estimated time: 45 min.

Instructor Note
- You can compare students' questions to the eight interview questions used in a study by Maxted et al. (2014) (see p. 348).

Activity 5: Assessing Cultural Factors in Patient Coping Strategies (Dyads or Small Groups)

Students work in dyads or small groups to develop a set of five to eight general questions they could ask to assess cultural aspects of grief for patients. Students should write the questions as if they are actually talking to the patient.

Instructor Note
- You can compare students' questions to the five questions from Gettig (2010) (see p. 118).

9.8 Written Exercises

Exercise 1: Grief and Loss

Describe a situation in your life where you experienced a significant loss. Do the aspects of grief described in this chapter accurately represent the process you went through to cope with your loss? How do they fit? Not fit? What sorts of things do you recall people saying to you at the time of your loss that were especially helpful? Unhelpful? Recommended length: one- to two-word-processed pages, double spaced.

Exercise 2: Anger

Part I: Describe the meaning of anger in your family of origin. For example, was it a socially acceptable emotion? What did it mean when someone became angry? How was anger expressed? How did others react to it? How does the meaning of anger within your family compare to the meaning within your culture? How do you currently react to anger? How do you currently express anger?

Part II: If you have had a genetic counseling patient become angry with you during a session, describe what happened, how you felt, and what you did. In retrospect, do you wish you had done something differently? If so, what? (If you have not actually had this experience, then make up a scenario, and use it to respond to these questions.)

Exercise 3: Defense Mechanisms

From the list of defense mechanisms in Table 9.1, identify two defenses that *you* are most likely to use in your personal life, and discuss how they might affect your work as a genetic counselor. Include a specific example of how each of your defense mechanisms might play out during a session and how they might affect the patient.

[*Hint*: Although Chap. 9 refers to patient defense mechanisms, the same defenses apply to genetic counselors.]

Exercise 4: Intellectual and Emotional Styles

Part I: Using the intellectual styles described in this chapter, identify your intellectual style, and discuss the advantages and disadvantages of your style for genetic counseling. Do you think that your style might be more effective for some patients and less effective for others? Why/how?

Part II: Using the emotional styles described in this chapter, identify your emotional style, and discuss the advantages and disadvantages of your style for genetic counseling. Do you think that your style might be more effective for some patients and less effective for others? Why/how?

[*Hint*: Think about how your intellectual and emotional styles might complement or clash with the patient's intellectual and emotional styles.]

Part III: Which patient intellectual and emotional styles will be most difficult for you? What makes them difficult?

Exercise 5: Spiritual Assessment[1]

Pretending they have a genetic condition, students select a partner from the class, and the dyads take turns interviewing each other (outside of the class) using the Anandarajah and Hight (2001, as cited in Reis et al. 2007) HOPE Tool for spiritual assessment questions. Upon completion of the interviews, students prepare reflection papers describing what it was like to answer the questions and what they learned about themselves as interviewee and as interviewer.

Questions from the HOPE Tool for Spiritual Assessment as Presented in the Survey Instrument

H: Sources of hope, meaning, comfort, strength, peace, love, and connection

- We have been discussing your support systems. I was wondering, what are your sources of hope, strength, comfort, and peace?
- What do you hold onto during difficult times?
- What sustains you and keeps you going?

[1]Adapted from Anandarajah and Hight (2001).

- For some people, their religious or spiritual beliefs act as a source of comfort and strength in dealing with life's ups and downs; is this true for you?
- If the answer is yes, go on to O and P questions.
- If the answer is no, consider asking: Was it ever? What changed? [then go on to O and P questions]

O: Role of organized religion

- Do you consider yourself part of an organized religion?
- How important is your participation in an organized religion in your life? What aspects of your religion are helpful and not so helpful to you at this difficult time?
- Are you part of a religious or spiritual community?
- How does being part of a religious or spiritual community help you?

P: Personal spirituality/practices

- Do you have personal spiritual beliefs that are independent of organized religion? What are they?
- Do you believe in God?
- What kind of relationship do you have with God?
- What aspects of your spirituality or spiritual practices do you find most helpful to you personally? (e.g., prayer, meditation, hiking).

E: Effects on medical care/end-of-life issues

- How has this experience affected your relationship with God?
- Is there anything that I can do to help you access the spiritual resources that usually help you?
- Are you worried about any conflicts between your beliefs and your medical situation/care/decisions?
- Would it be helpful for you to speak to a clinical chaplain/community spiritual leader?

References

Ahmed S, Hewison J, Green JM, Cuckle HS, Hirst J, Thornton JG. Decisions about testing and termination of pregnancy for different fetal conditions: a qualitative study of European white and Pakistani mothers of affected children. J Genet Couns. 2008;17:560–72.

Anandarajah G, Hight E. Spirituality and medical practice. Am Fam Physician. 2001;63:81–8.

Anderson RR. Religious traditions and prenatal genetic counseling. Am J Med Genet C Semin Med Genet. 2009;151C:52–61.

Arnold A, McEntagart M, Younger DS. Psychosocial issues that face patients with Charcot-Marie-tooth disease: the role of genetic counseling. J Genet Couns. 2005;14:307–18.

Batton B. Healing hearts. JAMA. 2010;304:1303–4.

Baty BJ. Facing patient anger. In: LeRoy BS, McCarthy Veach P, Bartels DM, editors. Genetic counseling practice. Hoboken: Wiley-Blackwell; 2010. p. 125–54.

Brasington CK. What I wish I knew then... Reflections from personal experiences in counseling about Down Syndrome. J Genet Couns. 2007;16:731–4.

Case DO, Andrews JE, Johnson JD, Allard SL. Avoiding versus seeking: the relationship of information seeking to avoidance, blunting, coping, dissonance, and related concepts. J Med Libr Assoc. 2005;93:353–62.

Cavanagh M, Levitov JE. The counseling experience a theoretical and practical approach. 2nd ed. Prospect Heights IL: Waveland Press; 2002.

Chaplin J, Schweitzer R, Perkoulidis S. Experiences of prenatal diagnosis of spina bifida or hydrocephalus in parents who decide to continue with their pregnancy. J Genet Coun. 2005;14: 151–62.

Cheston SE. Making effective referrals: the therapeutic process. New York: Gardner Press; 1991.

Clark AJ. The identification and modification of defense mechanisms in counseling. J Couns Dev. 1991;69:231–6.

Deatrick JA, Knafl KA, Murphy-Moore C. Clarifying the concept of normalization. Image J Nurs Sch. 1999;31:209–14.

Djurdjinovic L. Psychosocial counseling. In: Uhlmann WR, Schuette JL, Yashar B, editors. A guide to genetic counseling. 2nd ed. New York: John Wiley & Sons; 2009. p. 133–75.

Douglas HA. Promoting meaning-making to help our patients grieve: an exemplar for genetic counselors and other health care professionals. J Genet Couns. 2014;23:695–700.

Downing NR, Williams JK, Leserman AL, Paulsen JS. Couples' coping in prodromal Huntington disease: a mixed methods study. J Genet Couns. 2012;21:662–70.

D'Souza R. The importance of spirituality in medicine and its application to clinical practice. Med J Aust. 2007;186:S57.

Flynn M. A couple's devastating journey & my development as a genetic counselor. J Genet Couns. 2012;21:185–6.

Gettig E. Grieving: an inevitable journey. In: LeRoy BS, McCarthy Veach P, Bartels DM, editors. Genetic counseling practice. Hoboken: Wiley-Blackwell; 2010. p. 95–124.

Gold KJ. Navigating care after a baby dies: a systematic review of parent experiences with health providers. J Perinatol. 2007;27:230–7.

Greeson CJ, Veach PM, LeRoy BS. A qualitative investigation of Somali immigrant perceptions of disability: implications for genetic counseling. J Genet Couns. 2001;10:359–78.

Hallowell N, Lawton J, Badger S, Richardson S, Hardwick RH, Caldas C, et al. The psychosocial impact of undergoing prophylactic total gastrectomy (PTG) to manage the risk of hereditary diffuse gastric cancer (HDGC). J Genet Couns. 2017;26:752–62.

Helm BM. Exploring the genetic counselor's role in facilitating meaning-making: rare disease diagnoses. J Genet Couns. 2015;24:205–12.

Hurford E, Hawkins A, Hudgins L, Taylor J. The decision to continue a pregnancy affected by Down syndrome: timing of decision and satisfaction with receiving a prenatal diagnosis. J Genet Couns. 2013;22:587–93.

Kaimal G, Steinberg AG, Ennis S, Harasink SM, Ewing R, Li Y. Parental narratives about genetic testing for hearing loss: a one year follow up study. J Genet Couns. 2007;16:775–87.

Kessler S. Psychological aspects of genetic counseling. VII. Thoughts on directiveness. J Genet Couns. 1992a;1:9–17.

Kessler S. Psychological aspects of genetic counseling. VIII. Suffering and countertransference. J Genet Couns. 1992b;1:303–8.

Kessler S. Psychological aspects of genetic counseling. X. Advanced counseling techniques. J Genet Couns. 1997;6:379–92.

Klitzman RL. Misunderstandings concerning genetics among patients confronting genetic disease. J Genet Couns. 2010;19:430–46.

Klitzman R, Thorne D, Williamson J, Chung W, Marder K. Decision-making about reproductive choices among individuals at-risk for Huntington's disease. J Genet Couns. 2007;16:347–62.

Lafans RS, Veach PM, LeRoy BS. Genetic counselors' experiences with paternal involvement in prenatal genetic counseling sessions: an exploratory investigation. J Genet Couns. 2003;12:219–42.

Lazarus RS. Stress and emotion. Berlin: Springer; 1999.
Lindberg M. Monitoring and blunting styles in fluid restriction consultation. Hemodial Int. 2012;16:282–5.
Lobb EA, Butow P, Barratt A, Meiser B, Tucker K. Differences in individual approaches: communication in the familial breast cancer consultation and the effect on patient outcomes. J Genet Couns. 2005;14:43–53.
Lubinsky MS. Bearing bad news: dealing with the mimics of denial. J Genet Couns. 1994;3:5–12.
Maxted C, Simpson J, Weatherhead S. An exploration of the experience of Huntington's disease in family dyads: an interpretative phenomenological analysis. J Genet Couns. 2014;23:339–49.
McCarthy Veach P, Truesdell SE, LeRoy BS, Bartels DM. Client perceptions of the impact of genetic counseling: an exploratory study. J Genet Couns. 1999;8:191–216.
McCarthy Veach P, Bartels DM, LeRoy BS. Ethical and professional challenges posed by patients with genetic concerns: a report of focus group discussions with genetic counselors, physicians, and nurses. J Genet Couns. 2001;10:97–119.
Miller SM. Monitoring and blunting: validation of a questionnaire to assess styles of information seeking under threat. J Pers Soc Psychol. 1987;52:345–53.
Miller SM. Monitoring versus blunting styles of coping with cancer influence the information patients want and need about their disease. Implications for cancer screening and management. Cancer. 1995;76:167–77.
Morris BA, Hadley DW, Koehly LM. The role of religious and existential well-being in families with lynch syndrome: prevention, family communication, and psychosocial adjustment. J Genet Couns. 2013;2:482–91.
Ormerod JJ, Huebner ES. Crisis intervention: facilitating parental acceptance of a child's handicap. Psychol Sch. 1988;25:422–8.
Peters JA, Hoskins L, Prindiville S, Kenen R, Greene MH. Evolution of the colored eco-genetic relationship map (CEGRM) for assessing social functioning in women in hereditary breast-ovarian (HBOC) families. J Genet Couns. 2006;15:477–89.
Peters JA, Kenen R, Hoskins LM, Koehly LM, Graubard B, Loud JT, et al. Unpacking the blockers: understanding perceptions and social constraints of health communication in hereditary breast ovarian cancer (HBOC) susceptibility families. J Genet Couns. 2011;20:450–64.
Peters JA, Kenen R, Bremer R, Givens S, Savage SA, Mai PL. Easing the burden: describing the role of social, emotional and spiritual support in research families with li-fraumeni syndrome. J Genet Couns. 2016;25:529–42.
Pieterse K, van Dooren S, Seynaeve C, Bartels CC, Rijnsburger AJ, De Koning HJ, et al. Passive coping and psychological distress in women adhering to regular breast cancer surveillance. Psychooncology. 2007;16:851–8.
Quillin JM, McClish DK, Jones RM, Burruss K, Bodurtha JN. Spiritual coping, family history, and perceived risk for breast cancer—can we make sense of it? J Genet Couns. 2006;15:449–60.
Ramdaney A, Hashmi SS, Monga M, Carter R, Czerwinski J. Support desired by women following termination of pregnancy for a fetal anomaly. J Genet Couns. 2015;24:952–60.
Reeder R, Veach PM, MacFarlane IM, LeRoy BS. Characterizing clinical genetic counselors' countertransference experiences: an exploratory study. J Genet Couns. 2017;26:934–47.
Reis LM, Baumiller R, Scrivener W, Yager G, Warren NS. Spiritual assessment in genetic counseling. J Genet Couns. 2007;16:41–52.
Rhodes A, Rosman L, Cahill J, Ingles J, Murray B, Tichnell C, et al. Minding the genes: a multidisciplinary approach towards genetic assessment of cardiovascular disease. J Genet Couns. 2017;26:224–31.
Rich DE. When your client's baby dies. J Couples Ther. 1999;8:49–60.
Robinson CA. Managing life with a chronic condition: the story of normalization. Qual Health Res. 1993;3:6–28.
Roussi P, Miller SM. Monitoring style of coping with cancer related threats: a review of the literature. J Behav Med. 2014;37:931–54.
Sagaser KG, Hashmi SS, Carter RD, Lemons J, Mendez-Figueroa H, Nassef S, et al. Spiritual exploration in the prenatal genetic counseling session. J Genet Couns. 2016;25:923–35.

Schneider JL, Goddard KA, Davis J, Wilfond B, Kauffman TL, Reiss JA, Gilmore M, et al. "Is it worth knowing?" Focus group participants' perceived utility of genomic preconception carrier screening. J Genet Couns. 2016;25:135–45.
Schema L, McLaughlin M, Veach PM, LeRoy BS. Clearing the air: a qualitative investigation of genetic counselors' experiences of counselor-focused patient anger. J Genet Couns. 2015;24:717–31.
Sebold C, Koil C. Genetic library: grief and bereavement. J Genet Couns. 2009;18:200–3.
Seth SG, Goka T, Harbison A, Hollier L, Peterson S, Ramondetta L, et al. Exploring the role of religiosity and spirituality in amniocentesis decision-making among Latinas. J Genet Couns. 2011;20:660–73.
Sexton AC, Sahhar M, Thorburn DR, Metcalfe SA. Impact of a genetic diagnosis of a mitochondrial disorder 5–17 years after the death of an affected child. J Genet Couns. 2008;17:261–73.
Shaw A, Hurst JA. "What is this genetics, anyway?" Understandings of genetics, illness causality and inheritance among British Pakistani users of genetic services. J Genet Couns. 2008;17:373–83.
Sheets KM, Baty BJ, Vázquez JC, Carey JC, Hobson WL. Breaking difficult news in a cross-cultural setting: a qualitative study about Latina mothers of children with down syndrome. J Genet Couns. 2012;21:582–90.
Sheppard VB, Graves KD, Christopher J, Hurtado-de-Mendoza A, Talley C, Williams KP. African American women's limited knowledge and experiences with genetic counseling for hereditary breast cancer. J Genet Couns. 2014;23:311–22.
Shiloh S. Illness representations, self-regulation, and genetic counseling: a theoretical review. J Genet Couns. 2006;15:325–37.
Smart A. Impediments to DNA testing and cascade screening for hypertrophic cardiomyopathy and long QT syndrome: a qualitative study of patient experiences. J Genet Couns. 2010;19:630–9.
Tomlinson AN, Skinner D, Perry DL, Scollon SR, Roche MI, Bernhardt BA. "Not tied up neatly with a bow": professionals' challenging cases in informed consent for genomic sequencing. J Genet Couns. 2016;25:62–72.
Vos J, Asperen CJ, Oosterwijk JC, Menko FH, Collee MJ, Garcia EG, et al. The counselees' self-reported request for psychological help in genetic counseling for hereditary breast/ovarian cancer: not only psychopathology matters. Psychooncology. 2013;22:902–10.
Wakefield CE, Homewood J, Mahmut M, Taylor A, Meiser B. Usefulness of the threatening medical situations inventory in individuals considering genetic testing for cancer risk. Patient Educ Couns. 2007;69:29–38.
Weil J. Psychosocial genetic counseling. New York: Oxford University Press; 2000.
Weil J. Resistance and adherence: understanding the patient's perspective. In: LeRoy BS, McCarthy Veach P, Bartels DM, editors. Genetic counseling practice. Hoboken: Wiley-Blackwell; 2010. p. 155–74.
White MT. Making sense of genetic uncertainty: the role of religion and spirituality. Am J Med Genet C Semin Med Genet. 2009;151C:68–76.
Williams SR, Berrier KL, Redlinger-Grosse K, Edwards JG. Reciprocal relationships: the genetic counselor-patient relationship following a life-limiting prenatal diagnosis. J Genet Couns. 2017;26:337–54.
Williams-Piehota P, Pizarro J, Schneider TR, Mowad L, Salovey P. Matching health messages to monitor-blunter coping styles to motivate screening mammography. Health Psychol. 2005;24:58–67.
Wool C, Dudek M. Exploring the perceptions and the role of genetic counselors in the emerging field of perinatal palliative care. J Genet Couns. 2013;22:533–43.

Chapter 10
Providing Guidance: Advice and Influencing Skills

Learning Objectives
1. Define advice and influencing skills.
2. Differentiate between clinical recommendations and other types of advice.
3. Identify examples of types of advice and types of influencing responses.
4. Develop advice and influencing skills through self-reflection, practice, and feedback.

Genetic counselors are first and foremost health-care professionals. As such, in clinical practice, they are obligated to know and to share relevant clinical information and recommendations with their patients. This is not only an ethical responsibility [NSGC Code of Ethics (NSGC 2017)] but also a legal obligation (Schmerler 2007). It is crucial to differentiate between clinical information and recommendations and other types of advice and influencing responses in genetic counseling. Clinical information and recommendations are drawn from the relevant scientific and medical genetics literature as well as the collective clinical experience of practitioners in the field of medical/clinical genetics and genetic counseling as documented in published practice guidelines. Both the National Society of Genetic Counselors (www.nsgc.org) and the American College of Medical Genetics and Genomics (www.acmg.net) publish clinical practice guidelines that can be accessed through their public websites and/or peer-reviewed journals. Genetic counselors must also be aware of relevant clinical practice guidelines published by other medical professional organizations (e.g., American Academy of Pediatrics, American College of Obstetricians and Gynecologists, American Society of Clinical Oncology, etc.). A detailed discussion of these types of practice guidelines is beyond the scope of this text. The focus of this chapter is on other situations in genetic counseling where advice and influencing responses may be appropriate.

Refraining from providing advice that is not medically indicated and protecting patient autonomy have long been associated with the practice of genetic counseling. The value of protecting patient autonomy is reflected in Section II of the NSGC Code

P. McCarthy Veach et al., *Facilitating the Genetic Counseling Process*,
https://doi.org/10.1007/978-3-319-74799-6_10

of Ethics which states that "The counselor-client relationship is based on values of care and respect for the client's autonomy, individuality, welfare, and freedom" and that genetic counselors therefore work to "Enable their clients to make informed decisions, free of coercion, by providing or illuminating the necessary facts, and clarifying the alternatives and anticipated consequences" (NSGC 2017). This is also a major tenet of the Reciprocal-Engagement Model of genetic counseling—that "patient autonomy must be supported" (McCarthy Veach et al. 2007, p. 719).

Historically, the term "nondirectiveness" has been used to describe the approach used by genetic counselors to protect patient autonomy, specifically in decision-making. Strict, narrow definitions of nondirective genetic counseling emphasize what the genetic counselor should not do. This terminology is problematic, however, because it implies that genetic counselors never provide advice of any sort to a patient. This is not only inaccurate but also unachievable and, in many cases, inappropriate. A better way to conceptualize this approach is to consider how genetic counselors protect patient autonomy by providing balanced information, using value-neutral terminology, and responding to questions in a manner that addresses patients' underlying emotions and concerns (Weil 2000). Genetic counselors also use their counseling skills (e.g., primary and advanced empathy) to promote patient autonomy. As discussed by Resta (2010), although respect for patient autonomy should be maintained as an important value in genetic counseling, the extent to which autonomy is possible varies across patients. Active counseling strategies can also be used to address situations in which autonomy is limited due to economic, social, political, or cultural realities that confront patients (Resta 2010).

In this chapter, we discuss two genetic counseling skills that involve more directive behaviors: advice and influencing responses. Advice refers to the genetic counselor's professional recommendations, while influencing responses express the genetic counselor's opinions. Included in this chapter are several examples of genetic counselor responses obtained by Kao (2010) in a survey study of genetic counselor empathy in clinical practice. She asked genetic counselors to read slightly modified excerpts from actual patient statements reported in five qualitative studies published in the *Journal of Genetic Counseling* (Andersen et al. 2008; Gibas et al. 2008; Nusbaum et al. 2008; Phelps et al. 2007; Quaid et al. 2008). The patient statements reflect a variety of genetic disorders (long QT syndrome, Huntington disease, cleft palate, Fabry disease, and BRCA risk). Respondents were asked to pretend they were the genetic counselor in each scenario and then to provide a response as if they were actually speaking to the patient. Participant responses included advice and influencing statements.

10.1 Advice Giving

10.1.1 Definition of Advice

Advice is a type of response in which the genetic counselor attempts to direct patients by offering suggestions or recommendations about what they should do. Advice is intended to offer recommendations, to help advice seekers sort through the options they have already decided on, and/or to help them implement their decisions successfully (DeCapua and Dunham 1993). As opposed to information giving, which involves the communication of knowledge (see Chap. 7), advice involves a suggestion about a particular course of action and "…the counselor overtly attempts to shape and influence the counselee's behavior" (Kessler 1992, p. 10).

As Vehvilainen (2001) notes, advice involves "…a recommendation toward a course of action that the advice giver prefers, and it is given with the expectation that the recipient will treat it as relevant, helpful, or newsworthy and accept it. Advice implies that the adviser has knowledge or insight that the advisee lacks" (p. 373).

Advice varies along a continuum from directly expressed recommendations of what a patient should do [e.g., "You should share your test results with your adult children"] to indirect or implied suggestions [e.g., "Have you talked with your husband about your desire to have presymptomatic testing for HD?"]. Several authors propose that a less direct approach may be more effective because it can decrease resistance and promote patients' autonomy and authority over their actions. For instance, Couture and Sutherland (2006) suggest using collaborative, co-constructed advice. Specifically, genetic counseling practitioners frame advice within the patient's perspective and preferences and together figure out what to do. Consider, for example, a patient with a BRCA mutation who is indecisive about prophylactic surgery. Pt: "If I have the surgery I won't be very appealing to my husband." GC: "He's told you that?" (closed question) Pt: "No, but it just stands to reason." GC: "Is that something you'd like to know?" (closed question) Pt: "Yes, it would help me feel more certain about what to do." GC: "What do you think about discussing it with him?" (advice) Pt: "I could do that." GC: "What do you think you would say to him?" (open-question).

Butler et al. (2010) similarly suggest an indirect approach, using implied advice or questions that ask patients to evaluate the relevance or applicability of certain actions to their own situation. These questions allow the genetic counselor to avoid directly telling patients what to do, respect their experiences and perspectives, and allow them to retain authority over their own decisions and actions. An example of implied advice in genetic counseling is asking a patient, "What have you done in the past to make a major decision?" This question implies the patient may wish to consider taking similar actions about her or his current situation.

10.1.2 Advice Giving in Genetic Counseling

Genetic counseling patients may expect you to provide advice because they view you as an expert on genetic and medical topics and therefore assume you will give advice as you know what is "best" to do in a particular circumstance. As Kessler (1997) cautions, however, the provision of advice "is often a vote of no confidence in the client's own ability to sort things out for themselves and arrive at their own conclusions. It needs to be remembered that most of the people seen for genetic counseling are experienced decision makers; they have already made multiple decisions in the course of their lives without our help" (p. 383). In most situations, genetic counselors should employ their skills to facilitate patient decision-making, as discussed in Chap. 7, rather than offer specific "advice."

10.1.3 Advice Topics in Genetic Counseling

As mentioned in the introduction to this chapter, clinical recommendations (e.g., standards of care, management guidelines, etc.) are an appropriate and necessary component of genetic counseling. Other aspects of genetic counseling where advice may be particularly appropriate include (1) the genetic counseling process (e.g., "To help you come to a decision that works for you, I suggest that we talk through each of the different options") and (2) patient behavior (e.g., "Perhaps you should take a couple of days to think this over"; or "You might benefit from talking to some of the other parents in the local muscular dystrophy support group"). Genetic counseling, however, rarely involves telling a patient what decision to make (e.g., "I think having additional children might not be the best decision for you under the circumstances"; or "In light of your family history, you should definitely have carrier screening").

Patients may seek guidance and advice from genetic counselors about other issues related to genetic counseling or testing, such as strategies for disclosing test results to their relatives. Certain patient populations may be particularly desirous of advice. Two studies demonstrate that some parents desire advice about communicating with their children. Mac Dougall et al. (2007) interviewed couples who had used assisted reproductive technology to conceive, asking them about the timing and manner of their disclosure of this information to their child. Parents either endorsed early disclosure with subsequent conversations or waiting for the "right time" in the child's development. The parents who endorsed the "right time" approach reported uncertainty about how to share the information and about the outcome of the conversation, and they expressed a desire for more advice in that regard. Dennis et al. (2015) surveyed parents as well as individuals affected with a sex chromosome aneuploidy. They asked about the timing and content of parents' disclosure of that information to the affected child, resources parents used to prepare for the communication, parents' feelings of preparedness and their concerns, and recommendations for how to approach communicating with one's child. Like Mac Dougall et al. (2007), they found "parents utilizing the 'right-time' strategy reported greater feelings of uncertainty about the disclosure process and outcome, and expressed a desire for guidance or advice" (p. 90). The results of these investigations illustrate individual differences in parents' desire for advice, supporting the need to tailor your approach to each patient/family.

Patenaude and Schneider (2017) describe the major types of questions parents have about disclosing the results of their hereditary cancer testing to their children and conclude that "While psycho-educational aids can remind counselors of relevant topics to discuss with parents and can offer parents broad guidance about what children of different ages may be concerned about, families differ in so many ways that no "recipe" suffices to answer all parents' questions about how this important task should be approached in their family. Successful consultation to parents requires true counseling, matching parents' fears and questions with information, exploration and advice specific to their concerns, circumstances and strengths" (p. 259).

Examples of advice genetic counselors might give to patients are as follows:

- Some patients say they wish they had taken more time to make the decision to terminate a pregnancy. So, when counseling a patient(s) who is at the decision-making stage, the genetic counselor says, "I know it's natural to want to decide quickly and move on, but I would encourage you to take a few days."
- "Consider the issues very carefully. Take as much time as you need."
- A couple whose first child was affected with spinal muscular atrophy (SMA) was in conflict over whether to have preimplantation genetic diagnosis for a future pregnancy. After discussing the issue in the genetic counseling session, the counselor said, "I would encourage you to continue this conversation at home, and take some time to make the decision."
- "I think we should wait until your husband gets here and then maybe you will feel more comfortable about making a decision."
- Women who carry the gene for fragile X syndrome often feel alone, guilty, and burdened. Recognizing this, the counselor said: "I would encourage you to include your husband in decisions about having more children."
- "I think it's important that you know about all of the options available to you."
- "It sounds to me like you would prefer to have the ultrasound before we discuss prenatal testing options any further. So, I think it's a good idea to do that."
- "In making a decision about carrier testing, it's important to think about whether the information will be useful to you. If you know your child were at risk for cystic fibrosis (CF), would you do anything or plan anything differently?"
- "One thing you might consider is having an autopsy done to help you assess the risks of this happening again."
- The patient stated that she wanted predictive testing for early-onset Alzheimer disease because her doctor told her to have the test. The counselor said, "Perhaps you should focus on what is best for you and your family. Let's talk about that."
- "Many of my patients have found it very helpful to talk to other parents of children who have ___."
- "I recommend that you contact the national parent support organization for… to stay current about new developments, changes in health care management, etc. They have a great website."

10.1.4 Consequences of Advice Giving

Advice may have both positive and negative consequences within interpersonal relationships: "Advice may be seen as helpful and caring or as butting in; advice may be experienced as honest or supportive; and seeking and taking advice may enact respect and gratitude, yet recipients reserve the right to make their own decisions" (Goldsmith and Fitch 1997, p. 454).

Based on family therapy literature, when you give advice successfully, you may offer suggestions that patients perceive as helpful, you may present a new idea they had not considered before, and your advice may give permission to take an action they wanted to take anyway (Silver 1991). Advice may provide informational support and directive guidance, and it may demonstrate caring and give the impression that a problem is manageable (Goldsmith and Fitch 1997). Advice may also instill hope and confidence that the patient is capable of following a particular recommendation. In this regard, however, you should be sure your advice recommends actions the patient is capable of doing (that is, has the skills, resources, and opportunity to follow through on your recommendation). For instance, if you are advising patients to share relevant genetic test results with at-risk relatives, you might provide resources (e.g., a letter they can share with relatives) or engage in activities that will help patients build their skill or confidence in following through on the recommendation (e.g., role-play a conversation they might have with a relative).

Feng (2009) noted, "As research has shown, unwanted, irrelevant, or redundant advice is counterproductive in the sense that it tends to meet resistance from the recipient (e.g., Feng and MacGeorge 2006; Goldsmith 2000)" (p. 118). Patients may feel criticized because advice indicates they should be doing something differently, they may feel constrained to consider only the options you raise, they may feel pressured to follow your advice, and they may become oppositional (i.e., resisting everything you say for the remainder of the session) (Silver 1991). Additionally, your advice may imply patients lack the ability to come up with their own strategies or solutions, especially when given before you have sufficiently explored their situation. Advice may also be seen as an imposition of your values (Couture and Sutherland 2006). Finally, some advice may backfire because your patients are privy to reasons why it may not be feasible from their perspective, whereas you have only what they've told you so far, as well as more generic knowledge of how patients react and what they do (cf. Hepburn and Potter 2011).

10.1.5 Suggestions for Giving Advice

- *Make it clear that certain types of advice are not routinely part of genetic counseling*. At the beginning of the session, when you explain the process of genetic counseling, state that while you will provide information and relevant clinical recommendations, you otherwise tend to refrain from telling patients what to do because you prefer to help them come to a decision for themselves. This approach will tend to limit your advice giving and requests for advice from your patients.
- *Give advice later in the session*. You should offer advice only after you have demonstrated some expertise on the topic, after you've established rapport and have shown that you care, and only when the advice is appropriate to the situation. You should also wait until you have listened fully to the patient's situation

and have demonstrated accurate empathy (Feng 2009; Goldsmith and Fitch 1997; Hepburn and Potter 2011). It's important to assess what patients are thinking of doing and why (e.g., "Who is your family would be understanding of your decision to have testing?" This question could help you assess the extent to which the patient might be able to seek emotional support from family members).

- *Wait until asked.* Sometimes patients will ask you directly for advice (e.g., "How can I approach my family members about cascade testing?"). They may more readily accept your advice when they ask you for it. At times, however, you may need to approach a topic regardless of whether a patient has directly asked for advice.
- *Offer advice gently.* Avoid getting into arguments with patients. If patients resist, do not try to "argue [them] into backing down and accepting what you say" (Martin 2000, p. 63). Arguing is almost never effective for influencing patients to follow a suggested course of action. Instead, they will shut down, pretend to agree, leave prematurely, etc.
- *Mention decisions made by other patients.* Sometimes it's helpful to briefly and anonymously describe what other patients in similar situations have done (e.g., "Many people find it helpful to discuss their testing options with their close relatives before making a final decision").
- *Embed your advice.* Insert your advice within information provision (Hepburn and Potter 2011) (e.g., "I'd like to discuss our recommendations for sharing your test results with your close relatives, and share some strategies that other patients have used for doing this.").
- *Check out the impact of your advice.* Ask patients to discuss what they think and feel about your recommendations. This assessment also helps to ensure they accurately understood your advice.
- *Use questions instead of advice to facilitate decisions.* Use questions that get at what the patient considers to be the pros and cons of different options rather than suggesting what the patient should do. For example, you might say, "Which decision do you think you would feel more comfortable making?" Your questions will assist patients in thinking through their decision-making process to arrive at an outcome that is best for them rather than directing them to do what you think is best.
- *Use questions and advanced empathy to set the stage for advice.* Vehvilainen (2001) describes a stepwise entry method for advice giving through a question-answer format designed to align the advice with the patient's perspective and to minimize resistance. In this approach, the counselor first asks the patient what she/he is thinking of doing. The patient's answer to this question "…can be used as grounds for the counselor's advice, but the counselor can focus on the shortcomings of the [patient's] ideas and provide a revised plan" (p. 396). Consider this example. A patient with heart disease finds out she has a gene mutation that is responsible for her condition. When the genetic counselor asks if she plans to share these results with her brother and sister, the patient says "No, I don't want to worry them." The genetic counselor may then reply, "Earlier in the session,

when we were reviewing your family history, you mentioned how close you are to your brother and sister. I wonder if it might help to think about what it would do to your relationship if you don't tell them, and then they get sick? I think it would be good to tell them. Can we talk about how I can help you with this?"

- *Emphasize the decision-making process rather than the outcome.* "You've asked me if I think you should have carrier testing. From what you've said, these seem to be some of the reasons you might make that decision, and these are some of the reasons you might not..." This sort of response provides what Kessler (1997) refers to as a framework from which patients can view things more clearly.
- *Use primary empathy to reflect your understanding of your patient's view of the problem.* For example, regarding a patient at risk for Huntington disease: "It sounds like you would like to find a good way to talk to your children about your risk [primary empathy]. Maybe a family counselor could help you find the right time and way to discuss this with your children [advice]" (Kao 2010, p. 101).
- *Give advice in language that is consistent with the patient's view of the problem.* "You've said several times that you feel like you're 'being smothered' with the weight of this decision. What would you think about taking a couple of days to catch your breath? Could you put down the weight for a little while before you make your final decision?"
- *Be culturally sensitive.* Patients differ in their desire for advice. Sometimes these differences are due to cultural background. Two studies illustrate cultural differences in genetic counseling patients' reactions to advice. Barragan et al. (2011) interviewed women of Mexican origin regarding how they balance cultural practices with Western medicine. They noted that Mexican women expect to receive prescriptive medical advice and adhere to that advice. They found, however, that "More traditional women depended heavily on the advice of their mothers or other supportive women, while more acculturated women sought additional information from healthcare providers and written brochures" (p. 610). The authors also described a possible barrier to genetic counselors' understanding of patient reactions to advice, namely, *simpatía* or "the practice of demonstrating respect to healthcare providers by not questioning them and giving the appearance of understanding and agreeing with the provided advice even when this is not the case" (p. 620). They recommended genetic counselors use open-ended questions to assess patients' comprehension and their intention to comply, whether and how particular interventions may be potentially problematic, what patients think or feel about specific medical recommendations, and how comfortable they are discussing information with family members.

  Floyd et al. (2016) interviewed Spanish-speaking and English-speaking Latina, Asian, and White women who had received prenatal care about their opinions of cell-free DNA (cfDNA) screening. Among their results, they found more Spanish speakers referenced their doctor's advice as a reason to do prenatal testing as they respected and thus would follow the advice. English speakers more often critiqued the advice of care providers and more often disregarded the advice of

both doctors and genetic counselors. The researchers also speculated that even when they are critical of clinicians' advice, language barriers may prevent Spanish-speaking women from expressing their concerns.
- *Clarify your professional role.* When counseling patients who have a strong desire for advice, you may need to explain that, rather than offering advice, you will provide as much pertinent information as you can and possibly suggest the ways patients could go about using this information to arrive at a decision that is best for them. Such a statement can help to reduce misperceptions for any patient who expects you to be highly directive.

10.1.6 Advice-Giving Challenges

Several factors, some pertaining to the genetic counselor, some to the patient, and some to the situation, can make advice giving ineffective. It's important to be aware of the following:

Giving Advice to Satisfy Your Own Needs

As Kessler (1992) eloquently states, "Some [genetic] counselors have the fantasy and wish that if they could only exert their personal power of persuasion, others will begin to see the world the way they do.... Perhaps genetic counselors need to learn what others engaged in personal counseling and psychotherapy have had to resign themselves to and that is we are not very powerful when it comes to changing the behavior of others" (p. 16). Advice givers often feel powerful, helpful, and competent when they give advice (Silver 1991). As these outcomes feel quite good, you may be tempted to give more advice than you should.

Giving Advice Based on Faulty Assumptions

Silver (1991) suggests that mental health counselors who give advice may hold one or more of the following beliefs:

- Professionals know what is best.
- Patients do not know what is best.
- Professionals should take charge and make decisions for patients.
- Patients can't take responsibility for making their own decisions.
- There is one best view and solution, and the professional knows what these are.
- Patients want advice.
- Patients benefit from advice.
- An objective third party is in the best position to give advice.

Mistakenly Thinking Patients Are Seeking Your Advice

Often patients have already made up their minds before asking your opinion. They are not actually asking for advice; rather, they are seeking support for their decision (Goldsmith and Fitch 1997). They seldom come out and directly ask for this support, however. Instead, they will disguise it in the form of a request for advice [e.g., How do you think I should tell my sister she's at risk for breast cancer?]. Giving advice to these patients, especially advice that is discrepant with what they have decided, could be perceived as offensive, and they certainly would not consider it (Kessler 1992). Additionally, what sounds like a request for advice may actually be a request for information that would allow the patient to make her or his own decision (Kessler 1997): "Commonly this information concerns a way to think about a problem rather than a solution" (p. 383). For example, "What do you think I should do?" may be a request for information about the advantages and risks of undergoing whole genome sequencing rather than asking you to make the decision.

Thinking that Patients Will Listen to Your Advice

Patients usually will not take your advice. They might act as if they agree, but they will privately discount your suggestions. Or they might say, "Yes, but..." and go on to explain why your advice won't work. Fine and Glasser (1996) point out, "What a person tells himself is more valuable to him than anything you might tell him, even if what you tell him is better" (p. 66).

Not Realizing You May Appear to Be Taking Sides

Advice will probably lead you to be identified with the family member(s) or friend(s) who has made a similar suggestion (Silver 1991). For example, when counseling an adolescent, your advice may seem to reflect his or her parents' viewpoint.

Believing You Know Better Than Your Patients

While you may be an expert on genetic counseling, you are not an expert on your patient (Cavanagh and Levitov 2002). Consider for a moment how much you think a person would know about you after spending 1 hour together. Furthermore, "no amount of empathy can replace the fact that the counselee has to make and live with their decision" (Kessler 1992, p. 14). As you gain experience, you will begin to get a feel for typical or normative types of patient reactions and decisions. Remember, however, that a typical reaction may not fit for the patient sitting in front of you.

Forgetting that Patients Ultimately Are Responsible for Making Their Own Decisions

When you provide advice, you risk shifting the responsibility for the outcome to you, especially for patients who appear to be desperate for advice. Instead, try indicating that you understand their need for advice and are willing to help them figure out what's best for themselves (Couture and Sutherland 2006; Martin 2000). For instance, "I know you feel like you can't make this decision alone. Why don't we try together to figure out the best way to proceed?"; or with a patient affected with Long QT who wants to have a baby (which is life threatening for her), "… What we can do is talk about all of the possibilities and options that are available to you, to help you make the right decision for you" (Kao 2010, p. 85).

Thinking Your Behavior Is Advice-Free

Patients who want advice will believe you've given it even when you thought you were trying to support their autonomy. Be watchful for clues that patients are trying to pull a recommendation from you (e.g., patient says, "You probably think this is a bad idea..."; or "I suppose you think I'm making a mistake..." Think carefully about how you want to respond to such statements).

10.2 Influencing Responses

Influencing responses are expressions of the genetic counselor's opinion about the patient and/or topics relevant to genetic counseling processes and outcomes (e.g., the patient's feelings, thoughts, attitudes, actions, situation, plans, etc.). Some influencing statements express agreement/support, and, as such, they positively reinforce the patient (e.g., "Your decision seems to be well-thought out" or "You're going to get through this"). Other influencing statements express disagreement, and, as such, they provide a cautionary note to the patient (e.g., "Your decision seems a bit rushed" or, to the father in a prenatal session, "You say that this decision is up to your wife, but really, she is looking for your support"). Influencing responses are a form of persuasion as they are attempts either to affirm patients' feelings, attitudes, and behaviors or to modify them. Synonyms for influence are effect, inspire, impact, encourage, sway, manipulate, persuade, induce, prompt, and impel.

Often influencing responses are intended to provide encouragement to patients. Wong (2015) argues that "Encouragement is one of the most common ways through which individuals express support for one another…" (p. 179). He defines encouragement as: "the expression of affirmation through language or other symbolic representations to instill courage, perseverance, confidence, inspiration, or hope in a person(s) within the context of addressing a challenging situation or realizing a potential" (p. 180). Wong further notes that "...the instillation of courage reduces fear, perseveration combats a desire to give up, confidence addresses low self-efficacy, inspiration resolves a lack of motivation or creativity, and hope decreases pessimism" (p. 184).

Encouragement can include pointing out patients' strengths, validating their goals and decisions, and positively reframing their statements (Wong 2015). For example, your patient says, "I'm sorry to be asking so many questions." You might respond, "You care very much about your child and want to do what's best for him. Your questions are valid ones."

10.2.1 Guidelines for Using Influencing Statements

- *Establish rapport first.* Patients will be more likely to listen to and be affected by your influencing responses once they believe you know what you're talking about, that is, once you have demonstrated your expertise and credibility (Wong 2015).
- *Get to know the patient.* You may be off base with your opinions if you deliver them too early in the session, before you have a sense of who the patient is (strengths, needs, challenges). Even if you are correct in your opinion, patients may think you're "working from a script" and/or making generic statements that could apply to any patient. At best, they will disregard your opinion. At worst, they will feel disrespected and angry.
- *Consider individual and cultural differences.* "There is some preliminary evidence suggesting that encouragement might be relatively more important to the success and well-being of women, minority groups, and some non-Western cultures...individuals from non-Western collectivistic cultures might define themselves more strongly in terms of their relationships with others...[and perhaps be] more open to the influence of encouragement provided from significant others" (Wong 2015, p. 187).
- *Be genuine.* You must be sincere. It's important that you mean what you say and not simply attempt "to fill the silence," try to make patients feel better, or offer false reassurance. For example, to a patient who has just received an abnormal test result and is sobbing, you say, "I know it's difficult to get this news, but I'm sure that you will be able to handle this diagnosis." Although well-intentioned and likely related to a belief that you are empowering the patient, your influencing response will seem "hollow."
- *Provide evidence.* When you make an influencing statement, provide evidence to support it. If you tell a couple they are going to be great parents, include the reasons you believe that. If you tell a patient that keeping his test result a secret from everyone may be a mistake, explain why.
- *Build off patient comments.* A positive influencing statement may be "viewed as more credible by the [patient] if it is based on arguments endorsed or provided

by the [patient]" (Wong 2015, p. 193). For instance, "Your reasons to have testing make a lot of sense."

10.2.2 Reasons to Use Influencing Responses

- *To persuade patients to accept your advice.* One common way to use influence is when your offer advice to patients. In essence, you are attempting to "sell" your recommendation. For instance, you might say, "Here is the contact information for the local Alzheimer's support group. You might want to try attending a session." Then follow your advice with an influencing response: "This group can be very helpful for providing ongoing support to you and your family members." In one of Kao's (2010) scenarios, a patient talks about going through the process of genetic assessment for familial breast/ovarian cancer risk and expresses concern about the lengthy process. Some genetic counselors provided advice coupled with an influencing response. For example, "… Perhaps we can sit down and sort out pro's and con's to having surgery and give you something to think about while the testing is being performed [advice – counselor's professional recommendation]. That way hopefully by the time your results have come back you will have thought everything through and can make a well-informed decision [influence-counselor's opinion about why the advice is important] (p. 53)"; and "We can discuss all of your options for your future healthcare now [advice-counselor's professional recommendation] - so that as soon as the results return we can begin to implement which ever option you choose [influence- counselor's opinion about why the advice is important]" (p. 53).
- *To instill hope.* Wong (2015) suggests influencing strategies for instilling hope. The strategies include telling stories of how others have successfully coped with similar problems, asking questions about the patient's strengths (e.g., "I know that you have faced some difficult health issues in the past. What helped you then?"), and complimenting patients about their past actions and to explore their strengths (e.g., Imagine a couple who have just learned their second child is affected with PKU. They already have a child with PKU. The couple says they are overwhelmed and in despair. You say, "You've managed to take such good care of your other child and to remain positive. How have you done that?"
- *To guide patients away from ineffective attitudes or behaviors.* Influencing responses can help to shape patients' behaviors during the session (e.g., to a patient who seems stuck on the details of the risk figures rather than on the decisions that need to be made, "I think you're focusing on the numbers, rather than on the possible impact a positive or negative test result will have for your health"). They can also help to shape how patients are thinking about their situation and the information you have provided (e.g., "Talking through the reasons you would and would not have testing can help you come to a decision."). In the cancer scenario described in Kao (2010), some counselors provided a "reality check." For example: "… I think that…you're thinking several steps ahead of

where we are right now, which is [trying to determine your actual risk for developing breast cancer]…" (p. 53).

- *To express a medical opinion*. In the Kao (2010) cancer scenario, one counselor said: "… Having surgery is a big step that may or may not be appropriate, and it is not a decision that should be made rashly…" (p. 54); another counselor said "… Everyone on the team is interested in getting you the medical care you need. It is as important to go about this in an orderly fashion as it is to do everything quickly" (p. 54).
- *To normalize patient experiences*. In the Kao (2010) scenario involving a patient with Fabry disease, the patient described her intensely painful symptoms of the disease. Examples of differently nuanced genetic counselor influencing responses include normalizing responses—"We go through life wanting to live and be happy, but this can be a very complicated thing to do when we are suffering through chronic and intense pain…" (p. 70); "… Pain is one of those things that you can't accurately imagine experiencing until it happens to you…" (p. 70); and "I think it's very normal to feel scared of the pain and to not know what will happen after you pass out…" (p. 70).
- *To acknowledge the patient's resiliency and ability*. In the Kao (2010) Fabry disease scenario, some counselors said, "… It really is an act of bravery to get through it each and every time you have an episode of pain" (pp. 70–71); "You must be a very strong person to be able to endure that kind of pain…" (p. 71); and "… You have actually done a very good job of explaining the pain…" (p. 71).

10.3 Closing Comments

Keep in mind that medical recommendations and advice are necessary and appropriate in genetic counseling. In this chapter, we focused on other situations in genetic counseling where you might consider using advice and influence. These are powerful skills because they can be quite directive. Therefore, we recommend that before using either advice or influencing responses, you ask yourself: "How can I best be responsive to this patient's needs?"

10.4 Class Activities

Activity 1: Advice (Think-Pair-Share Dyads)

Students think about a time that someone gave them advice that was very ineffective. What was it like? How did the person present the advice? Now, think about a time when they received advice that was very effective. What was it like? How did the person present the advice? Have students discuss their experiences with a partner.

Then the class discusses the following: What are ineffective ways to give advice? What are effective ways to give advice? The instructor summarizes their responses on the board.

Estimated time: 15–20 min.

Activity 2a: Low-Level Advice and Influencing Skills Model

The instructor and a volunteer genetic counseling patient engage in a role-play in which the counselor demonstrates poor advice giving and influencing responses. Students observe and take notes of examples of poor behaviors.

Estimated time: 10 min.

Process

Students discuss their examples of poor behaviors and the impact of the counselor's poor skills on the patient. The patient can offer her or his impressions of the counselor's behaviors after the other students have made their comments. The instructor could divide the group of students and have half focus on counselor behaviors and half focus on patient behaviors.

Estimated time: 15 min.

Instructor Notes

- One option is to continue with a role-play used earlier in the class so the genetic counselor can more quickly move to advice and influencing skills.
- Students may have difficulty differentiating advice from influencing skills, as advice is often accompanied by an influencing response. The instructor should assist students in categorizing the responses they observe in the role-play. One issue that may come up is the genetic counselor's intended response may be perceived differently by the patient and/or the observers.

Activity 2b: High-Level Advice and Influencing Skills Model

The instructor and the same volunteer repeat the same role-play, only this time the genetic counselor displays good advice and influencing skills. Students take notes of examples of good behaviors.

Estimated time: 15 min.

Process

Students discuss their examples of good advice and influencing behaviors and the impact of the counselor's behaviors on the patient. They also contrast this role-play to the previous role-play. The instructor could divide the group of students and have half focus on counselor behaviors and half focus on patient behaviors.

Estimated time: 15 min.

Instructor Note

- Students could work together in Think-Pair-Share dyads to identify examples of counselor advice and influencing skills and their impact on the patient.

Activity 3: Role-Plays (Small Groups)

Working in small groups, students volunteer to be patient and genetic counselor. The students read their roles silently. Then the student playing the genetic counselor reads her or his role aloud. Next the students engage in a 10- to 15-min role-play. If the student playing the genetic counselor gets stuck, stop the role-play and ask the group [except for the patient] to brainstorm possible ways to handle the situation. Resume the role-play, so the student can try out some of the group's suggestions. Ask the group to provide feedback to the counselor at the end of the role-play and have a general discussion about how to handle each type of situation. Allow about 10–15 min to process each role-play.

Patient Role I

You are a 25-year-old woman who is discussing an abnormal prenatal test result with the genetic counselor. During this session, you say to the counselor, "What should I do?"

Genetic Counselor Role I

Your patient is a 25-year-old woman who is discussing an abnormal prenatal test result with you.

Patient Role II

You are a 35-year-old who is talking about whether to pursue testing for Huntington disease. You should repeatedly ask the counselor for advice, and each time the counselor gives you advice, you should say, "Yes, but…" and then go on to explain why the advice wouldn't work.

Genetic Counselor Role II

Your patient is a 35-year-old who is discussing whether to pursue testing for Huntington disease. The patient does not have a clear idea of what she/he wishes to do.

Patient Role III

You are a graduate student from China who is 18 weeks pregnant. Ultrasound in your doctor's office showed some abnormalities, and you were referred for genetic counseling to discuss your options. Although you have been able to understand everything the counselor says, you remain silent when the counselor asks you what you think you will do if further testing confirms the suspected diagnosis of trisomy 13. After all, the counselor is an expert and should tell you what to do. Although you know what you want to do if the pregnancy is affected, you withhold your opinion.

Genetic Counselor Role III
Your patient is a graduate student from China who is 18 weeks pregnant. She is referred for follow-up of an abnormal ultrasound indicating possible trisomy 13. You are trying to assess what she would do with the information if additional testing confirms this diagnosis. You suspect she knows but is uncomfortable telling you, the expert, her opinion.

Patient Role IV
You are a 25-year-old prenatal patient who has been told by the counselor that there is a problem with the pregnancy. You cried when she/he gave you this information. You are feeling overwhelmed and alone and completely uncertain of what you will do. Do not disclose these feelings unless the counselor encourages you to. Instead, continue to cry a bit and in a shaky voice say, "I'm fine. It's ok."

Genetic Counselor Role IV
Your patient is a 25-year-old prenatal patient. You have just told her that there is a problem with the pregnancy. As you tell her this information, she begins to cry. You suspect she is embarrassed about crying.

Patient Role V
You are a 30-year-old woman whose father was recently diagnosed with Huntington disease. Your genetic counselor has just explained that there is a test that could reveal whether you also carry the gene for this condition. You say, "I just couldn't handle hearing that I have it, too. I'll take my chances. My husband and I are trying to have a baby, and I want to concentrate on that. That's, the right thing to do, isn't it?"

Genetic Counselor Role V
Your patient, a 30-year-old woman has a father who was recently diagnosed with Huntington disease. You have just explained that there is a test that could reveal whether she also carries the gene for this condition.

Estimated time: 20–30 minutes per role play.

Instructor Note
- The instructor may want to encourage students to attempt advice and/or influencing responses during the role-plays, as they otherwise may exhaust the time allotted with other sorts of responses.

Activity 4: Advice and Influencing (Triad Role Plays)

Students practice advice and influencing skills in 15-min role-plays taking turns as counselor, patient, and observer. The scenarios can be of the instructor or the students' choosing. Allow 10 min of feedback after each role-play. The students should focus on using good helping behaviors.

Criteria for Evaluating Counselor Advice and Influencing Behaviors
Well-timed

Used sparingly
Concise
Non-argumentative
Intended to meet patient goals
Genuine versus falsely reassuring
Relevant to patient's situation
Followed up with empathy
Estimated time: 75 min.

Instructor Note

- The observer or counselor may wish to stop the role-play if the counselor is obviously stuck. The students [except the patient] can then engage in a brief conversation about the patient's dynamics, issues, etc., to help the counselor. Then the counselor and patient resume the role-play.

Process

Discuss in the large group: How was it to do this exercise? What are you learning about advice and influencing behaviors in general? About yourself? What questions do you still have about these skills?

Estimated time: 20 min.

10.5 Written Exercises

Exercise 1: Advice

Refer to Silver's (1991) eight beliefs of counselors who give advice described in this chapter under the heading, "Giving Advice Based on Faulty Assumptions". Provide one or two written arguments against each belief.

Exercise 2: Advice and Influencing Responses

Read each of the 14 patient statements listed in Chap. 8, Exercise 2, and give one advice response and one influencing response for each statement. Write your responses as if you were actually talking to the patient.

[*Hint*: You may need to infer more knowledge about the patient in order to formulate your responses. It may be helpful to follow up on the empathy statements you developed previously for Chap. 8, Exercise 2.]

Example

For the example of the 40-year-old man at risk for Huntington disease cited in Chap. 8, Exercise 2:

Advice: "Perhaps you should reconsider what having the testing done will mean for you."

Influence: "It's good that you are seeking as much information as you can because of how frightened you are about testing positive."

Exercise 3: Role-Play

Engage in a 30-min role-play of a genetic counseling session with a classmate. The role-play can be based on a patient you saw in a clinic or it can be a made-up patient situation. During the role-play, focus on all of the helping skills you've learned so far. Try to include at least one advice and one influencing response. Audio record the role-play. Next transcribe the role-play and critique your work. Use the following method for transcribing the session:

Counselor	Patient	Self-critique	Instructor
Key phrases of dialogue	Key phrases	Comment on your own responses	Will provide feedback on your responses

Create a brief summary:

1. Briefly describe patient *demographics* (e.g., age, gender, ethnicity, socioeconomic status, relationship status) and *reason* for seeking genetic counseling.
2. Identify *two* things you said/did during the role-play that were effective and *two* things you could have done differently:

Give the recording, transcript/self-critique, and summary to the instructor who will provide feedback.

[*Hint*: This assignment encourages self-reflective practice regarding your clinical performance. The goal is not to do a perfect session. Rather the goal is to assess the extent to which you can accurately assess your psychosocial counseling skills. You will gain more from this exercise if you refrain from scripting what you plan to say as the counselor.]

References

Andersen J, Øyen N, Bjorvatn C, Gjengedal E. Living with long QT syndrome: a qualitative study of coping with increased risk of sudden cardiac death. J Genet Couns. 2008;17:489–98.

Barragan DI, Ormond KE, Strecker MN, Weil J. Concurrent use of cultural health practices and Western medicine during pregnancy: exploring the Mexican experience in the United States. J Genet Couns. 2011;20:609–24.

Butler CW, Potter J, Danby S, Emmison M, Hepburn A. Advice-implicative interrogatives: building "client-centered" support in a children's helpline. Soc Psychol Q. 2010;73:265–87.

Cavanagh M, Levitov JE. The counseling experience a theoretical and practical approach. 2nd ed. Prospect Heights IL: Waveland Press; 2002.

Couture SJ, Sutherland O. Giving advice on advice-giving: a conversation analysis of Karl Tomm's practice. J Marital Fam Ther. 2006;32:329–44.

DeCapua A, Dunham JF. Strategies in the discourse of advice. J Pragmat. 1993;20:519–31.
Dennis A, Howell S, Cordeiro L, Tartaglia N. "How should I tell my child?" Disclosing the diagnosis of sex chromosome aneuploidies. J Genet Couns. 2015;24:88–103.
Feng B. Testing an integrated model of advice giving in supportive interactions. Hum Commun Res. 2009;35:115–29.
Feng B, MacGeorge EL. Predicting receptiveness to advice: characteristics of the problem, the advice-giver, and the recipient. South Commun J. 2006;71:67–85.
Fine SF, Glasser PH. The first helping interview. Thousand Oaks, CA: Sage; 1996.
Floyd E, Allyse MA, Michie M. Spanish-and English-speaking pregnant women's views on cfDNA and other prenatal screening: practical and ethical reflections. J Genet Couns. 2016;25:965–77.
Gibas AL, Klatt R, Johnson J, Clarke JT, Katz J. Disease rarity, carrier status, and gender: a triple disadvantage for women with Fabry disease. J Genet Couns. 2008;17:528–37.
Goldsmith DJ. Soliciting advice: the role of sequential placement in mitigating face threat. Commun. Monogr. 2000;67:1–9.
Goldsmith DJ, Fitch K. The normative context of advice as social support. Hum Commun Res. 1997;23:454–76.
Hepburn A, Potter J. Designing the recipient: managing advice resistance in institutional settings. Soc Psychol Q. 2011;74:216–41.
Kao JH. Walking in your patient's shoes: an investigation of genetic counselor empathy in clinical practice. Minneapolis, MN: University of Minnesota; 2010. Retrieved from the University of Minnesota Digital Conservancy, http://hdl.handle.net/11299/96724.
Kessler S. Psychological aspects of genetic counseling. VII. Thoughts on directiveness. J Genet Couns. 1992;1:9–17.
Kessler S. Psychological aspects of genetic counseling. X. Advanced counseling techniques. J Genet Couns. 1997;6:379–92.
Mac Dougall K, Becker G, Scheib JE, Nachtigall RD. Strategies for disclosure: how parents approach telling their children that they were conceived with donor gametes. Fertil Steril. 2007;87:524–33.
Martin DG. Counseling and therapy skills. 2nd ed. Prospect Heights, IL: Waveland Press; 2000.
McCarthy Veach P, Bartels DM, LeRoy BS. Coming full circle: a Reciprocal-Engagement Model of genetic counseling practice. J Genet Couns. 2007;16:713–28.
National Society of Genetic Counselors. National society of genetic counselors code of ethics. J Genet Couns. 2017. https://doi.org/10.1007/s10897-017-0166-8. [Epub ahead of print].
Nusbaum R, Grubs RE, Losee JE, Weidman C, Ford MD, Marazita ML. A qualitative description of receiving a diagnosis of clefting in the prenatal or postnatal period. J Genet Couns. 2008;17:336–50.
Patenaude AF, Schneider KA. Issues arising in psychological consultations to help parents talk to minor and young adult children about their cancer genetic test result: a guide to providers. J Genet Couns. 2017;26:251–60.
Phelps C, Wood F, Bennett P, Brain K, Gray J. Knowledge and expectations of women undergoing cancer genetic risk assessment: a qualitative analysis of free-text questionnaire comments. J Genet Couns. 2007;16:505–14.
Quaid KA, Sims SL, Swenson MM, Harrison JM, Moskowitz C, Stepanov N, et al. Living at risk: concealing risk and preserving hope in Huntington disease. J Genet Couns. 2008;17:117–28.
Resta RG. Complicated shadows: a critique of autonomy in genetic counseling. In: LeRoy BS, McCarthy Veach P, Bartels DM, editors. Genetic counseling practice. Hoboken: Wiley-Blackwell; 2010. p. 13–30.
Schmerler S. Lessons learned: risk management issues in genetic counseling. New York: Springer; 2007.
Silver E. Should I give advice? A systematic review. J Fam Thpy. 1991;13:293–309.
Vehvilainen S. Evaluative advice in educational counseling: the use of disagreement in the "stepwise entry" to advice. Res Lang Soc Interact. 2001;34:371–98.
Weil J. Psychosocial genetic counseling. New York: Oxford University Press; 2000.
Wong YJ. The psychology of encouragement: theory, research, and applications. Couns Psychol. 2015;43:178–216.

Chapter 11
Counselor Self-Reference: Self-Disclosure and Self-Involving Skills

Learning Objectives

1. Define self-disclosure and self-involving skills.
2. Differentiate self-disclosure from self-involving responses.
3. Determine guidelines for effective self-disclosure and self-involving responses.
4. Describe potential benefits and risks of each type of response.
5. Identify examples of counselor-patient themes appropriate for self-involving responses.
6. Develop self-disclosure and self-involving skills through self-reflection, practice, and feedback.

Two types of genetic counseling skills involve self-reference by genetic counselors: self-disclosure and self-involving responses. Self-disclosure is the genetic counselor's communication to the patient of information about herself or himself. Self-disclosure includes a range of information including demographics, beliefs, attitudes, perceptions, experiences, desires, and actions, as well as feelings about people and/or situations other than the patient (McCarthy Veach 2011). Self-involving responses are direct communications of the counselor's feelings about and reactions to the patient in the here-and-now situation (McCarthy Veach 2011). These responses vary in the extent to which they are *I-focused* (i.e., self-disclosure about one's self, "My mother had breast cancer, so I understand a bit of what you are going through.") versus *we-focused* (i.e., self-involving statements about the counselor-patient relationship, "I'm feeling uncomfortable that you are not answering my questions.") (McCarthy Veach 2011).

P. McCarthy Veach et al., *Facilitating the Genetic Counseling Process*,
https://doi.org/10.1007/978-3-319-74799-6_11

11.1 Self-Disclosure

Self-disclosure is a multidimensional skill that affects genetic counseling processes and outcomes. Self-disclosures vary with respect to intimacy level, content, timing, and length, disclosure of present experiences or past situations, their relative similarity or dissimilarity to the patient's experiences, counselor motivations for disclosing, cultural considerations, whether the disclosure is patient-requested or counselor-initiated, intentional versus unavoidable revelations, and counselor and patient characteristics (McCarthy Veach 2011).

11.1.1 To Disclose or Not to Disclose?

Counselor self-disclosure is a controversial behavior. Within genetic counseling, some authors (e.g., Kessler 1992) suggest caution in its use, arguing that self-disclosure is highly directive (e.g., telling a patient what you would do if you were in her or his situation, thereby implying what the patient should do). Some mental health authors (e.g., Simone et al. 1998) caution that self-disclosure may reflect the therapist's unconscious needs (e.g., for intimacy), blur relationship boundaries (are you my counselor or my friend?) (Audet 2011), shift focus from the patient (Audet and Everall 2003; Dewane 2006), confuse patients about the nature of counseling (Audet and Everall 2003), and even reverse roles such that the patient is caretaking the counselor (Audet and Everall 2003; McCarthy Veach 2011).

As described in different disciplines, such as psychotherapy and genetic counseling, general reasons for using self-disclosure include to "respond to client requests for disclosure (Peters et al. 2004; Thomas et al. 2006); help client feel s/he is not alone; convey understanding of client's situation; decrease client anxiety; build rapport/working alliance; normalize client's feelings/reactions; encourage client and instill hope; increase clinician's credibility; build trust; suggest/model coping strategies; encourage client disclosure; increase client awareness of alternative viewpoints; provide a rationale for clinician-initiated topics; connect with clients whose cultural background encourages such disclosure; encourage client to express emotions; challenge the client; and prevent client idealization of the counselor (Henretty and Levitt 2010; Peters et al. 2004; Simone et al. 1998; Thomas et al. 2006)" (McCarthy Veach 2011, pp. 351–352).

Conversely, reasons for refraining from self-disclosure are to avoid blurring boundaries, remain patient-centered, prevent the patient from becoming concerned about the counselor's welfare, avoid giving the patient information to manipulate the counselor, and avoid counselor discomfort (Balcom et al. 2013; McCarthy Veach 2011). Additional reasons include to prevent undermining patient autonomy, and viewing self-disclosure as generally not relevant/helpful to the patient (Thomas et al. 2006). Balcom et al. (2013) investigated genetic counselor responses to prenatal patients' requests for self-disclosure: "Particularly noteworthy, counselors avoided disclosure they judged to be highly directive, either because of its content (e.g., personal opinions and pregnancy decisions) and/or because of perceived patient motives for asking the question (e.g., wanting the counselor to make their decision)" (p. 370).

Self-disclosure is not always a response that you will initiate, as patients will often ask you to disclose. Some research suggests patient requests comprise a prevalent reason for genetic counselors to self-disclose. Peters et al. (2004) investigated the effects of being a recipient of genetic counseling services on genetic counselors' own practice. A large percentage of their survey respondents reportedly had self-disclosed about their experiences to their patients, and the most common reason was because their patients asked them to disclose. Thomas et al. (2006) interviewed practicing genetic counselors who had previously received genetic counseling services about their general self-disclosure practices. Similar to Peters et al. (2004), they found that the most prevalent reason to self-disclose was because patients asked them to do so, although not every counselor disclosed about her or his receipt of genetic counseling services.

We believe self-disclosure, when used strategically and sparingly, is acceptable to some patients. You must always make a conscious decision of whether to disclose and how much and in what ways to directly share yourself in the genetic counseling relationship (McCarthy Veach 2011). Moreover, "an 'immutable rule' regarding the use of self-disclosure (e.g., 'never disclose,' or 'always disclose' certain information) is not feasible. Genetic counselor self-disclosures and non-disclosures should be done skillfully and only in the patient's best interests" (Balcom et al. 2013, p. 371).

11.1.2 Indirect versus Direct Self-Disclosures

A certain amount of self-disclosure is always present in genetic counseling sessions, as it's impossible to avoid revealing some information about yourself. Every behavior you engage in with a patient (your facial expressions, posture, voice tone, etc.) reveals something about you (McCarthy Veach 2011). Furthermore, patients may *read into* your behaviors. They may determine (not always accurately) whether you approve or disapprove of their actions, whether you would or would not make the same decision, etc.

Your personal characteristics also communicate information that patients will actively interpret:

- Gender (e.g., a prenatal patient may believe you can understand her situation if you are a woman, and question your ability to understand if you are a man).
- Age (e.g., you appear to be too young to know what it's like to have experienced years of infertility.)
- Race/ethnicity (e.g., the patient may feel some distance if you appear to be of a different racial or ethnic group).

- Relationship status (e.g., if you wear a wedding ring, you may be perceived as someone who understands the conflict a couple is experiencing).
- Physical appearance (e.g., if your physical characteristics suggest you have a genetic condition, this might make some patients reluctant to discuss termination of an affected pregnancy). Being obviously pregnant may evoke any number of reactions from patients (e.g., Clark 2010, 2012; Menezes 2012). Balcom et al. (2013) found that patient requests for self-disclosure increase when the counselor is pregnant. The most prevalent questions asked are "When are you due?," "How do you do this job while being pregnant?," and "How is your pregnancy going?"

This type of *indirect* disclosure is not something you can or necessarily should try to control or manipulate. It *is* important, however, to reflect upon what your characteristics and actions may convey to the patients. Depending on the given situation and circumstances, you may need to directly discuss your unintentional disclosures (McCarthy Veach 2011).

There are other types of indirect disclosures, however, that you can control. For example:

- Office decorations [e.g., pictures of your children may lead some patients to perceive you as understanding about pregnancy but perhaps less about pregnancy loss; the presence of LGBT-friendly literature in your office may reflect your openness and comfort with patients who self-identify as LGBT (VandenLangenberg et al. 2012)].
- Accessories/jewelry (e.g., expensive jewelry and clothes may cause a patient with fewer resources to think you would not be able to relate to their circumstances or situation; religious jewelry may cause a patient to draw conclusions about your attitudes or beliefs that may or may not be accurate).

In contrast to indirect self-disclosure, direct self-disclosure refers to intentional communications about yourself. You may sometimes deliberately choose to reveal information about yourself, and sometimes your disclosures will be in response to patient questions (e.g., "Have you ever worked with patients who have a genetic condition like mine?"). Direct disclosures are the primary focus of this chapter.

11.1.3 Self-Disclosure Intimacy Levels

Self-disclosures vary along a continuum from low, to moderate, to high intimacy. In Table 11.1 we describe and illustrate different levels of disclosure intimacy.

Generally speaking, sharing information about one's personal experiences (e.g., history of infertility) is higher in intimacy than sharing information about one's professional experiences (e.g., what other patients you've counseled have felt or done).

Table 11.1 Self-disclosure levels of intimacy

Lower intimacy			Higher intimacy		
Self-disclosure topic	Situationally required	Beliefs	Facts about yourself	Personal feelings and perceptions not generated by the present relationship	Expressions of feelings experienced in the past toward the patient
Self-disclosure example	*I am a second-year genetic counseling student*	*I believe it's important to take your time making a decision like this*	*I am married*	*I feel frustrated when test results are inconclusive*	*I was concerned after talking with you last week*

11.1.4 Functions of Self-Disclosure

As mentioned earlier, there are several reasons mental health counselors, genetic counselors, and other human service professionals might disclose:

Enhances Social Influence

Like most other health-care professionals, genetic counselors appear to be more human when they self-disclose; they may be regarded as more receptive, warm, capable, and trustworthy (McCarthy Veach 2011; Paine et al. 2010). For example:

- "I have been working in this clinic more than 10 years."
- Patients often ask about the pictures on a counselor's desk. "Do you have children?" or "Are these your children?" The counselor acknowledges the question and reveals a small amount of information—the children's ages, for example.
- Patient: "I'm worried about what these test results will do to my children." Counselor: "I have children of my own and can understand why you feel that your decision also affects them."
- "You look uncomfortable/anxious. I sometimes feel that way, too, when I have a medical appointment."
- "I have a strong family history of heart disease, too. I've been working on changing my diet and exercise, but it sure isn't easy!"

Builds the Relationship

Self-disclosure can communicate your interest and concern, suggest you are genuine, and imply that you trust the patient with the information you reveal about yourself. Self-disclosure can strengthen the connection between you and the patient (Simone et al. 1998; Ziv-Beiman 2013). For example:

- "When I was pregnant, I was anxious/worried all the time."
- "So, you are from Chicago. I grew up there. I really miss___."
- Identifying with your patient as a parent: "I think it's natural for us as parents to struggle when deciding what's best for our families."
- Patient: "This pregnancy is so important to me. We spent 5 years getting pregnant and had to do an in vitro fertilization. Counselor: "Infertility can color your perspective and make any type of risk to the pregnancy seem unacceptable. I felt that way, too, when I was deciding about prenatal testing."

Reinforces Patient Self-Disclosure

There is a give and take, in that both the patient and you are risking being open (cf. Henretty and Levitt 2010).

- Pt: "It's hard to explain what's going through my mind right now."
- Co: "Sometimes I have a hard time explaining myself when my feelings are so mixed. I wonder if that's how it is for you?"

Reassurance that the Patient Is Not Alone

This type of disclosure tends to normalize or validate patient feelings and decreases patient anxiety and isolation.

- Pt: "I feel so mixed up right now; I should be able to make this decision."
- Co: "I'd have a difficult time, too, if I were in your situation."

Provides Reality Testing

Self-disclosure can point out that decisions are not always clear-cut (Dewane 2006; McCarthy Veach 2011).

- Pt: "I can't believe I'm waffling on this! I mean, I told you before that I was having BRCA testing so I'd be able to let my daughters know if they were at increased risk. Now I'm afraid of telling them my results."
- Co: "It's been my experience that many people in a similar situation initially feel as conflicted as you do."

Generates New Perspectives

You may be able to assist patients in decision-making by providing a different viewpoint or strategy.

- Pt: "What would you do if you were me?"
- Co: "I'm not sure, but when I've had a big decision to make, I think things over for a while and talk with my family. I try not to rush into a decision before I feel ready. How would that work for you?"

Elicits Strong Feelings

Patients may become sad, angry, and/or frightened during the session. You may need to give them permission to express their feelings. One way to do this is with self-disclosure. For example:

- Co: "As a parent too, I know I would be very anxious if someone told me my baby's newborn screening test was abnormal. Is that how you're feeling?"
- Co: "It looks like you want to cry and that you're holding yourself back. Sometimes I feel uncomfortable crying, but it helps me to let it out."

Provides Education

Self-disclosure can be educational when done hypothetically. For example, a clinician might say, "I can't tell you what you should do, but here is what I would be thinking about if I were you… (McCarthy Veach 2011, p. 353).

Paine et al. (2010) surveyed 151 undergraduate and graduate students who completed surveys describing a hypothetical genetic counseling session with a patient at risk for FAP who was deciding to pursue testing or surveillance procedures. The patient asked, "What would you do if you were me?" The counselor either shared what she would do (Personal Disclosure) or what other patients have done (Professional Disclosure), or she deflected the question (No Disclosure). Participants rated the *non-disclosing* counselor significantly lower in social attractiveness (warmth, likeability) than either of the disclosing counselors, and less satisfying than the professional *disclosing* counselor. Ratings of satisfaction with the information provided in the genetic counseling session were higher for the professionally disclosing genetic counselor than for the non-disclosing counselor. The findings suggest self-disclosure may enhance perceptions of the counselor, and sharing one's clinical experience (e.g., what other patients have done) provides useful information.

11.1.5 Guidelines for Using Self-Disclosure

Several authors offer suggestions for using self-disclosure:

Examine your reasons for disclosing. Self-disclosure should help patients accomplish their goals for genetic counseling and should not be for reasons such as reducing your own anxiety or to avoid disappointing, frustrating, or angering the patient (Dewane 2006; Henretty and Levitt 2010; McCarthy Veach 2011). Before disclosing, ask yourself: Will my disclosure help the patient open up, see a different perspective, or move toward a decision?

Thomas et al.'s (2006) genetic counselor participants identified certain situations in which they felt "obliged to disclose" including when they were obviously pregnant, when they strongly identified with the patient, when patients requested them to self-disclose, and obvious counselor characteristics (e.g., an accent).

Menezes et al. (2010) interviewed prenatal genetic counselors about the personal impact of their work and similarly found that genetic counselors were faced with "inadvertent" or "unavoidable" self-disclosure about their pregnancy. Nine of 11 counselors who had been pregnant while working in the prenatal setting reported having disclosed the type of testing they had during pregnancy. Yet, the counselors experienced conflicts about self-disclosure, including feeling "forced" to disclose about their very personal experience of pregnancy. The authors concluded the counselors "…were aware that they were relating to clients differently, perhaps more on a personal level, and realizing the need to keep a professional distance. This seems to be where the worry of self-disclosure lies, as counselors were more aware of how their client may be relating to them because they too were pregnant" (p. 649).

Be intentional. Keep your disclosure brief and focused. A useful technique is to make a disclosure and then immediately follow it with a question, "Is that how it is for you?" or "What do you think (or how do you feel) about what I just said?" This brings the focus back to your patient and helps the patient use the information for his or her own situation (McCarthy Veach 2011).

Choose an appropriate intimacy level. As self-disclosures range on a continuum from demographics to highly personal experiences, you must be sensitive enough to choose a level that will not overwhelm or alienate your patient. For example, Balcom et al. (2013) found that prenatal genetic counselors' use of self-disclosure was sometimes unsuccessful when patients viewed it as "oversharing" personal information. One way you might gauge the intimacy of a disclosure is to ask yourself how many other individuals you have told this information to in the past (McCarthy and Oakes 1998).

Choose an appropriate time. If you disclose too soon, you allow patients to avoid the painful work of making decisions for themselves. You risk having them grab onto your experiences and solutions or those of your previous patients. They do not work it through, and they risk selecting an option that is not the best for themselves. For example, some patients know exactly how they are going to handle a situation; others will tell you they don't know what they would do. Well-timed self-disclosure in decision-making situations ideally is after patients have described where they are in the decision-making process and directly or indirectly ask for help in making a decision.

Be conservative. When disclosures are too frequent, too intense, and/or too lengthy, they can shift the focus to you, burden your patient with your problems, be distracting (Audet and Everall 2003; McCarthy Veach 2011), and cause patients to experience your disclosures as oversharing (Balcom et al. 2013).

Be purposeful and relevant. Your self-disclosure should pertain to the session goals and should be expressed in a way that makes its relevance obvious to the patient (Audet and Everall 2003; Henretty and Levitt 2010).

Keep more personal disclosures non-immediate. It's generally less risky to disclose information from your past experiences rather than from your current experiences (McCarthy Veach 2011). For example, patients might be distressed to learn you currently are undergoing BRCA testing, but they might benefit from learning that you underwent testing 5 years ago.

Be prepared. Bonovitz (2006) asserts "We personally reveal much more about ourselves on those occasions when we are thrown into a situation unprepared" (p. 295). Therefore, it's a good idea to reflect in advance about the sorts of information you would never disclose to patients and the reasons why you would not disclose, as well as the sorts of information you might share and why.

Relatedly, remember that although you are required to maintain patient confidentiality, your patients are not under the same imperative (Sweezy 2005). Patients can reveal anything that they care to, and with anyone. So, "…be aware of choices and possible consequences before this question [of whether to self-disclose] arises in session" (Sweezy 2005, p. 90). When thinking about topics that you might disclose, you should consider how you would feel if patients passed this information along to others. Furthermore, patients vary in how sensitive and nonjudgmental they will be about your situation.

Know your own reactions. You should anticipate how you will feel as you disclose certain information and generally avoid topics that would cause you to be highly emotional, such as information that would make you quite distressed, anxious, or angry.

Assess what a patient is really asking and respond accordingly. Thomas et al.'s (2006) genetic counselor participants perceived patients' motivations for requesting self-disclosure as to seek guidance about a decision, out of respect for the counselor and her/his expertise and trustworthiness, to seek validation, to build the relationship/establish a connection with the counselor, to determine whether the counselor can understand them/their situation, and to avoid responsibility for their decision and its outcomes.

It's always a good idea to consider the possible motivation for a patient's question and to ask about it in a noncritical/nondefensive way. For example, a patient might ask a genetic counseling student, "How old are you?" The question could simply be a desire to know more about the student. It might also be an indirect way for the patient to ask if the student is experienced enough to meet her or his needs. It is not uncommon for patients to ask students a lot of questions about their training (e.g., How long is your program?, When are you going to graduate?, Where do you hope to get a job?, Why did you choose genetic counseling?, etc.). Consider that a patient may just genuinely be interested in getting to know more about you or about the profession. Conversely, the patient may be trying to deflect the discussion away from more sensitive topics.

When the patient's question is about a relatively low-intimacy topic, you could answer the question, observe the patient's nonverbal reaction, and then decide whether to follow up with a question such as "Can you tell me more about why you are asking?"

When patient questions are about more highly intimate topics, try to determine the "latent question" behind their request before deciding whether to self-disclose. Does your patient really want the information? Is she hoping for a particular answer? Is the patient looking for your support? Is your patient actually saying she doesn't trust her own judgment? Is she questioning your ability to be helpful? Questioning whether you can truly understand her situation? Wanting you to tell her what to do? Wanting to know what your other patients do so she can do the same? Wanting to make you responsible for the outcome of her decisions? Wishing to "lighten the tone"/take a break from her intense feelings by shifting the focus to you? Hoping you will side with her when she disagrees with her partner or other family member who attends the session?

Sarangi et al. (2004) noted that "Typically the clients' framing of the question to counselors—"what would you do if it were you"—is often referred to as the 'infamous question' in genetic counseling. It is very likely that whatever the counselor says in response to such a question may be heard as potential advice… This means that the counselor has to work hard—interactionally speaking—so as to avoid an advisory role if s/he did not want it" pp. 137–138).

Depending on the patient's question and motivation for asking, one of the following responses might be appropriate:

- "I'd be happy to tell you what my experience has been, but first, I'd like to know a little bit more about why you're asking."
- "What are you hoping I will say?"
- "Perhaps you're hoping that I'll be able to give you the right answer? What I would do in your situation may not be appropriate for you. Let's try together to figure out which option is best for you."
- "Many of my patients ask this question. Here are some of the issues they consider in making their decision. Let's see if any of these apply to you."
- It seems that by asking what my other patients do, you're wanting to know if your decision makes sense.
- This is such a difficult decision. In some ways, it would be nice if someone could just tell you what to do.

Thomas et al.'s (2006) genetic counselor participants suggested genetic counselors should follow up self-disclosure by "…variously asking, 'What were you hoping I would say?'; 'I'm guessing that's not the response you were hoping for'; 'Do you think my answer means I can't understand you?'; or, 'What does my answer mean for you and your situation?'…[and] when genetic counselors disclose, they should clarify differences between their and the patient's situation" (p. 178).

Observe patient reactions. Bonovitz (2006) stresses the importance of "hearing the personal impact" (p. 298) of your self-disclosure on the patient, rather than assuming you know what its effect will be.

Consider patients' individual characteristics. Some patients are dependent decision-makers who rely on others to make their decisions for them. Be watchful for this motivation if a patient asks you what you would do. If you decide not to disclose, you might try using a strategy recommended by Kessler (1992). He suggests that genetic counselors avoid answering questions about what to do by redirecting attention to process issues (e.g., a young genetic counselor responded to questions about whether she had children by saying that perhaps the patient was wondering if she would be able to understand). If you do choose to disclose, consider not only saying what you would do, but also describing your decision-making process in order to help patients understand (and possibly use) a similar process. For example, "When I decided to have BRCA testing, I first discussed the decision with my sisters and my daughters, because I knew the results could directly affect them. I found it helpful to have their perspective, even though it may not have changed my decision to be tested." Relatedly, patient cognitive functioning may be an important consideration. Individuals with intellectual disability may be more inclined to imitate the behaviors of the expert.

Additional individual characteristics include the patient's age. Peterson (2002) notes that in psychotherapy, self-disclosing with adolescents "…can model openness and authenticity" (p. 27).

Consider patients' cultural characteristics. You should consider answering some direct questions if you think it will help to build a trusting relationship. Conversely, self-disclosure may be contrary to the basic values of some cultural groups. Try to familiarize yourself with the disclosure norms of different cultures. When you sense there is a cultural "disconnect" between you and the patient, self-disclosure that acknowledges the differences may help to build rapport/trust (Burkard et al. 2006). Also, disclosing your own "unique cultural influences and ethnicity is one example of self-disclosure that demonstrates willingness to include and respect diverse cultural influences" (Dewane 2006, p. 556).

Glessner et al. (2012) surveyed genetic counselor attitudes and practices when counseling GLBT patients. Forty-six counselors (23.6%) reported having disclosed their own orientation to a patient, either directly or indirectly by mentioning a partner or displaying a wedding photo. The most common reasons to disclose were patient inquiry, normalization of patient feelings and reactions, rapport building, and trust building. The GLB counselors in the sample also mentioned helping the patient to not feel alone, conveying that they understood the patient, and decreasing patient anxiety as motivations for self-disclosure.

Be honest. Tell the truth when you share information about yourself and why you are sharing it with patients as well as why you do not share certain information (McCarthy Veach 2011). Skillfully explaining your behavior seems to have a stronger effect on the counseling process than whether you actually disclose or refrain from disclosing (Balcom et al. 2013; Hanson 2005; Redlinger-Grosse et al. 2013). For instance, Balcom et al.'s (2013) prenatal genetic counselor participants noted that nondisclosure responses to patient requests were successful when they included an explanation of the reason they did not disclose. So, for example, in response to the question "Did you have prenatal testing?," a genetic counselor might say, "The decision I made about testing may not apply to your situation, but some of the things I thought about were…".

11.1.6 Examples of Self-Disclosure Topics and Genetic Counselor Self-Disclosures

Topics genetic counselors have reported disclosing include whether they had children, if they had received genetic counseling services, common life experiences, and religious/spiritual beliefs (Thomas et al. 2006); sexual orientation (Glessner et al. 2012); and, in prenatal genetic counseling, responses to patient questions about counselor demographics (e.g., "How many children do you have?"), personal opinions regarding patient decisions (e.g., "What would you do in my situation?"), genetic counselor's personal pregnancy experiences/decisions (e.g., "Have you ever been pregnant? and "Did you have amniocentesis during your pregnancy?"), and professional experiences/opinions regarding patient decisions (e.g., "Do you see lots of other people with this result/situation?") (Balcom et al. 2013).

In Balcom et al.'s (2013) study of genetic counselor responses to prenatal patients' disclosure requests, counselors either typically responded with: (1) *personal self-disclosure* (e.g., "If people ask me if I have children I will say, 'Yeah, I have a little girl,' or I'll say, 'Yeah, I have a baby'." (p. 364), (2) *professional self-disclosure* (e.g., "Typically when [patients] ask about what I have done when I was pregnant I will give sort of a group disclosure… Like if we're talking about the first trimester screen, [I'll tell patients], 'There are four groups of people…One group never wants the amnio and this might not be the best test for them. Some people want the diagnostic information; they don't want a new number. And, the screen may not be right for them either; they go straight to the amnio. Or the middle two groups kind of want to avoid it or kind of want it but want more information. And after talking to you, I'm really getting the feeling that you are in blank group. Is that a fair assessment'?" (p. 364), and (3) *redirection* (e.g., "There have been times when [patients] have asked me ['What did you do during your pregnancy?'] and I've said, 'Let's really focus on what's most important for you'." (p. 364), or they (4) *decline to answer the question*" (e.g., "When I'm asked what I would do…I usually just tell them that my circumstances would be different from [theirs], and that they know themselves and what they can handle much better than I can after a 1 h. consultation" (p. 364).

Redlinger-Grosse et al. (2013) studied genetic counseling students' and genetic counselors' responses to a hypothetical prenatal patient's request for self-disclosure. Survey participants read a scenario about a patient who was referred for prenatal counseling due to advanced maternal age. She was hesitant about having an amniocentesis and asked the genetic counselor either "What would you do if you were me?" or "Have you ever had an amniocentesis?" Participants wrote a response to the patient as if they were the genetic counselor and then explained their response. Rates of self-disclosure were significantly higher for "What would you do if you were me?" than for "Have you ever had an amniocentesis?" Similar to Balcom et al. (2013), responses included *personal disclosure*, *professional disclosure*, or a *mixture* of the two. Prevalent reasons to self-disclose were to promote decision-making, remain patient focused, build the relationship, enhance counselor credibility, and counselor comfort with disclosure.

Nondisclosure responses included *declining to answer* [e.g., "This is an individual situation and what would be best for me may not be what is best for you. What information have I given to you today that has you questioning your original plan?" and "I understand that you are struggling with this decision, but whether or not I've had an amniocentesis isn't important. We should discuss what your thoughts and feelings are and what I can do to help you make the decision" (p. 462)], and *redirection* [e.g., "I am wondering if you are asking what I would do because you are feeling unsure about wanting an amniocentesis?" and "How do you think that knowing if I had underwent [sic] amniocentesis may or may not influence your decision?" (p. 462)]. Prevalent reasons for not disclosing were nondirectiveness, to remain patient-focused, to support/empower the patient, to maintain the counselor's privacy, and self-disclosure was not relevant.

The researchers categorized both disclosure and nondisclosure responses according to their emphasis. Some were corrective and literal responses, in which participants took the patient's questions at "face value" without attempting to get at the motivation behind her questions. Other responses were interpreting statements in which participants tried to explore the patient's motivations. Redlinger-Grosse et al. (2013) also noted some responses were *nondirective self-disclosures*. Nondirective self-disclosures are responses that avoided influencing the patient's decision (e.g., disclosing that they had never been pregnant and therefore could not answer the patient's question; or disclosing that they did not wish to influence the patient's decision). The researchers noted that nondirective disclosures have a potential drawback "…patients could easily shift their question to, 'But what if you *were* pregnant?' Thus, nondirective self-disclosure of this sort might lead to further patient self-disclosure requests" (p. 465).

Here are several additional examples of the types of self-disclosures genetic counselors have made to their patients:

- "I think that, too. Sometimes all the technology we have today just makes things more difficult. It sure would have been simpler to be pregnant 100 years ago."
- "I think that I would also have a difficult time deciding what to do."
- "I am also a very fact-oriented/information-seeking person, so I can understand your need to know everything possible before making a decision."
- "I don't have children yet, so I don't know first-hand what it's like to have to make a pregnancy decision. But I have walked through similar situations with my patients in the past."

- "I know how hard it can be to deal with insurance companies, too. I've run into roadblocks with them myself. I can help you make some progress in getting this procedure/test covered."
- "My mother had breast cancer, and I remember how difficult it was to live with uncertainty. How is it for you?"
- "I understand that considering religious beliefs is an extremely important part of this process for you. My religion is important to me as well. So, tell me more about what you're thinking."
- Regarding cancer testing: "…I assure you that I'll do everything I can to make the process go as quickly and smoothly as possible…" (Kao 2010, p. 54).
- Regarding a cleft palate scenario in which a mother described the traumatic experience of finding out at birth that her baby was diagnosed with clefting: "… I can imagine that I would feel the same way…" (p. 68); and "From what you shared, it sounds like everyone else in the room was surprised and concerned and you didn't know what was going on [primary empathy]. In this type of situation, my imagination always works overtime [self-disclosure]. Do you think that is what you were doing? [question]" (Kao 2010, p. 69).
- Regarding a patient with Fabry disease: "…I know a little about this kind of pain, from knowing people with sickle cell…" (p. 77); and "I can't imagine dealing with that. It sounds like it affects every part of your life. I would be so afraid and worried about when it was going to happen" (Kao 2010, p. 77).
- Regarding a patient with Long QT: "…Hopefully I can help in any way that I can with your decision and if possible put you in contact with other women with Long QT who have had successful pregnancies" (Kao 2010, p. 87).
- Regarding a patient who is at risk for Huntington disease: "Whenever I see someone to talk about HD, the difficult decision about how and when to tell children is one of the greatest struggles they face …" (p. 100); and "…I would think that if so many people in my family were affected with Huntington's disease that I would be a little afraid to talk about it, too…" (Kao 2010, p. 100).

11.2 Self-Involving Responses

As we said earlier, self-involving responses are direct communications of the genetic counselor's feelings about and reactions to the patient and the counselor-patient relationship in the here-and-now situation. Self-involving responses deal with the immediate counselor/patient relationship, and they are a type of communication about how the relationship is personally affecting either or both the counselor and patient(s). As such, they are more intimate responses. Self-involving responses can be particularly helpful when there are issues preventing the patient from disclosing deeper feelings and thoughts (Hill et al. 2008; Hill et al. 2014; Novotney 2008); they can reduce patient anxiety (McCarthy Veach 2011; Shafran et al. 2017) and help the patient feel cared for (Hill et al. 2014); they are an effective way to enhance your genuineness, likability, and trustworthiness; and they can enhance the relationship (Dewane 2006).

11.2.1 Counselor-Patient Situations that May Prompt Self-Involving Responses

There are several situations in which a genetic counselor may consider using a self-involving response:

- *Session is losing direction.* "I'm concerned we're getting off track here. Can we stop for a minute and see if we can figure out what's going on?"
- *Tension exists between patient and counselor.* Anxiety is a very contagious emotion, that is, it's easy to become anxious when you are with an anxious patient. First, recognize the anxiety, second remain as calm as possible, and then talk about it in a composed and accepting manner. For example, a patient may become very anxious in response to the information you are sharing. In this situation you might say, "I'm concerned that this information is making you very anxious. Can we talk about what's going on?" Some signs that the patient may be tense include behaving dependently, seeking continual reassurance from you, repeating the same questions, shifting the topic when you raise sensitive issues, making jokes, and frequently interrupting you.
- *Trust has not developed.* "I'm concerned that you seem reluctant to talk with me." In cases where trust issues may be due to cultural differences: "I'm concerned that because we are from different cultures, I might unintentionally say something offensive. Please tell me if that happens or if there are other things I can do to help you."
- *There are conflicting agendas.* "I know your sister is here to provide you with support, but right now, I'm concerned that I cannot meet both of your needs at the same time. I wonder if we might speak privately for a few minutes." Or, for example, a patient may be expressing a lot of anger at his primary care provider for failing to recognize early symptoms of cancer. The counselor may say "I can understand your frustration that your cancer was not diagnosed early. But I feel like we're getting stuck here, and I'd like to take some time to talk with you about how genetic testing can help you move forward."
- *You have just given the patient bad news.* After allowing them some time to react initially to the news, say, "I'm sorry. I know this is not what you wanted to hear." This is a time when there's nothing you can say that seems to be adequate for the situation. Let your patient regain some composure and then ask, "Is there something I can do right now?"
- *You sense the patient is under pressure to decide.* "I'm concerned that you may be rushing into a decision before you're ready."
- *The patient seems angry.* "It seems like you might be angry, and I'm concerned that it's getting in the way of our talking right now."
- *The patient shares a painful experience.* For example, a patient is describing her perinatal hospice experience. You may find yourself becoming tearful and could say, "I feel myself tearing up as I listen to you. You must have been in so much pain." In an example from the Kao (2010) study, in which a mother learned in a traumatic way that her baby had clefting, two counselor participants, respectively,

said, "…I'm sorry you had to go through that experience…" (p. 65); and "I'm so sorry that you had that experience with the birth of your child [self-involving response]. Hearing those words from the mouth of the doctor must have been awful [advanced empathy]" (p. 62)
- *When you have made an error*: "This makes me feel terrible. I thought I had [scheduled that appointment for you, included that information in the letter I sent you, etc.]. Please accept my apology" (Klinger et al. 2012).

11.2.2 Some Cautions About Using Self-Involving Responses

Self-involving responses can be risky because they require you to express *your* feelings. You must be aware of what you are feeling and comfortable enough with your reactions to discuss them with your patients. Patients may react negatively to your feelings, or they may ignore them because they're uncomfortable discussing emotions. You may need to redirect patients to your self-involving statement if they move on without commenting (e.g., "Can you tell me what you think about what I just said?"). This will help to clarify confusion or concerns the patient may have about what you expressed.

Moreover, when you are considering using self-involving responses in difficult situations (e.g., a patient is angry with you), you need to first reflect on your reactions including potential countertransference (see Chap. 12), such as taking the anger personally (cf. Schema et al. 2015), before deciding whether sharing your feelings is appropriate (Hill et al. 2014, p. 313; Novotney 2008).
Remember also that some members of certain cultural groups (e.g., Chinese patients) may be uncomfortable discussing feelings directly. In those situations, you might try discussing feelings indirectly (e.g., "Some individuals might feel reluctant talking to a genetic counselor because they would not trust her").

11.2.3 Examples of Genetic Counselor Self-Involving Responses

Here are several examples of the types of self-involving responses genetic counselors have made during sessions:

- "I sense you're angry at something. Is there anything I can do to help you?"
- "I get the feeling there's something I'm not understanding. Can you tell me what's upsetting you?"
- "I hope you've found this information helpful."
- "I'm sorry that we can't be more certain about your risk."
- "I'm concerned about you."

- "I'm sorry this conversation is making you very uncomfortable. I know that you've been given a lot of information all at once."
- "I can see now that termination of your pregnancy is not an option for you, and I apologize if my bringing it up has made you uncomfortable. I just wanted to be sure you were aware of all of your options."
- "I'm terribly sorry to hear that your son died." (This was not related to the consult; he did not die of a genetic condition. You should comment on issues that are extremely important to the patient but are unrelated to the topic at hand).
- The genetic counseling session involved a prenatal patient and her partner. The ultrasound revealed a neural tube defect. Her partner was very hostile and distrustful. The counselor said, "I sense that you're having difficulty believing the information I'm giving you."
- The patient and her partner were seen for genetic counseling to discuss prenatal diagnosis. Her partner was reading a magazine during the session. The counselor said, "I feel somewhat uncomfortable with your reading a magazine. Your input is important in this discussion."
- "I'm worried that you're blaming yourself for your child's condition."
- "I'm concerned that you are not willing to share this information with your sister. I know you do not want to upset her, but I worry about how she might feel if she develops breast cancer and learns that she could have prevented it or found it early. Is there something I can do to help make this easier for you?"
- Regarding cancer testing: I'm sorry the process takes a long time. I can see why you would be anxious" (Kao 2010, p. 60).
- Regarding a patient with Long QT: "… I wish we had a window into knowing for you if it would all work out fine…." (Kao 2010, p. 86).

11.3 Closing Comments

Self-disclosure and self-involving responses are powerful skills that occur less frequently than many of the other counseling skills we've discussed in this text. Because self-referent responses can be quite directive, we recommend that before self-disclosing or expressing your here-and-now reactions to the patient, you ask yourself two questions: "Whose needs are being served by my response?" and "Could I achieve the same results with a less directive intervention?"

Self-referent responses are advanced helping skills. You can expect to become more comfortable and more effective using these skills after you have established solid attending, primary empathy, and questioning skills. Also, your self-reference skills should improve as you see more genetic counseling patients. As with all counseling skills, the most important thing is to genuinely care for your patients.

11.4 Class Activities

Activity 1: Self-Disclosure Vs. Self-Involving Responses (Group Discussion)

Students talk about what they think self-disclosure and self-involving responses are and how the two skills are similar to and differ from each other. Students can first respond to these questions in dyads in order to start the discussion.

Estimated time: 10–15 min.

Activity 2: Self-Disclosure Boundaries (Small Group Discussion)

Students in a small group discuss the following question: What do you think we should sometimes, never, and always disclose to our patients? The instructor summarizes their comments in three columns on the board:

Never	Always	Sometimes

Estimated time: 10–15 min.

Activity 3: Self-Disclosure (Small Group Discussion)

Students discuss each of the following questions. Students can first respond to these questions in dyads in order to begin the discussion.

- When is it ok, if ever, to use a personal story to illustrate an idea to a patient?
- How do you think self-disclosure in genetic counseling differs from self-disclosure outside of genetic counseling?
- What are the potential benefits of self-disclosure?
- What are the potential risks of self-disclosure?
- Have you experienced patients who seemed very interested in your training, or asked a lot of questions about you? How did you respond? How did their questions make you feel?
- Describe additional questions you have been asked by patients that necessitated a self-disclosing response. How did you respond to these questions? How did it make you feel?
- How do you feel about answering a patient's question asking you to self-disclose? What if you have not gone through an experience similar to theirs? What if you have?

- Is genetic counselor self-disclosure a counseling technique or a counseling "mistake" (adapted from Hanson 2005)?

  Estimated time: 30–45 min.

Instructor Note
- This activity could also be done as a journaling exercise.

Activity 4: Self-Involving Responses (Small Group Discussion)

Students discuss each of the following questions. Students can first respond to these questions in dyads in order to start the discussion.

- What would you do if you made a mistake with a patient?
- What would you do if you did not know the answer to a patient's question?
- What would you do if you became tearful/cried with a patient?

  Estimated time: 20 min.

Instructor Note
- This activity could also be done as a journaling exercise.

Activity 5: Brainstorming Nondisclosure Responses to Patient Requests for Self-Disclosure (Group Discussion)

Respond to each of the following patient questions in a non-disclosing way. Formulate three non-disclosing responses for each patient question.

Patient asks:

- Do you go to church?
- Do you have children?
- Are you married?
- What do you think about abortion?
- Do you believe in God?
- Do you think it's wrong to wish my disabled child had never been born?
- Did you drink when you were pregnant?
- Don't you think my doctor should have told me more about the prenatal screening test?
- Do you think I'm being too hasty in my decision to terminate this pregnancy?
- Would you have this test if your family history looked like mine?
- Would you have a mastectomy if you knew you had the "BRCA gene"?

  Estimated time: 20–30 min.

Activity 6a: Low-Level Self-Reference Skills Model

The instructor and a volunteer genetic counseling patient engage in a role-play in which the counselor demonstrates poor self-disclosure and self-involving behaviors. Students observe and take notes of examples of poor self-reference behaviors.

Estimated time: 10 min.

Process

Students discuss their examples of poor behaviors and the impact of the counselor's poor skills on the patient. The patient can offer her or his impressions of the counselor's behaviors after the other students have made their comments. The instructor could divide the group of students and have half focus on counselor behaviors and half focus on patient behaviors.

Estimated time: 15 min.

Instructor Notes

- One option is to continue with a role-play used earlier in the class so the genetic counselor can more quickly move to self-reference skills.
- Students may have difficulty differentiating self-disclosure from self-involving responses. The instructor should assist them in categorizing the responses they observe in the role-play. One issue that may come up is that the genetic counselor's intended response is perceived differently by the patient and/or the observers.

Activity 6b: High-Level Self-Reference Skills Model

The instructor and the same volunteer repeat the same role-play; only this time the genetic counselor displays good self-reference skills. Students take notes of examples of good behaviors.

Estimated time: 15 min.

Process

Students discuss their examples of good self-reference behaviors and the impact of the counselor's behaviors on the patient. They also contrast this role-play to the previous role-play. The instructor could divide the group of students and have half focus on counselor behaviors and half focus on patient behaviors.

Estimated time: 15 min.

Instructor Note

- Students could work together in think-pair-share dyads to identify examples of counselor self-reference and their impact on the patient.

Activity 7: Small Group Role-Plays

Working in small groups, students volunteer to be patient and genetic counselor. The students read their roles silently. Then the student playing the genetic *counselor* reads her or his role aloud. Next the students engage in a 10- to 15-min role-play. If the student playing the genetic counselor gets stuck, stop the role-play and ask the group [except the patient] to brainstorm possible ways to handle the situation. Resume the role-play, so the student can try out some of the group's suggestions. Ask the group to provide feedback to the counselor at the end of the role-play and have a general discussion about how to handle each type of situation. Allow about 10–15 min to process each role-play.

Patient Role I
You are a 37-year-old woman who is discussing a positive BRCA result with the genetic counselor. During this session, you say to the counselor, "Well, would you wait to have surgery until after you are done having children?"

Genetic Counselor Role I
Your patient is a 37-year-old woman who is discussing a positive BRCA result with you. During this session, she says….

Patient Role II
You are a 35-year-old who is talking about whether to pursue testing for familial colon cancer. You are afraid that you will die of cancer just like your father (but are embarrassed to admit this unless the counselor brings it up). Instead you repeatedly ask the counselor for advice about what you should do.

Genetic Counselor Role II
Your patient is a 35-year-old who is discussing whether to pursue testing for familial colon cancer. The patient does not have a clear idea of what she/he wishes to do, and you suspect this is connected to some underlying issue. You say...

Patient Role III
You are here to see the genetic counselor for cancer counseling as you have a strong family history of breast cancer. Your educational background is very limited and you have not been able to understand everything the counselor is telling you. However, you nod your head and smile and pretend that you do. If the counselor brings this up with you, don't admit right away that you do not understand.

Genetic Counselor Role III
Your patient is here to see you for cancer counseling as she has a strong family history of breast cancer. Your patient has a very limited educational background, and you do not believe she has understood everything you've told her. You say...

Estimated time: 90 min.

Instructor Note

- The instructor may want to encourage students to attempt self-disclosure and/or self-involving responses during the role-plays, as they otherwise may exhaust the time allotted with other sorts of responses.

Activity 8: Triad Role-Plays

Students practice self-disclosure and self-involving skills in 15–20-min role-plays taking turns as counselor, patient, and observer. Allow another 15 min of feedback after each role-play. The students should focus on using good helping behaviors. In these role-plays, the counselor and observer will not have advanced knowledge of patient-counselor dynamics. As with triad role-plays in other chapters, only the person playing the patient will fully know patient background and issues.

Criteria for Evaluating Counselor Self-Reference Behaviors
Well-timed
Used sparingly
Concise
Intended to meet patient goals
Appropriate depth/intimacy
Follow-up with empathy
Estimated time: 90–105 min.

Instructor Note

- The observer or counselor may wish to stop the role-play if the counselor is obviously stuck. The triad [except the patient] can then engage in a brief conversation about the patient's dynamics, issues, etc., to help the counselor. Then the counselor and patient resume the role-play.

Process
Discuss in the large group: How was it to do this exercise? What are you learning about self-reference behaviors in general? About yourself? What questions do you still have about these skills?

Estimated time: 20 min.

11.5 Written Exercises

Exercise 1: Patient Self-Disclosure Questions

For each of the following patients, generate a list of all the questions you can think of that the patient might ask you to disclose about:

Pregnant adolescent—pregnancy affected with multiple anomalies.
30-year-old patient—tested positive for HD.

Parents whose 4-year-old son was diagnosed with autism.
35-year-old woman whose mother and sister died from ovarian cancer.

Next select five of the questions you generated, and write a self-disclosure response to each one as if you were speaking to the patient(s) directly. Then write a nondisclosure response to each of the same five questions as if you were speaking directly to the patient(s).

Exercise 2: Indirect Self-Disclosure

Write three or four paragraphs responding to these questions:

- What do patients see when they look at you?
- What might your physical characteristics mean to different patients?
- What do you think your characteristics and actions might communicate to patients?

Exercise 3: Self-Disclosure and Self-Involving Responses

Read each of the 14 patient statements listed in Chap. 8, Exercise 2, and give one self-disclosure response and one self-involving response for each statement. Write your responses as if you were actually talking to the patient.

[*Hint*: You may have to infer more knowledge about the patient in order to formulate your responses].

Example
For the example of the 40-year-old man at risk for Huntington disease cited in Chap. 8, Exercise 2:

Self-disclosure: "I'd be very scared to learn that I had the gene. I wonder if that's how you are feeling, too?"
Self-Involving: "I'm concerned that you may be pursuing testing before you're ready."

Exercise 4: Role-Play

Engage in a 30-min role-play of a genetic counseling session with a classmate. The role-play can be based on a patient you saw in a clinic, or it can be a made-up patient situation. During the role-play focus on all the helping skills you've learned so far. Try to include at least one self-disclosure and one self-involving response.

Audio-record the role-play. Next transcribe the role-play and critique your work. Use the following method for transcribing the session:

Counselor	Patient	Self-critique	Instructor
Key phrases of dialogue	Key phrases	Comment on your own responses	Will provide feedback on your responses

Create a brief summary:

1. Briefly describe patient *demographics* (e.g., age, gender, ethnicity, socioeconomic status, relationship status), and *reason* for seeking genetic counseling.
2. Identify *two* things you said/did during the role play that were effective, and *two* things you could have done differently:

Give the recording, transcript/self-critique, and summary to the instructor who will provide feedback.

[*Hint*: This assignment encourages self-reflective practice regarding your clinical performance. The goal is not to do a perfect session. Rather the goal is to assess the extent to which you can accurately assess your psychosocial counseling skills. You will gain more from this exercise if you refrain from scripting what you plan to say as the counselor].

References

Audet C, Everall RD. Counsellor self-disclosure: client-informed implications for practice. Couns Psychother Res. 2003;3:223–31.

Audet CT. Client perspectives of therapist self-disclosure: violating boundaries or removing barriers? Couns Psychol Q. 2011;24:85–100.

Balcom JR, Veach PM, Bemmels H, Redlinger-Grosse K, LeRoy BS. When the topic is you: genetic counselor responses to prenatal patients' requests for self-disclosure. J Genet Couns. 2013;22:358–73.

Bonovitz C. The illusion of certainty in self-disclosure: commentary on paper by Helen K. Gediman. Psychoanal Dialogues. 2006;16:293–304.

Burkard AW, Knox S, Groen M, Perez M, Hess SA. European American therapist self-disclosure in cross-cultural counseling. J Couns Psychol. 2006;53:15–25.

Clark K. Life as a pregnant genetic counselor. J Genet Couns. 2010;19:235–7.

Clark K. Life as a pregnant genetic counselor: take two. J Genet Couns. 2012;2:27–30.

Dewane CJ. Use of self: a primer revisited. Clin Soc Work J. 2006;34:543–58.

Glessner HD, VandenLangenberg E, Veach PM, LeRoy BS. Are genetic counselors and GLBT patients "on the same page"? An investigation of attitudes, practices, and genetic counseling experiences. J Genet Couns. 2012;21:326–36.

Hanson J. Should your lips be zipped? How therapist self-disclosure and non-disclosure affects clients. Couns Psychother Res. 2005;5:96–104.

Henretty JR, Levitt HM. The role of therapist self-disclosure in psychotherapy: a qualitative review. Clin Psychol Rev. 2010;30:63–77.

Hill CE, Sim W, Spangler P, Stahl J, Sullivan C, Teyber E. Therapist immediacy in brief psychotherapy: case study II. Psychother Theory Res Pract Train. 2008;45:298–315.

Hill CE, Gelso CJ, Chui H, Spangler PT, Hummel A, Huang T, et al. To be or not to be immediate with clients: the use and perceived effects of immediacy in psychodynamic/interpersonal psychotherapy. Psychother Res. 2014;24:299–315.

Kao JH. Walking in your patient's shoes: An investigation of genetic counselor empathy in clinical practice. University of Minnesota; 2010. Retrieved from the University of Minnesota Digital Conservancy, http://hdl.handle.net/11299/96724.

Kessler S. Psychological aspects of genetic counseling. VIII. Suffering and countertransference. J Genet Couns. 1992;1:303–8.

Klinger RS, Ladany N, Kulp LE. It's too late to apologize: therapist embarrassment and shame. Couns Psychol. 2012;40:554–74.

McCarthy Veach P. Reflections on the meaning of clinician self-reference: are we speaking the same language? Psychotherapy. 2011;48:349–58.

McCarthy P, Oakes L. Blank screen or open book? A reminder about balancing self-disclosure in psychotherapy. Voices: Art Sci Psychother. 1998;34:60–8.

Menezes MA. Commentary on "life as a pregnant genetic counselor: take two". J Genet Couns. 2012;21:31–4.

Menezes MA, Hodgson JM, Sahhar MA, Aitken M, Metcalfe SA. "It's challenging on a personal level"—exploring the 'lived experience' of Australian and Canadian prenatal genetic counselors. J Genet Couns. 2010;19:640–52.

Novotney A. Go ahead, let it out: how to find the right moment to express emotions with clients. Monit Psychol. 2008;39:44–6.

Paine AL, Veach PM, MacFarlane IM, Thomas B, Ahrens M, LeRoy BS. "What would you do if you were me?" effects of counselor self-disclosure versus non-disclosure in a hypothetical genetic counseling session. J Genet Couns. 2010;19:570–84.

Peters E, Veach PM, Ward EE, LeRoy BS. Does receiving genetic counseling impact genetic counselor practice? J Genet Couns. 2004;13:387–402.

Peterson ZD. More than a mirror: the ethics of therapist self-disclosure. Psychother Theory Res Pract Train. 2002;39:21–31.

Redlinger-Grosse K, Veach PM, MacFarlane IM. What would you say? Genetic counseling graduate students' and counselors' hypothetical responses to patient requested self-disclosure. J Genet Couns. 2013;22:455–68.

Sarangi S, Bennert K, Howell L, Clarke A, Harper P, Gray J. (2004). Initiation of reflective frames in counseling for Huntington's disease predictive testing. J Genet Couns. 2004;13:135–55.

Schema L, McLaughlin M, Veach PM, LeRoy BS. Clearing the air: a qualitative investigation of genetic counselors' experiences of counselor-focused patient anger. J Genet Couns. 2015;24:717–31. https://doi.org/10.1007/s10897-014-9815-3.

Shafran N, Kivlighan DM, Gelso CJ, Bhatia A, Hill CE. Therapist immediacy: the association with working alliance, real relationship, session quality, and time in psychotherapy. Psychother Res. 2017;27:734–48.

Simone DH, McCarthy P, Skay CL. An investigation of client and counselor variables that influence likelihood of counselor self-disclosure. J Couns Dev. 1998;76:174–82.

Sweezy M. Not confidential: therapist considerations in self-disclosure. Smith Coll Stud Soc Work. 2005;75:81–91.

Thomas BC, Veach PM, LeRoy BS. Is self-disclosure part of the genetic counselor's clinical role? J Genet Couns. 2006;15:163–77.

VandenLangenberg E, Veach PM, LeRoy BS, Glessner HD. Gay, lesbian, and bisexual patients' recommendations for genetic counselors: a qualitative investigation. J Genet Couns. 2012;21:741–7.

Ziv-Beiman S. Therapist self-disclosure as an integrative intervention. J Psychother Integr. 2013;23:59–74.

Chapter 12
Genetic Counseling Dynamics: Transference, Countertransference, Distress, Burnout, and Compassion Fatigue

Learning Objectives

1. Define patient transference.
2. Identify ways to respond to transference.
3. Define genetic counselor countertransference.
4. Identify strategies for managing countertransference.
5. Define distress, burnout, and compassion fatigue.
6. Distinguish compassion fatigue from distress and burnout.
7. Identify distress, burnout, and compassion fatigue-coping strategies.

To be an effective genetic counselor, you must be aware of issues that impact your relationship with patients. This chapter discusses several critical issues that affect genetic counseling relationships: (1) transference and countertransference, (2) counselor distress and burnout, and (3) compassion fatigue. Transference and countertransference are primarily (but not always) unconscious dynamics, and they emerge within the relationship itself, while distress, compassion fatigue, and burnout are conditions that develop in the counselor and spill over into genetic counseling relationships. You will see that strategies for addressing these issues share several similarities, in particular, self-awareness and self-reflection.

12.1 Transference and Countertransference

The primary focus of this section is countertransference, a phenomenon in which your own needs and experiences can affect your clinical work. Sometimes countertransference occurs in response to patient transference. Therefore, we begin by briefly discussing patient transference.

P. McCarthy Veach et al., *Facilitating the Genetic Counseling Process*,
https://doi.org/10.1007/978-3-319-74799-6_12

12.1.1 Definition of Patient Transference

Transference is an unconscious way patients relate to the genetic counselor based on their own history of relating to others (Djurdjinovic 2009; Weil 2010). Transference concerns how the patient perceives the counselor and how the patient behaves toward the counselor. For instance, patients may project onto the counselor attitudes, roles, and expectations based on previous encounters with others. Transference is a patient's misperception of the counselor that can occur from the first moment of contact and even in anticipation of the genetic counseling session. An important aspect of transference is that the patient's feelings and reactions tend to be overreactions to the reality of the situation. Because transference often is an unconscious process, patients are unaware they are experiencing it (Djurdjinovic 2009). It's normal to have transference (e.g., experiencing an immediate attraction to or dislike of someone for no apparent reason). Upon some reflection, however, you realize it's because the individual reminds you of a family member or friend.

Transference tends to be stronger when the counseling relationship is longer, more in-depth, and/or particularly distressing; and it may involve positive affect (e.g., feelings of affection or dependency), negative affect (e.g., feelings of hostility and aggression), or mixed affect (e.g., ambivalence toward those in authority). Patients may also experience cultural transference, relating to you by transferring positive or negative feelings from prior experiences with individuals from your cultural group. Indeed "…transference and countertransference always take place between two or more people who have a culture, ethnic and racial identity, class status, and the like" (Lewis 2010 p. 215).

Patients who have transference reactions toward you may perceive you in one or more of five ways (Watkins 1985):

- Counselor as an ideal: You are the perfect individual. Patient behaviors may include excessively complimenting you, and/or agreeing with everything you say. Similarly aged patients, for instance, may identify with your seemingly perfect life.
- Counselor as seer: You have all the right answers. Patient behaviors may include repeatedly asking you what you would do. Keep in mind, however, that patients may have cultural values which lead them to place health-care providers in a position of authority (cf. Cura 2015). In such cases, their behaviors may not be transference but rather a reflection of common attitudes from their culture.
- Counselor as nurturer: You are their source of strength. Patient behaviors may include acting helpless, displaying excessive crying and emotionality, and making urgent requests/demands for solutions to their problems.
- Counselor as frustrater: You are the spoiler of their experience. Patients may be excessively defensive, have minimal to no self-disclosure, and inappropriately blame you for the bad news you communicate (cf. Schema et al. 2015).
- Counselor as nonentity: You are an inanimate figure with no feelings, unique perspectives, or needs. Patient behaviors may include topic shifting, talking

nonstop, and dismissing/ignoring your interpretations and reactions. For instance, sometimes in prenatal genetic counseling with couples, one of the partners will use their cell phone or laptop computer during the session (cf. Lafans et al. 2003).

In summary, patient transference is based on patient misperceptions, and it results in overreactions to the reality of the situation. Keep in mind, however, that not all "first impressions" are transference (invalid perceptions). For example, when you nonverbally and verbally express interest, care, and acceptance, most patients will accurately view you as someone to whom they can relate.

Examples of Patient Transference

- A 40-year-old patient had prenatal testing that revealed Down syndrome. The patient terminated the pregnancy by induction of labor. The genetic counselor gave the patient the test results and provided some initial counseling over the phone. The patient made an excessive number of phone calls to the counselor and wrote her several letters. She requested a follow-up session but would not come into the building, asking instead that the genetic counselor have lunch with her. None of the genetic counselor's suggestions or referrals to other health professionals would work. The patient continued to be helpless and was not open to any suggestions.
- A patient was seen for genetic counseling regarding a positive family history of breast cancer. The genetic counselor called to give the patient the results of her BRCA testing, and the patient acted as if she did not remember meeting with the counselor. The counselor gave the patient some information about their last visit and then asked if the patient remembered her. The patient replied in a very hostile manner, "How could I forget you!" The patient was defensive and would not disclose any feelings about the test results.
- A patient was the mother of a 2 1/2-year-old child newly diagnosed with Angelman syndrome. The child had a history of moderate-to-severe developmental delay, no speech and language, and seizures. The mother was a single parent and was managing a career and this child fairly well. She had, however, an exceptionally intense reaction to the diagnosis, especially the mental impairment component. She displayed excessive crying and emotionality and wanted the genetic counselor to be a nurturer. She called several times with urgent questions and had a need to go over the information repeatedly. She requested another appointment to go over the information yet again.
- A couple had an intensely negative reaction to a geneticist who was present during their counseling session in which a postnatal diagnosis of achondroplasia was given. They wrote a letter to the head of the hospital complaining bitterly about his lack of compassion, when in fact he had behaved appropriately and in a caring manner.

- A 33-year-old patient was referred because her prenatal screening showed that her risk for Down syndrome was 1 in 44. The risk for Down syndrome in her last pregnancy was 1 in 180, but she reported that everything "turned out perfect." Although she had never met with a genetic counselor before, she assumed the genetic counselor was a "spoiler" of her experience. She hardly listened during the session and kept saying, "Those blood tests are always wrong anyway." She even refused to have an ultrasound because she didn't want to be told any more "fake bad news."
- A fairly common transference situation involves patients who come to the clinic completely exhausted or enraged due to a difficult commute or difficulty parking at the clinic. Although the travel experience is not without tribulations, the patients usually have transferred their concerns about undergoing a genetic consultation. They may later say that getting to the office was not that big of a deal; they were just nervous about the visit.

12.1.2 Responding to Patient Transference

There is no single way to respond to patient transference. Depending on the situation and patient, you might try one of the following strategies:

- *Simply accept it*. Handle transference feelings as you would any type of patient feeling. Let patients express the feelings and allow them to either take back their feelings or continue to express them (Schema et al. 2015).
- *Recognize it*. Recognizing that transference may be happening allows you to understand it and avoid overreacting to patient distortions (Djurdjinovic 2009; Schema et al. 2015). Clues that transference is happening include your feelings of confusion and discomfort and your belief that the patient's behavior contains some amount of distortion and misperception (Djurdjinovic 2009).
- *Decide whether to address it*. You should be careful about drawing patient attention to transference because, "A hasty decision to correct can be disruptive to the working relationship…the resulting confusion may elicit a more intense response from the counselee" (Djurdjinovic 2009, p. 145). Given your time constraints and the scope of what you must accomplish, genetic counseling may not be the appropriate venue for dealing with transference. You might, however, choose to gently address mild expressions of transference in order to decrease their impact on the session. For example, a patient says she's angry that you cannot absolutely ensure a healthy child based on prenatal test results. You might respond, "I wonder if part of what you're angry about is that you think I'm giving you the run-around, just like the other medical professionals you've seen."
- *Ask clarifying questions*. For example, "You seem really angry. Can you tell me what's bothering you?" This response is a prelude to advanced empathy (see Chap. 8), but first explore the patient's attitudes and give the patient the opportunity to do her or his own interpreting.

- *Reflect transference feelings*. For example, "You said you don't want to discuss your infertility history because you think it may make *me* uncomfortable?" Further discussion might prompt the patient to acknowledge that negative reactions from family members have made her wary of talking about it with anyone. You could then assure her you can handle whatever she wishes to disclose.
- *Interpret transference feelings directly*. For example, "Sometimes when people feel they've been sharing too much, they get uncomfortable about their relationship with that person. Do you suppose this is happening here?"

While some authors believe transference (and countertransference) is a part of every relationship, including the genetic counseling relationship (e.g., Kessler 1992; Reeder et al. 2017), others believe its occurrence depends more upon the depth of the relationship that forms and on the interplay of the personalities of the genetic counselor and patient (Djurdjinovic 2009). Regardless of whether transference occurs in all relationships, it's important to keep in mind that not every patient reaction is transference. Patients may be responding appropriately to the situation and to you (e.g., feeling annoyed if you're late to the session, feeling confused if your presentation of information is too complicated or rushed), and/or behaving in accordance with their cultural beliefs (e.g., that health-care providers are authorities who will tell them what to do). If, however, you have not made a mistake, cultural differences are not apparent, and the patient's reaction is greatly exaggerated (e.g., being furious because you're a couple of minutes late), transference may be occurring.

12.1.3 Definition of Counselor Countertransference

Countertransference has been described as the same phenomenon as patient transference, but in the opposite direction (Cerney 1985). Countertransference is "an inevitable and potentially valuable aspect of clinical interactions…[and it] refers to conscious and unconscious emotions, fantasies, behaviors, perceptions, and psychological defenses that the genetic counselor experiences as a response to any aspect of the genetic counseling situation" (Weil 2010, p. 176). Countertransference can include emotional reactions and projections toward patients that may not be particularly appropriate to the current genetic counseling relationship (Djurdjinovic 2009; Reeder et al. 2017; Weil 2010). For example, you might find yourself feeling angry with a patient who took drugs during a pregnancy when you have struggled with infertility. Or, when a patient who is around your age tells you she was diagnosed with ovarian cancer, you may find yourself asking questions because of your own anxiety—"Did you have any symptoms? How did you find out you had it?" Similar to transference, countertransference involves misperceptions (e.g., viewing a patient as too dependent when he or she is not) and overreactions (e.g., anger over a patient behavior that most counselors would be able to take in stride).

Causes of Countertransference

Why does countertransference occur? You and your patients may be similar or different in any number of ways such as your values, behaviors, attitudes, language, physical appearance, age, gender, etc. These similarities and differences affect the ways in which you identify with the patient. Countertransference can occur when you have extreme over-identification with a patient (you perceive the patient as "just like me"). When you over-identify, you become wrapped up in your patient's situation and have difficulty distinguishing where the patient's feelings stop and yours begin. For example, you may find yourself thinking about and feeling very involved with a patient whose child is affected with muscular dystrophy and is the same age as your son. The more you perceive yourself as similar to a patient, the greater the chance of over-identification.

Countertransference can also occur when you experience extreme disidentification (you perceive the patient as "nothing like me") (Watkins 1985). When you disidentify, you feel disconnected, disengaged, and possibly even become hostile and rejecting toward the patient. For instance, a patient declines testing for colon cancer, despite a very suggestive family history. You may consider his decision to be irresponsible and find yourself pulling away from him. The more you perceive yourself as dissimilar to a patient, the greater the chance of dis-identification.

Counselor countertransference is sometimes a reaction to patient transference. For example, some patients may expect you to be a nurturer, and their demands prompt you to engage in rejecting countertransference. In addition, countertransference may be prompted by a particular type of patient (e.g., terminally ill or cognitively impaired) and/or by certain genetic counseling situations that "push your buttons" (e.g., sex selection, presymptomatic testing of minors), or it may be a more habitual type of reaction you have toward all or most of your patients (e.g., distancing from patients' strong emotions, being overly protective, etc.).

A growing literature in genetic counseling suggests many potential triggers of genetic counselor countertransference. These include the patient characteristics such as behavior or appearance (Reeder et al. 2017; Weil 2010); general similarity to the patient as well as medical/genetic similarity (Reeder et al. 2017); patient emotional responses (Weil 2010) such as anger (Reeder et al. 2017; Schema et al. 2015); patient's use of defenses (Weil 2010); discomfort with disease, disability, and loss (Geller et al. 2010; Reeder et al. 2017; Weil 2010; Wells et al. 2016); patient behaves differently from genetic counselor expectations (Reeder et al. 2017); giving bad news (Mathiesen 2012; Reeder et al. 2017; Weil 2010); discomfort asking patients about certain topics such as psychiatric conditions (Monaco et al. 2010); personal life events that are similar to patients' situations, such as pregnancy (Menezes 2012; Menezes et al. 2010; Sahhar 2010); pregnancy termination (e.g., Anonymous 2008); birth of a child with a disability (e.g., Bellcross 2012); personal health issues (e.g., Glessner 2012); and health issues in a loved one (e.g., Matloff 2006).

Cultural issues may also lead to countertransference reactions. "Working with patients who differ from the genetic counselor with respect to ethnicity, culture, religion, sexual orientation, socioeconomic status, and/or disability may raise issues of countertransference. Stereotypes, fears, misunderstanding, or misinterpretation may occur when the genetic counselor confronts a situation in which, to a greater or lesser extent, his or her own background and experience provide less of a guide for understanding the patient's beliefs, values, expectations, and responses (Weil 2010, pp. 183–184). For instance, a female genetic counselor may respond negatively to the authoritarian role of the male in some cultures (e.g., English-speaking husband dismisses the translator saying that it's not important for his wife to understand the conversation as he makes medical decisions for her).

Effects of Countertransference

Countertransference can have both negative and positive consequences. You should be particularly concerned about negative effects. One possible negative consequence is that countertransference can interfere with your empathy for a patient. You may learn something from a patient that triggers your own experiences, and soon you have stopped listening to your patient and are busy thinking and feeling about your own situation (Kessler 1992). You may believe your thoughts and feelings are about your patient, but they are actually (and usually unconsciously) about you. Additionally, your patient's situation may reopen current or old hurts, and because this is painful, you may avoid exploring the patient's feelings, especially if your typical coping style is to distance yourself emotionally (Kessler 1992; Reeder et al. 2017). One possible positive consequence of countertransference is that the triggering of experiences from your past might give you increased empathy for patients (to the extent that your experiences are similar to theirs). As already stated, however, there is always the risk that you may listen less carefully to patients and instead impose your experience on them.

As with transference, you must be careful to distinguish countertransference from situations in which your reactions are a realistic response to your patient and her or his behavior (Cerney 1985). For example, it's natural to feel sad when a patient is grieving over a pregnancy loss. If you become quite distraught over your patient's situation, however, it might indicate that you have unresolved feelings about a past loss. It's also natural to feel irritated at a patient who lies about being at risk in order to get a genetic test. But if you become very angry with this patient, it might suggest you're acting from past experiences where you felt manipulated or controlled by others (see self-involving responses in Chap. 11, for a more extensive discussion of realistic counselor reactions). It's also important to distinguish countertransference from your natural, empathic response to patients. Empathy, as discussed in Chaps. 4 and 8, involves the ability to experience patient feelings as if they were your own while maintaining enough distance to realize they are not your feelings. Empathy also involves the ability to listen to the patient's story without imposing your own assumptions.

Reeder et al. (2017) surveyed clinical genetic counselors about their countertransference experiences. They identified four types of negative effects: disruption in rapport building, over-identification, conversation does not reach its fullest potential, and counselor is drained emotionally. They also identified one positive type of effect, namely, repaired empathy (a better relationship develops between the genetic counselor and patient).

Types of Countertransference

Kessler (1992) describes two primary types of countertransference in genetic counseling:

- Projective identification: Projective identification occurs when you mistakenly believe your feelings are your patient's feelings. So, for instance, if you feel a great deal of discomfort, but you think this is what your patient is feeling, you might encourage the patient to focus on less distressing ideas or images. When this happens, you will only, at best, have shallow empathy, because you will avoid going deeply into feelings that are too upsetting to you. Projective identification also occurs whenever you have the misperception that you understand exactly what a patient is going through because you've had a similar experience.
- Associative countertransference: In associative countertransference, your patient's experience taps into your inner self, and you begin to focus on your own thoughts, feelings, and sensations. Like projective identification, associative countertransference is triggered by your own past or current problems or situations that are similar to your patient's. A major difference, however, is that you do not think your feelings are the patient's feelings. You know they are your feelings. When you experience associative countertransference, you find yourself losing focus. Your attention shifts from the patient to yourself. You may find yourself daydreaming about your situation and realize you haven't fully heard anything the patient has said for a few seconds or longer. Associative countertransference can be quite common. As Kessler (1992) points out, genetic counselors must deal with patients whose situations are similar to difficulties and problems the counselors are currently experiencing or experienced in the past. He further states, "Bad things do happen to genetic counselors. But even if they do not, we are as vulnerable as the next person to experience loss and pain. Disappointment, loss, feelings of being rejected and misunderstood, of failure, embarrassment, hurt, and so on are ubiquitous human phenomena. No one is exempt" (p. 304).

Watkins (1985) identified four types of countertransference that can either occur occasionally, with some patients, or can be more pervasive, occurring with many patients:

- Overprotective countertransference: You regard some or most patients as child-like and in need of great care and protection, so you cushion the information you give ("Most of the time the results of this test will be normal."), or you qualify your interpretations ("You told me that you are very angry, but I wonder if you are also sad. I'm probably off base with that. It was just a guess. Forget I even mentioned it."), or you don't allow patients to experience and express their painful feelings ("Everything will be OK. It will be fine.") (Watkins 1985). Other evidence that you may be overprotective includes talking in a low voice and using physical gestures such as patting patients on the back, hugging them, or patting their hands, all of which can be perceived as infantilizing (Watkins 1985). An additional aspect of overprotective countertransference is worrying excessively about a patient, even to the point of obsession (dreaming about the patient, looking for reasons to contact the patient, etc.).

- Benign countertransference: This type of countertransference is often due to an intense need to be liked by patients or to a fear of strong patient affect, especially anger (Watkins 1985). To prevent being disliked or to avoid strong affect, you create an atmosphere that is the same across all patients and situations, one that is characterized by shallow exploration of emotions; by optimistic, cheerful interchanges; and by limited consideration of negative information or issues (Watkins 1985). There may also be a lot of extraneous chitchat as you attempt to be more like a friend than a genetic counselor or focus on facts and figures rather than exploring emotional issues.
- Rejecting countertransference: Like overprotective countertransference, you may regard some or most patients as dependent and needy, but you react punitively, becoming aloof or cold, and behave in ways that create distance between you, either because you fear the demands patients might place on you or you're afraid of being responsible for their welfare (Watkins 1985). Examples of distancing behaviors are blunt explanations ("You know that you should be having screening because your family history puts you at a really high risk for developing cancer."), and dismissive responses to patient requests ("That's your decision. I'm not you."). The following two examples of rejecting countertransference involve genetic counseling student statements made during supervision: "My explanation of the genetic condition wouldn't have been so confusing if the patient had just given me a chance to explain!"; and "I don't know where she got the idea that I wanted her to terminate her pregnancy… She was just looking for someone to tell her what to do." In the first example, it's important to note that the patient did give the counselor the chance to explain, and in the second example, the patient gave no indication that she wanted to be told what to do.
- Hostile countertransference: This type of countertransference occurs when you dislike something about your patient (e.g., a mannerism, a physical characteristic, an attitude, a value), and attempting to be as unlike the patient as possible, you try to distance yourself in both overt and covert ways (Watkins 1985). You go even further than with rejecting countertransference, perhaps making harsh statements (e.g., "I already told you that I'm not the one making this decision!"). Your attitude is that the patient deserves what she/he is getting (Watkins 1985). Even if you would never say these sorts of things to the patients, if you are thinking them, you probably are experiencing countertransference, and it may "leak out" in subtle ways. Hostile countertransference may be more common in genetic counselors who are experiencing some degree of distress and/or burnout. Perhaps

they are working repeatedly with a patient population that is very needy and for whom there is little room for change in the system (e.g., a medical assistance population, new immigrant populations).

Reeder et al. (2017) conducted the first comprehensive study solely focused on clinical genetic counselors' countertransference tendencies. They found three types of countertransference:

- *Control*: "counselor reactions motivated by a desire to exert undue influence over ambiguity, affect (patient's emotions or one's own emotions), and/or the genetic counseling process" (p. 938)
- *Conflict Avoidance*: "counselor actions motivated by a desire to prevent conflict due to emotions that might be triggered in patients (e.g., anger) and/or in the counselor (e.g., insecurity)...the genetic counselor may avoid being direct, respond defensively to perceived criticism, omit certain topics, skip over certain topics, and/or minimize certain topics" (p. 938)
- *Directiveness*: "pertaining to actions motivated by a counselor's desire to 'push' patients regarding how quickly to decide or what to decide, and to either press them to decide on their own or to step in and do some of the decisional work for them" (p. 940)

They also found one type of strategy for managing countertransference:

- *Self-regulation*: "counselor actions motivated by a desire to manage [countertransference] through intentional self-reflection/awareness of ones' [countertransference] and through setting boundaries" (p. 940)

12.1.4 Behaviors that May Indicate Countertransference

Countertransference (and transference) can be very difficult to identify and resolve, especially because it occurs primarily at an unconscious level. You may have to carefully observe and explore your overt and covert behaviors to detect its occurrence.

The following genetic counselor behaviors may indicate countertransference, especially if you exhibit more than one of them:

- Engage in compulsive advice giving (Weil 2010).
- Have unusually strong feelings toward a particular patient (Reeder et al. 2017; Weil 2010).
- Have "rescuer" fantasies, that is, believing you will be able to help a patient, even when others have failed (Weil 2010), or when there is no resolution for the situation (e.g., patient is at risk for a familial cancer).
- Dread a session or are overly eager for a session with a particular patient (Hofsess and Tracey 2010).
- Feel sleepy during the session (Hofsess and Tracey 2010).
- Avoid or dislike patient feelings, especially negative feelings directed toward you. You may avoid feelings by showing disapproval (frowning, interrupting, etc.), using fewer reflections, and/or giving excessive information (Weil 2010).

- Engage in self-disclosure that is of questionable value/relevance to the genetic counseling goals (Balcom et al. 2013; Menezes 2012; Peters et al. 2004; Redlinger-Grosse et al. 2013; Thomas et al. 2006; Weil 2010). For example, Thomas et al. (2006) investigated genetic counselor self-disclosure and concluded that "Evidence of possible countertransference is suggested by some participants' comments that they 'tried not to give in' to disclosure when it was prompted by their identification with a patient" (p. 174).

Reeder et al.'s (2017) sample of clinical genetic counselors described six major types of behaviors that demonstrated their countertransference: being self-focused, projecting feelings onto the patient, experiencing intense emotional reactions to patients, being overly invested, counselor disengagement, and counselor physical reactions (e.g., sweating).

Hofsess and Tracey (2010) identified a variety of therapist behaviors that suggest countertransference. Most applicable to genetic counseling are the following:

- Daydreams about relationships or events related to client
- Loses all neutrality and sides with a client
- Treats client in a punitive manner during session
- Acts flirtatious or feels sexual attraction to a client
- Engages in too much self-disclosure
- Expresses hostility toward or about a client
- Acts in a submissive way with the client during session
- Dreads seeing a client
- Feels protective of a client
- Expresses a need to be respected, appreciated, and liked by the client
- Acts defensive when discussing a client with a supervisor
- Rushes in to solve a client's problem
- Behaves as if he or she were "somewhere else" during the session
- Is apathetic toward a client in session
- Feels hurt by something a client says or does during the session
- Experiences anger and frustration when with a client
- Experiences envy, guilt, or pity when with a client

Remember, generally speaking, any behaviors, thoughts, feelings, or attitudes, that either are out of character for you or are considered by others (e.g., your supervisor, the patient) to be ineffective or inappropriate, could signal countertransference.

Countertransference Examples

- The genetic counselor saw a family with whom she shared many similarities. She knew that she was over-identifying with this family and the counseling (for her) was much more intense emotionally. The patient was a 14-year-old healthy girl. The patient had a brother who died at age 10 of Hunter syndrome (MPSII). The patient's mother brought the patient to a clinic for carrier testing for Hunter syndrome.

The genetic counselor also had a 14-year-old daughter and a 10-year-old son. The counselor felt very strongly that this patient should not be tested, but she tried to present the pros and cons objectively. She felt a need and desire to protect this 14-year-old girl. The patient's mother was clearly still struggling with her grief and was very fragile. The mother's reasons for testing all seemed to relate to her own needs rather than to her daughter's needs.

- A genetic counselor with a history of infertility met with a patient who went through infertility treatment, and the counselor asked the patient several questions about procedures, feelings, and how the patient got pregnant—all unrelated to the indication for genetic question but of interest to the genetic counselor.
- A genetic counselor who recently had a baby met with a patient who had a 6-month-old baby and was pregnant again. The genetic counselor commented that it must be a shock to be pregnant again and that the patient must be very tired. The patient informed the counselor that this was a planned pregnancy and that she was not shocked.
- The genetic counselor had a patient who was a 23-year-old single woman whose fetus had just been diagnosed by ultrasound as having Achondroplasia. The patient struggled with the decision about whether or not to continue the pregnancy. The genetic counselor had an abortion as a teenager and now regrets that decision. The genetic counselor viewed the patient's indecision as wanting someone to tell her that it's OK to keep the baby and to raise it as a single mother. The patient repeatedly asked the genetic counselor if she should keep her pregnancy. The counselor explained that the baby would most likely still have a very good quality of life.
- A genetic counselor who had struggled with 18 months of active infertility treatment believed her patient's attitude toward pregnancy was all wrong. The 16-year-old patient, who came to clinic with her mother, was immature, naive, and afraid of needles, so she refused to have any of the available screening/testing options that might help identify if there was a genetic problem in the pregnancy (anomalies had been seen on the ultrasound). The genetic counselor shifted her focus and talked primarily with the patient's mother.
- Whenever patients have refused to have a student attend a counseling session, the supervising genetic counselor suspects a transference issue is present. For instance, the patient wishes to exert control over the session, as a reaction to possibly feeling powerless in the exchange. The genetic counselor's countertransference in these situations is sometimes to assess the patients as manipulative even though she has not explored their reasons for limiting student contact. Maybe they have had a bad experience with students in the past, or are simply private people, or any variety of other explanations.
- The genetic counselor has a bit of a problem with authority, so counseling lawyers and judges is a challenge for her. She comes to these sessions with some uneasiness. She had one judge offer to examine her clinic's consent form outside of the session, and he produced a three-page brief on the form's merits and limitations. This simply confirmed her uneasiness in these sessions.
- The genetic counselor had a particularly grueling session discussing first trimester screening results with a patient who was a statistician. The algorithm for

value calculation was dissected, and the issue became the process, and not the implications of testing. It was as if there was no baby in the equation, just a risk assessment problem. Since this session, the genetic counselor found herself dreading sessions with statisticians.

- Some pregnant prenatal counselors worry about self-disclosing in ways that would unduly direct their patients' decisions (Menezes et al. 2010).
- Lafans et al. (2003), in a study of genetic counselors' experiences of problematic paternal involvement in prenatal counseling, noted this example: "One participant finds it difficult to deal with a father's over-involvement that elicits countertransference due to her own family of origin issues (...hardest for me are the really domineering [fathers]—"I'm going to tell the little wife what she should do"—because that kind of is the setting I grew up in, and it's kind of hard to deal with—to get him to back down a little bit...My tendency is to just say, 'Would you just shut up a minute!' and, obviously, we can't do that)" (p. 239).

- In some instances, your patients' behaviors may provide you with a clue that you are experiencing countertransference (Cerney 1985). For example, your patient says, "You sound just like my mother…"; or "You look so upset! I'll be OK"; or "I know you want me to make a decision, but I just can't yet!" (One caution in interpreting these patient comments as signs of your countertransference is that they may be due to the patient's transference!).

12.1.5 Management of Countertransference Feelings

There are several strategies you can consider using to recognize and manage your countertransference:

- Accept the inevitability of countertransference. It happens to everyone sometimes. It does not mean you are a bad genetic counselor or a bad person. An accepting, nondefensive attitude is essential.
- Locate the source of feelings. Weil (2010) describes three potential origins of one's emotions: "(1) it is a normal response to the situation [this is not countertransference]; (2) it involves the counselor's personal issues; and/or (3) it is a response to the patient's emotions and behaviors" (p. 189). To locate the source, ask yourself, "I wonder why this is so. Why did I make this particular response to this person's remark? What was behind it? What was I reacting to when making this remark? Why did I ask that question? Was it really to help my patient?"
- Practice self-regulation, that is, intentional self-reflection and awareness of your countertransference, and set and maintain appropriate boundaries in genetic counseling (Reeder et al. 2017).
- Seek supervision assistance/consultation/feedback (Geller et al. 2010; McCarthy Veach 2006; Peters et al. 2004; Reeder et al. 2017; Weil 2010; Zahm et al. 2008). As countertransference can be mostly unconscious, it may not be detected until after it has happened (Reeder et al. 2017). Therefore, self-reflection and

supervision are so crucial. You might realize after a genetic counseling session that you were acting out of character, or your supervisor or another colleague might comment on the intensity of your feelings about a patient or situation (either intense liking or dislike, intensely defensive, etc.). These are clues to countertransference. After a challenging genetic counseling session, it may be useful to ask yourself what, if anything, was out of character for you (Cerney 1985).
- Analyze sessions with your supervisor. Seek personal counseling/psychotherapy if your countertransference is fairly pervasive and you are unable to manage it with the preceding strategies (Hyatt 2012; Reeder et al. 2017; Weil 2010).

12.2 Distress and Burnout

12.2.1 Distress

Genetic counseling requires intense involvement with patients on a highly personal level. Both technical expertise and sound emotional health are necessary to meet the demands of the profession. The practice of genetic counseling can be very stressful. Often patients have genetic conditions and situations for which there is no remedy. Additionally, whether you are at the beginning of your career or have been in the genetic counseling profession for many years, you face the continuing challenge of remaining involved and satisfied with your work (Miranda et al. 2016; Zahm et al. 2016). This can be difficult because distress and burnout are common in the genetic counseling profession (Bernhardt et al. 2009; Johnstone et al. 2016; Werner-Lin et al. 2016).

What is distress? It is physical, emotional, and cognitive reactions to overload. There are several signs and symptoms, including feeling emotionally drained, overwhelmed, and out of control; physical, mental, and emotional fatigue; feeling reluctant or dreading going to work and seeing patients; physical reactions such as headaches, stomach complaints, and back pain; having a cynical attitude toward patients and/or feeling too detached from them; lack of satisfaction; and questioning whether you are being helpful or are doing anything meaningful (Geldard and Anderson 1989).

One factor that leads to distress (and burnout) is taking on too many commitments to the point where you feel as if you are always working and always behind (Volz 2000). Another common risk factor is working alone or in isolation from others (Lee et al. 2015; Udipi et al. 2008; Volz 2000). The less time you make for yourself and the more isolated you become in dealing with your reactions to your work, the more likely you are to develop symptoms of distress. Another factor involves difficulties maintaining appropriate boundaries in your counseling work. Although you must develop an empathic connection with patients in order to be effective, you must be careful about becoming overly involved: "With experience you will learn how to walk beside the client with empathy and also how to protect yourself from the excesses of emotional pain by at times moving back a little, grounding yourself, and then joining with the client again" (Geldard and Anderson 1989, p. 177).

Genetic counselors can experience distress and burnout at any time in their career (Jungbluth et al. 2011; Zahm et al. 2016), and so you must develop ways to alleviate the symptoms and either reduce or remove the underlying causes.

Managing Distress as a Novice

Although distress can occur at any time in your career (e.g., Zahm et al. 2016), you may be experiencing unique stressors because you are in the process of learning how to become an effective genetic counselor (Jungbluth et al. 2011; MacFarlane et al. 2016). Studies of genetic counseling students have identified stressors that include professional uncertainty (e.g., about one's competency), impact of personal life events (e.g., finances, family situations), interpersonal demands (e.g., challenging interactions), academic demands (e.g., school performance), and isolating circumstances (loneliness) (Jungbluth et al. 2011).

How can you deal with the stresses of being a novice? The following strategies may be effective:

- Discuss how things are going with your peers and with friends.
- Talk with supervisors, as they can provide helpful support and guidance (MacFarlane et al. 2016).
- Really "hear" positive feedback about your work, and don't dwell solely on negative feedback.
- Engage in positive self-talk (e.g., "Here is what I did well. I made this mistake, but it's a common mistake for beginners."). As a genetic counseling student in a study by Jungbluth et al. (2011) said, "'If you really focus on learning and gaining experiences for the pure enjoyment and the importance/relevance of the information for your future work, you naturally will find yourself less stressed than students who worry more about 'making the grades'" (p. 281).
- Maintain a sense of humor.
- Observe others providing genetic counseling, so you have multiple models from which to develop your own style (Hendrickson et al. 2002).
- Take risks: volunteer to do role-plays, disclose your concerns in supervision and in classroom discussions, etc.
- Keep a journal for recording your thoughts and feelings. Periodically review earlier entries, so you can see how you are developing as a genetic counselor.
- Practice in simulated genetic counseling sessions with a classmate or friend and record your sessions. Play them back and critique your work (what went well and not so well).
- Seek personal counseling if your anxiety is having a negative impact on your clinical work and/or your responsiveness to supervision.

- Set your genetic counseling priorities. Decide which are the most important things to accomplish during a session and what things are less important. This requires strategic and conscious decisions (Osborn 2004).
- Try to focus more on the patient and less on yourself during sessions, and work to trust your feelings and instincts about the right way to respond to patients.
- Practice self-care such as finding personal time and developing healthy outlets (Jungbluth et al. 2011).
- Optimize your living arrangements—"Make sure that 'home' is as stress free as possible" (Jungbluth et al. 2011, p. 282).
- Manage your responsibilities—prioritize, organize, and keep up with requirements (Jungbluth et al. 2011).
- Maintain realistic expectations—of yourself, your academic and clinical experiences, and your program (Jungbluth et al. 2011). And pace yourself. As one genetic counselor recommended in a study of lessons learned on the job, "Fight your natural inclination to want to impress your colleagues and supervisors by overworking yourself when you first start out. It is like a marathoner who has set too fast a pace in the initial few miles, and tries to keep it up for the whole race—it can lead to fatigue and burnout" (Runyon et al. 2010, p. 380).

12.2.2 Burnout

Burnout is "…a critical disruption in an individual's relationship with work, resulting in a state of exhaustion in which one's occupational value and capacity to perform are questioned. Burnout can negatively affect an individual's personal life, as well as employers in terms of decreased work quality, patient/client satisfaction, and employee retention" (Johnstone et al. 2016, p. 731). Burnout involves "…a prolonged response to chronic emotional and interpersonal stressors on the job and is characterized by exhaustion, depersonalization, and lack of personal accomplishment" (Bernhardt et al. 2009, p. 527). Burnout is a more chronic condition than distress, which typically is more acute; however, the same signs and symptoms of distress may be indicators of burnout.

Burnout Prevalence and Triggers

Johnstone et al. (2016) studied genetic counselor burnout and occupational stress. They found more than 40% of their sample "had either considered leaving or left their job role due to burnout" (p. 731). Factors contributing to burnout included "role overload (job demand/resource balance), role boundary (level of conflicting role demands/loyalties), vocational strain (problems in work quality/output/attitude), psychological strain (psychological/emotional problems), physical strain (health worries/physical symptoms), role switching (switched or considered switching job role due to burnout), marital status, and patients seen per week" (Johnstone et al. 2016, p. 735). Additional factors found to contribute to genetic counselor burnout are larger patient caseloads, logistical demands, stress from administrative tasks, lack of workplace support, poor quality of professional relationships, and extra professional responsibilities (Benoit et al. 2007; Lee et al. 2015), and having fewer years of experience and experiencing less meaning from patient care (Bernhardt et al. 2009).

12.2.3 General Strategies for Managing Distress and Preventing Burnout

Regardless of whether you are a beginning genetic counselor or have practiced for many years, the following strategies may help you manage distress and avoid burnout, thus allowing you to remain actively engaged in your professional growth:

- Recognize and acknowledge what you are experiencing (this strategy alone may reduce some symptoms) (Warren et al. 2010).
- Engage in self-monitoring and self-reflection activities such as mindfulness meditation, reflective writing, peer support groups, and additional communication skill-based training (Bernhardt et al. 2009; Bernhardt et al. 2010).
- Talk with someone (a supervisor, colleague, trusted friend) about your feelings, so you can gain perspective (Bernhardt et al. 2009).
- Establish clear job roles and expectations (Johnstone et al. 2016).
- Practice self-care (Warren et al. 2010). For instance, try to lead a balanced life that includes leisure and relationships, as well as work (Runyon et al. 2010). Peters (2010) notes that "…one important foundation of good self-care is attending to the body: becoming mindful about getting enough sleep, eating healthy foods and finding time for recreation" (p. 327)
- Practice relaxation exercises (cf. Peters 2010).
- Address negative emotions prompted by your work (Warren et al. 2010). "Positive emotions promote discovery of novel and creative actions, ideas, and social bonds, which in turn expand personal resources" (Peters 2010, p. 327).
- If you have perfectionistic standards, you may need to adjust the expectations you have of yourself, your patients, your peers, and your employer (Jungbluth et al. 2011).
- Maintain a curiosity about people, developments in the profession, and yourself (Osborn 2004).
- Enjoy life, and cultivate and use your sense of humor.
- Keep work and non-work activities separate. For example, one counselor in a study of lessons learned on the job commented: "'I learned that I can separate work life and personal life, but it takes a conscious effort. I learned I can be good at my job, make a difference at work, but not let it define my whole life. Having other things in my life is important to me, especially if I don't want to burn out in 5 years. Upon graduation, I had this idea that the best genetic counselors let their

job take over all aspects of their life. But then I met other counselors who showed me how to 'have it all,' and I realized I could do it too. You can be a good counselor and leave work at work when you leave at 5 pm'" (Runyon et al. 2010, p. 376).

- Do not take your problems home with you. Use thought-stopping techniques to prevent worrying about patients when you are not at work. For instance, if you catch yourself worrying, try distracting yourself, or tell yourself that you will deal with the worry tomorrow at work at a specific time, and then focus on what you are doing in the here and now.
- Draw upon a religious or philosophical belief system for support (Wells et al. 2016).
- Schedule the first 30 min of each day to collect your thoughts and prepare for the events ahead of you.
- Participate in peer supervision. Peer supervision can act as a buffer against stress and burnout, can help you manage your genetic counseling cases, and can strengthen your clinical skills (Middleton et al. 2007; Peters 2010; Zahm et al. 2008).
- Seek personal counseling or psychotherapy to deal with crises you are experiencing at work (Reeder et al. 2017; Runyon et al. 2010; Volz 2000; Weil 2010).
- Build a support system (Runyon et al. 2010; Peters 2010). Make friends with people who are outside of the genetic counseling field (Volz 2000).
- Give yourself some real downtime where you turn off the computer and put away the paperwork (Volz 2000).
- If at all possible, schedule time during the day (midmorning, midafternoon) that is just for you to take a walk, relax your muscles, meditate, etc. (Fine and Glasser 1996; Miller and Sprang 2017).
- Think in sane ways (Fine and Glasser 1996; Miller and Sprang 2017). To a great extent, distress comes from what we tell ourselves about what we experience rather than from the experience itself. For example, "I must say 'yes' to every request made of me."; "I can't make any mistakes or everyone will think I'm incompetent."; "If I were a good genetic counselor, I wouldn't be feeling so overwhelmed."; "If I were a good counselor, I would have all the information in my head." Try to replace these irrational ideas with more reasonable ones.

12.3 Compassion Fatigue

> "the expectation that we can be immersed in suffering and loss daily and not be touched by it is as unrealistic as expecting to be able to walk through water without getting wet" (Remen 1996, p. 52, as cited in Miller and Sprang 2017).

Have you ever lost sleep over the distressing experiences of someone you counseled? Avoided certain activities or situations because they remind you of your patients' distressing experiences? Suffered the distress of someone you counseled? Because of genetic counseling, felt "on edge" about various things? If you answered "yes" to any of these questions, you may have experienced compassion fatigue.

As Peters (2010) notes, "…genetic counselors clearly do witness much pain and suffering, and may fall prey to compassion fatigue" (p. 314). Compassion fatigue is a type of distress that comes from repeated exposure to patient suffering (Benoit et al. 2007; Bernhardt et al. 2010; Injeyan et al. 2011; Udipi et al. 2008). When you experience compassion fatigue, you feel overwhelmed by patient suffering and feel as if you have cared to the point where you are "drained of empathy." You may feel depressed, tired, disillusioned, and worthless regarding your ability to care for your patients (Zeidner et al. 2013). Compassion fatigue is believed to be caused either by feeling and expressing empathy without being able to "let go" of the "emotional residue" that stays with you (Figley 1995, 2002) or by fear and avoidance of empathic engagement with patients that cause you to expend a great deal of effort pretending to empathize (Miller and Sprang 2017). In either case, lack of effective coping strategies compounds compassion fatigue's effects (Miller and Sprang 2017; Udipi et al. 2008; Zeidner et al. 2013).

The risk for compassion fatigue is prevalent among genetic counselors. As many as 39–57% of genetic counselors may be at moderate risk, and 26–61% at high risk (Lee et al. 2015; Udipi et al. 2008). This risk is not surprising, as "Genetic counseling sessions across settings are often brimming with intense emotion: fear, worry, anger, sadness, and frustration about the limits of information. Witnessing such intensity, and working with it in a concentrated time frame, takes a toll on providers" (Werner-Lin et al. 2016, p. 865).

Although compassion fatigue may be an inevitable part of caring for patients, it only becomes problematic when it is not recognized and managed effectively. Unchecked compassion fatigue can compromise patient care, damage one's professional self-confidence, and even lead to leaving the profession (Lee et al. 2015).

12.3.1 Differences Between Compassion Fatigue and Distress and Burnout

Before describing compassion fatigue in greater detail, it may be helpful to distinguish it from distress and burnout. Although compassion fatigue and distress share similar signs and symptoms and certain coping strategies, distress can arise from all aspects of your genetic counseling roles and responsibilities, whereas compassion fatigue is exclusive to empathy for patient suffering. Burnout is a reaction to excessive amounts of work and feeling disempowered to make positive work-related changes. Burnout can occur in any type of work, and it involves a gradual "wearing out" physically and emotionally. In contrast, compassion fatigue is prompted by intense interactions with distressed patients and grieving for the tragedies that occur in their lives. Compassion fatigue is unique to individuals in human services professions, and it can come on suddenly in response to a single intense experience, or from multiple exposures (Figley 1995, 2002). Any of these three phenomena (i.e., distress, burnout, compassion fatigue), however, can place you at risk of experiencing the others (Lee et al. 2015; Udipi et al. 2008).

12.3.2 Recognizing Compassion Fatigue

Figley (1995, 2002) developed a framework for characterizing compassion fatigue symptoms. His model is useful for helping you recognize your own tendencies to experience compassion fatigue. In this section, we describe eight categories of symptoms and illustrate them with examples from genetic counselors who participated in research on compassion fatigue.

- *General Symptoms*: avoidance, hypervigilance, hyperarousal, and flashbacks
- *Example*:

> "A patient was diagnosed with a neurologic condition of relatively quick onset and the partner was struggling with both the diagnosis and the effects of the condition on everyday responsibilities and the couple's relationship. The partner contacted me repeatedly to discuss her frustrations and wasn't comfortable talking with professionals to whom I referred her. I found myself not answering my phone in case she was calling so that she would get my voicemail. It was exhausting, though I really wanted to be sure that she was safe and that she spoke with a professional" (Udipi 2007, pp. 129–130).

- *Physical Symptoms*: exhaustion, sluggishness, and lack of enthusiasm
- *Example*:

> "I work in both cardiology and neurology clinics and work with support groups for both. I find that in doing so I am starting to feel what I consider compassion fatigue in that every one of the patients who come to the group wants to speak with me separately before or after because I am so involved in their ongoing care, their families, etc. and when you constantly have your empathy on, it gets exhausting!" (Udipi 2007, pp. 143–144).

- *Emotional Symptoms*: irritability, angry outbursts, and crying and sadness
- *Example*:

> "I find myself having heightened irritability, and a quick temper - with occasional angry outbursts - and I am immediately frustrated and angry with myself - because I do not want to be like this. I also do wake up in the night and start thinking about cases/patients/situations that I am dealing with and what I could possibly do additionally, or should have done to the point that I can't sleep. This happens probably once a week at least" (Udipi 2007, p. 134).

- *Cognitive Symptoms*: quitting the profession, or moving to nonclinical work
- *Example*:

> "We were seeing a patient in follow-up (another counselor had seen her for the initial appointment) for twin to twin transfusion syndrome. Ultrasound revealed that both twins were deceased, and I was the person who told the family. I relive this moment even now, 7 years later. From that point on, I was intensely sensitive to high stress situations of my patients and my role in them. This was a main reason I stopped seeing patients" (Udipi 2007, p. 132; Udipi et al. 2008, p. 467).

- *Behavioral Symptoms*: avoidance
- *Examples*:

> "One of my patients recently died. He was 23 months old. A couple days later, a family member [of mine] died. I decided to not attend the funeral because I didn't want to think about death anymore" (Udipi 2007, p. 132).

> "I find myself avoiding people socially who are currently pregnant or in emotionally needy states. I also find myself responding in close ended statements with defensive body language when faced with 'counseling' type situations outside of work" (Udipi 2007, p. 138).

- *Interpersonal symptoms*: short temper, irritable reactions, and inability to meet life's demands
- *Example*:

> "...work stress most negatively impacts my life when I feel I can't perform home tasks for being 'wiped out' by work emotions. Especially when it comes to helping my children with their drama" (Lee 2013, p. 48).

12.3.3 Genetic Counselor Compassion Fatigue Triggers and Risk Factors

Several studies have identified one or more triggers and risk factors for compassion fatigue (Benoit et al. 2007; Bernhardt et al. 2010; Injeyan et al. 2011; Lee et al. 2015; Miller and Sprang 2017; Udipi et al. 2008; Zeidner et al. 2013). Compassion fatigue triggers include working with difficult patients, delivering bad news, feeling responsible for patient suffering, feeling burdened by the information you must convey, being emotionally invested in patients, and feeling helpless. Risk factors include personality characteristics (high trait anxiety, high compassion satisfaction, self-blame, desire to be in control, low dispositional optimism, low trait emotional intelligence, and low emotion management/regulation), ethnicity/race (identifying as other than Caucasian), experiencing burnout, having a larger caseload and a greater variety of difficult clinical situations, and high job-related interpersonal stress.

12.3.4 Coping Strategies for Managing Compassion Fatigue

Compassion fatigue risk is a "by-product" of the services you provide to patients and their families. Therefore, it's important that you have a variety of coping strategies for minimizing its impact on your services and on your professional development. A growing body of research has identified strategies that vary in their effectiveness for managing compassion fatigue symptoms. The most *ineffective* strategies are (Benoit et al. 2007; Miller and Sprang 2017; Peters 2010; Udipi et al. 2008; Zeidner et al. 2013) avoiding engaging empathically with patients, shutting down/off with patients, ruminating excessively, pretending you are fine, isolating yourself —not sharing your feelings and thoughts with others—blaming yourself inappropriately, losing confidence in yourself, and becoming cynical (about patients, genetic counseling, your role, and responsibilities). These strategies are especially ineffective if you use them excessively and over a long period.

Many of the strategies for managing compassion fatigue effectively are similar to strategies for alleviating distress and preventing burnout. These include a range of "in-session" and "out of session" actions (Benoit et al. 2007; Burgess et al. 2015; Middleton et al. 2007; Miller and Sprang 2017; Miranda et al. 2016; Peters 2010; Udipi et al. 2008; Wells et al. 2016; Werner-Lin et al. 2016; Zahm et al. 2008; Zeidner et al. 2013):

- Remind yourself that empathy is a critical aspect of genetic counseling and is meaningful and effective "in and of itself."
- Fight the urge to let fear keep you from having feelings during sessions. Some master practitioners have noted the importance of letting themselves feel: "'… sometimes I just go with whatever I'm feeling. If something is following me home, if I'm feeling sad, I just need the space to kind of dwell on it a little bit. I may not try to dispel it'" (Miranda et al. 2016, p. 779).
- Use emotion management skills before, during, and after a genetic counseling session. For example, when you don't feel empathy, take a stance of curiosity to help you understand.
- Reflect upon the meaningfulness of the work you do.
- Develop and use problem-focused skills with patients.
- Engage in mindfulness activities.
- As students, use supervision and consultation to describe and debrief about your experiences.
- Engage in peer group supervision and consultation after graduation—commit to making supervision a lifelong activity.
- Balance patient care with other professional activities.
- Seek outside support when necessary.
- Take a brief "time-out"—take a walk around the block, sit quietly for a few minutes. If feasible, take some time off from work, even if only a couple of hours.
- Work on developing a range of coping strategies. That way, you will be able to "pick and choose" among them, as needed.

12.4 Impact of Personal Counseling on Genetic Counseling Practice

Personal counseling can be an effective way to address general distress, burnout, compassion fatigue, and transference and countertransference (Lee et al. 2015; Reeder et al. 2017; Weil 2010) and to cope with the unique stressors of being a novice. In addition to helping you resolve these situations, personal counseling or psychotherapy can have other positive effects (e.g., Osborn 2004; Weil 2010):

- Leads to greater empathy, acceptance, and genuineness, possibly because therapy increases one's ability to be aware of feelings and makes one more comfortable discussing affect
- Allows you to know how it feels to be a patient

- Provides a role model of how to counsel on psychosocial issues (e.g., using skills and techniques your therapist used with you)
- Allows you to learn to be yourself
- Helps you learn your own limits and boundaries
- Helps you learn what not to do (i.e., therapist behaviors that were not helpful for you)
- Helps you learn how to separate your own feelings from your patients' feelings
- Helps you address issues on a deeper level with your patients
- Provides a venue for identifying and exploring transference and countertransference
- Can increase personal resilience. "The antithesis of compassion fatigue and burnout is resilience…[Resilience] involves several important core elements: self-knowledge and insight; sense of hope; healthy coping styles; strong relationships; personal perspective; and a sense of greater purpose and meaning" (Peters 2010, p. 326).

12.5 Closing Comments

The counseling dynamics discussed in this chapter are common occurrences. You are not the only one to have a countertransference reaction or to feel distress, burnout, or compassion fatigue; and you are not odd or incompetent because of these experiences. The worst thing you can do is pretend you are not experiencing one or more of these phenomena. Unacknowledged, they will only get worse. The best thing you can do is to be proactive—recognize and reflect upon what is going on; deal with the issue by consulting with others, a supervisor, a professor, a genetic counselor, and peers; and proactively build and maintain effective coping strategies. These actions will assist you in "thriving" as opposed to "surviving" in your work and throughout your career.

12.6 Class Activities

Activity 1: Transference (Think-Pair- Share Dyad Discussion)

Students discuss the following situation: Your patient expresses unrealistic expectations about what you should be able to do for her. She tells you that you should be able to test for everything possible to guarantee her baby will be ok and that if you cared more about her situation, you would tell her what she should do if abnormal test results come back.

- How would you deal with her unrealistic expectations?
- Would you try convincing her that her demands are unrealistic? How would you do this?

- Would you be inclined to give her advice by telling her what you think she should do if she receives abnormal test results?

Process
The whole group discusses their responses to the situation.
Estimated time: 30 min.

Activity 2: Transference Role-Play I (Triads or Small Groups)

Using the situation in Activity 1, engage in a 5- to 10-min role-play in which the genetic counselor attempts to respond to patient expectations.

Process
Discuss in triads or in the whole group the counselor's reactions and responses to the patient, the patient's reactions to the counselor's interventions, and how transference can be managed in genetic counseling sessions.
Estimated time: 45 min.

Activity 3: Transference Role-Play II (Triads or Small Groups)

Engage in a series of 5–10-min role-plays in which the patient selects one of the types of transference described in this chapter (counselor as an ideal, counselor as seer, counselor as nurturer, counselor as frustrater, counselor as nonentity). The student should not tell anyone what type of transference she/he selected. The genetic counselor attempts to manage the patient's transference.

Process
Discuss in triads or in the whole group the counselor's reactions and responses to the patient, the type of transference students believe the patient acted out during the role-play, and different ways transference can be managed in genetic counseling sessions.
Estimated time: 45–60 min.

Activity 4: Countertransference (Think-Pair-Share Dyad Discussion)

Students discuss with a partner their countertransference triggers, using the types of triggers listed in written Exercise 3. They can have this discussion either before or after completing the written exercise or in lieu of the written exercise.

Process

The whole group discusses how they felt discussing their countertransference triggers. Next the group generates ideas about ways to anticipate and manage their countertransference reactions.

Estimated time: 30 min.

Activity 5: Countertransference (Triad Role-Plays)

In triads, the student who will be the counselor selects one of Watkins' four types of countertransference and plays this out in a 10–15-min role-play. The student should not tell the other members of the triad which type of countertransference will be demonstrated, and she/he should be subtle in showing the countertransference.

Estimated time: 30–45 min.

Process

Triads discuss the type of countertransference they thought the counselor demonstrated and the counselor behaviors that indicated the countertransference. Next, they should discuss the patient's reaction to the counselor's behaviors. They can also discuss what the counselor could have said or done differently to manage the countertransference and counsel more effectively.

Estimated time: 45 min.

Instructor Note

- The instructor could conduct a large group discussion of student reactions to the role-plays on transference and countertransference as well as their thoughts about these two counselor-patient dynamics.

Activity 6: Distress and Burnout (Think-Pair-Share Dyads)

Students take turns talking about a situation from their past where they experienced distress and a situation where they experienced burnout and what they did to cope with each experience. Next, they discuss what aspects of a career in genetic counseling might make them vulnerable to distress and burnout.

Estimated time: 30 min.

Process

The whole group offers strategies for dealing with distress and burnout. The group can also discuss what aspects of genetic counseling may make them personally vulnerable to distress and burnout.

Estimated time: 30 min.

Instructor Note

- This activity could also be turned into a written exercise—either as a follow-up to this activity or in place of the activity.

12.7 Written Exercises

Exercise 1: Irrational Beliefs

List all the irrational beliefs you have about being a genetic counselor, a supervisee, and a professional in the genetic counseling field. Then dispute each belief by writing down a more reasonable idea.

Example

Irrational belief: "I must be very helpful with all of my patients or I am not a good genetic counselor." Disputing belief: "I should try to be helpful to my patients while recognizing that some will find what I have to say more helpful than others will."

Exercise 2: First Impressions

Go to a shopping mall or some other public place and write a description of an individual you see there. Alternatively, you could select a photo of an individual from a newspaper or magazine. Include the following in your description:

- Your first impressions of the person.
- Do you think you would like this person if you met them? Why or why not?
- What assumptions do you have about the person (personality, likeability, attractiveness, intelligence, education, hobbies, etc.)?

Discuss what led to your impressions and the assumptions you made about the person you are describing. How confident are you about your impressions? In what ways might you be wrong?

Exercise 3: Countertransference Issues

What types of patients (e.g., terminally ill, highly emotional, authoritarian, etc.) and genetic counseling situations (e.g., sex selection, patients who refuse to reveal information to at-risk relatives, ambiguous test results, lethal conditions) "push your buttons" or are particularly hard for you to work with as a genetic counselor? What makes these patients/situations so challenging? What type(s) of countertransference reactions would you be likely have in response to these patients and situations?

Exercise 4: Countertransference and Compassion Fatigue Checklist[1]

Place a check in the space to indicate whether you have had this tendency or believe you might be likely to have this tendency in future genetic counseling work:

___I am likely to become overly involved on an emotional level with certain patients.
Comment:
___I might find a number of ways to avoid patients who prompt strong negative feelings in me.
Comment:
___I worry that I may have a strong need to give lots of advice and that I will manipulate patients to think and act the way I think they should.
Comment:
___I might fall back on giving excessive amounts of information to patients in order to keep the session structured and emotionally safe.
Comment:
___I am concerned that I may bring home some patients' problems, and I will over-identify with some of my patients.
Comment:
___I can imagine myself getting angry and upset over patients who do not appreciate me.
Comment:
___I tend to respond very defensively to certain types of people or certain kinds of remarks.
Comment:
___There are some topics I would feel very uncomfortable exploring with patients, and I am likely to steer away from talking about them.
Comment:
___I am afraid that I will feel responsible if a patient does not understand, cannot make a decision, or makes a bad decision.
Comment:
___I worry that I will pity my patients who have disabling or terminal conditions.
Comment:
___I am afraid that I would break down and cry with some patients.
Comment:
___I usually do whatever I can to avoid negative or angry encounters.
Comment:

[1]Adapted from Corey et al. (1984).

References

Anonymous. A genetic counselor's journey from provider to patient: a mother's story. J Genet Couns. 2008;17:412–8.

Balcom JR, Veach PM, Bemmels H, Redlinger-Grosse K, LeRoy BS. When the topic is you: Genetic counselor responses to prenatal patients' requests for self-disclosure. J Genet Couns. 2013;22:358–73.

Bellcross C. A genetic counselor's story of birth, grief, and survival. J Genet Couns. 2012;21:169–72.

Benoit LG, Veach PM, LeRoy BS. When you care enough to do your very best: genetic counselor experiences of compassion fatigue. J Genet Couns. 2007;16:299–312.

Bernhardt BA, Rushton CH, Carrese J, Pyeritz RE, Kolodner K, Geller G. Distress and burnout among genetic service providers. Genet Med. 2009;11:527–35.

Bernhardt BA, Silver R, Rushton CH, Micco E, Geller G. What keeps you up at night? Genetics professionals' distressing experiences in patient care. Genet Med. 2010;12:289–97.

Burgess M, Tai G, Martinek N, Menezes M, Delatycki M. AB117. An exploration of Australasian genetic counsellors' attitudes towards compassion fatigue, mindfulness and genetic counselling. Ann Transl Med. 2015;3(Suppl 2):AB117.

Cerney MS. Countertransference revisited. J Couns Dev. 1985;63:362–4.

Corey G, Corey M, Callanan P. Issues and ethics in the helping professions. Pacific Grove, CA: Brooks/Cole; 1984.

Cura JD. Respecting autonomous decision making among Filipinos: a re-emphasis in genetic counseling. J Genet Couns. 2015;24:213–24.

Djurdjinovic L. Psychosocial counseling. In: Uhlmann WR, Schuette JL, Yashar B, editors. A guide to genetic counseling. 2nd ed. New York: Wiley; 2009. p. 133–75.

Figley CR. Compassion fatigue: secondary traumatic stress disorders from treating the traumatized. New York: Brunner/Mazel; 1995.

Figley CR. Compassion fatigue: Psychotherapists' chronic lack of self care. J Clin Psychol. 2002;58:1433–41.

Fine SF, Glasser PH. The first helping interview. Thousand Oaks, CA: Sage; 1996.

Geldard D, Anderson G. A training manual for counsellors: basic personal counselling. Springfield, IL: Charles C. Thomas; 1989.

Geller G, Rushton CH, Francomano C, Kolodner K, Bernhardt BA. Genetics professionals' experiences with grief and loss: implications for support and training. Clin Genet. 2010;77:421–9.

Glessner HD. Will my voice be heard? J Genet Couns. 2012;21:189–91.

Hendrickson SM, Veach PM, LeRoy BS. A qualitative investigation of student and supervisor perceptions of live supervision in genetic counseling. J Genet Couns. 2002;11:25–49.

Hofsess CD, Tracey TJ. Countertransference as a prototype: the development of a measure. J Couns Psychol. 2010;57:52–67.

Hyatt J. Countertransference in the genetic counseling setting: one counselor's personal journey. J Genet Couns. 2012;21:197–8.

Injeyan MC, Shuman C, Shugar A, Chitayat D, Atenafu EG, Kaiser A. Personality traits associated with genetic counselor compassion fatigue: the roles of dispositional optimism and locus of control. J Genet Couns. 2011;20:526–40.

Johnstone B, Kaiser A, Injeyan MC, Sappleton K, Chitayat D, Stephens D, et al. The relationship between burnout and occupational stress in genetic counselors. J Genet Couns. 2016;25:731–41.

Jungbluth C, MacFarlane IM, Veach PM, LeRoy BS. Why is everyone so anxious? An exploration of stress and anxiety in genetic counseling graduate students. J Genet Couns. 2011;20:270–86.

Kessler S. Psychological aspects of genetic counseling. VIII. Suffering and countertransference. J Genet Couns. 1992;1:303–8.

Lafans RS, Veach PM, LeRoy BS. Genetic counselors' experiences with paternal involvement in prenatal genetic counseling sessions: an exploratory investigation. J Genet Couns. 2003;12:219–42.

Lee W. Role of anxiety in genetic counselors' risk for compassion fatigue. Minneapolis, MI: University of Minnesota; 2013.

Lee W, Veach PM, MacFarlane IM, LeRoy BS. Who is at risk for compassion fatigue? An investigation of genetic counselor demographics, anxiety, compassion satisfaction, and burnout. J Genet Couns. 2015;24:358–70.

Lewis L. Honoring diversity: Cultural competence in genetic counseling. In: LeRoy BS, McCarthy Veach P, Bartels DM, editors. Genetic counseling practice. Hoboken: Wiley-Blackwell; 2010. p. 201–34.

MacFarlane IM, Veach PM, Grier JE, Meister DJ, LeRoy BS. Effects of anxiety on novice genetic counseling students' experience of supervised clinical rotations. J Genet Couns. 2016;25:742–66.

Mathiesen AM. Counseling the "angry patient": a defining moment of changing focus from myself to the patient. J Genet Couns. 2012;21:209–10.

Matloff ET. Becoming a daughter. J Genet Couns. 2006;15:139–43.

McCarthy Veach P. Commentary on becoming a daughter: trauma is a powerful teacher. J Genet Couns. 2006;15:145–8.

Menezes MA. Commentary on "life as a pregnant genetic counselor: take two". J Genet Couns. 2012;21:31–4.

Menezes MA, Hodgson JM, Sahhar MA, Aitken M, Metcalfe SA. "It's challenging on a personal level"—exploring the 'lived experience' of Australian and Canadian prenatal genetic counselors. J Genet Couns. 2010;19:640–52.

Middleton A, Wiles V, Kershaw A, Everest S, Downing S, Burton H, et al. Reflections on the experience of counseling supervision by a team of genetic counselors from the UK. J Genet Couns. 2007;16:143–55.

Miller B, Sprang GA. Components-based practice and supervision model for reducing compassion fatigue by affecting clinician experience. Traumatology. 2017;23:53–64.

Miranda C, Veach PM, Martyr MA, LeRoy BS. Portrait of the master genetic counselor clinician: a qualitative investigation of expertise in genetic counseling. J Genet Couns. 2016;25:767–85.

Monaco LC, Conway L, Valverde K, Austin JC. Exploring genetic counselors' perceptions of and attitudes towards schizophrenia. Public Health Genomics. 2010;13:21–6.

Osborn CJ. Seven salutary suggestions for counselor stamina. J Couns Dev. 2004;82:319–28.

Peters E, McCarthy Veach P, Ward EE, LeRoy BS. Does receiving genetic counseling impact genetic counselor practice? J Genet Couns. 2004;13:387–402.

Peters JA. Genetic counselors: Caring mindfully for ourselves. In: LeRoy BS, McCarthy Veach P, Bartels DM, editors. Genetic counseling practice. Hoboken: Wiley-Blackwell; 2010. p. 307–52.

Redlinger-Grosse K, Veach PM, MacFarlane IM. What would you say? Genetic counseling graduate students' and counselors' hypothetical responses to patient requested self-disclosure. J Genet Couns. 2013;22:455–68.

Reeder R, Veach PM, MacFarlane IM, LeRoy BS. Characterizing clinical genetic counselors' countertransference experiences: an exploratory study. J Genet Couns. 2017;26:834–47.

Remen RN. Kitchen table wisdom: stories that heal. New York: Riverhead; 1996.

Runyon M, Zahm KW, Veach PM, MacFarlane IM, LeRoy BS. What do genetic counselors learn on the job? A qualitative assessment of professional development outcomes. J Genet Couns. 2010;19:371–86.

Sahhar MA. Commentary on "life as a pregnant genetic counselor". J Genet Couns. 2010;19:238–40.

Schema L, McLaughlin M, Veach PM, LeRoy BS. Clearing the air: a qualitative investigation of genetic counselors' experiences of counselor-focused patient anger. J Genet Couns. 2015;24:717–31.

Thomas BC, Veach PM, LeRoy BS. Is self-disclosure part of the genetic counselor's clinical role? J Genet Couns. 2006;15:163–77.

Udipi S. An investigation of the personal and demographic predictors of compassion fatigue among genetic counselors. University of Minnesota; 2007. Available from Dissertations & Theses @ CIC Institutions; ProQuest Dissertations & Theses A&I. (304822912). Retrieved from http://

login.ezproxy.lib.umn.edu/login?url=https://search-proquest-com.ezp3.lib.umn.edu/docview/304822912?accountid=14586.
Udipi S, Veach PM, Kao J, LeRoy BS. The psychic costs of empathic engagement: personal and demographic predictors of genetic counselor compassion fatigue. J Genet Couns. 2008;17:459–71.
Volz J. Clinician, heal thyself. Amer Psych Assoc Monitor. 2000;31:46–7.
Warren J, Morgan MM, Morris LN, Morris TM. Breathing words slowly: creative writing and counselor self-care—the writing workout. J Creat Ment Health. 2010;5:109–24.
Watkins CE. Countertransference: its impact on the counseling situation. J Couns Dev. 1985;63:356–9.
Weil J. Countertransference: making the unconscious conscious. In: LeRoy BS, McCarthy Veach P, Bartels DM, editors. Genetic counseling practice. Hoboken: Wiley-Blackwell; 2010. p. 175–95.
Wells DM, McCarthy Veach P, Martyr MA, LeRoy BS. Development, experience, and expression of meaning in genetic counselors' lives: an exploratory analysis. J Genet Couns. 2016;25:799–817.
Werner-Lin A, McCoyd JL, Bernhardt BA. Balancing genetics (science) and counseling (art) in prenatal chromosomal microarray testing. J Genet Couns. 2016;25:855–67.
Zahm KW, Veach PM, LeRoy BS. An investigation of genetic counselor experiences in peer group supervision. J Genet Couns. 2008;17:220–33.
Zahm KW, Veach PM, Martyr MA, LeRoy BS. From novice to seasoned practitioner: a qualitative investigation of genetic counselor professional development. J Genet Couns. 2016;25:818–34.
Zeidner M, Hadar D, Matthews G, Roberts RD. Personal factors related to compassion fatigue in health professionals. Anxiety Stress Coping. 2013;26:595–609.

Chapter 13
Professionalism: Ethically Based Reflective Practice

Learning Objectives

1. Examine one's motivations for being a genetic counselor and how they influence practice.
2. Describe principles guiding students' and health-care professionals' ethical behavior.
3. Recognize ethical challenges that arise when patients have genetic concerns.
4. Apply ethical principles and models to cases involving genetic concerns.
5. Describe key aspects of professional development in genetic counseling.
6. Recognize the role of self-reflective practice in professional development.

Acting as a professional means responsibly addressing patients' needs and expectations. This requires first an understanding of yourself and the personal characteristics you bring with you into genetic counseling sessions. For instance, examining your motivations for being a genetic counselor can help you to identify the strengths you bring to clinical situations as well as shed light on situations where your needs or values might impede your ability to provide adequate care for patients. This chapter addresses motivations for being a genetic counselor, describes several ethical principles and models for ethical decision-making, identifies some of the major ethical and professional challenges you may encounter, and includes resources you can call upon to meet these challenges.

As you transition from being a student to assuming the responsibilities of a genetic counseling professional, it is also helpful to explore issues related to professional development. A commitment to lifelong learning and self-reflective practice and taking care of your emotional and physical health greatly enhance your ability to grow professionally.

P. McCarthy Veach et al., *Facilitating the Genetic Counseling Process*,
https://doi.org/10.1007/978-3-319-74799-6_13

13.1 Genetic Counselor Motivations, Culture, and Values

You've probably been asked by a number of people why you want to become a genetic counselor. What do you usually say? Your response to this question contains clues about your motivations for becoming a genetic counselor. These may include the need to feel a sense of accomplishment, the need for stimulation (intellectual, emotional, etc.), the need to have hope, the need to have fun, the need to have an existential purpose in life (Cavanagh and Levitov 2002; Wells et al. 2016), the need to help others, the need to feel powerful and in control, the need to feel competent, the need to be altruistic, the need for security (financial, social, etc.), the need to be liked, and the need to be respected. This is not an exhaustive list. You may have other motivations as well.

According to the National Society of Genetic Counselors (NSGC), "There are many paths to genetic counseling, and the motivations for choosing genetic counseling are diverse. Many people start with an interest in genetics, but want something more personal than laboratory work. Some individuals desire to be in the medical field but do not think medical school is the best fit for them. Other students are drawn to the counseling sides of genetic counseling, and enjoy the unique topics genetic counselors cover (e.g., facilitating decision-making, reducing guilt, grief and bereavement). Other reasons for choosing genetic counseling include an interest in clinical research, genomic technologies, patient advocacy and education, and the desire to be in a field that is always changing" (http://www.nsgc.org/page/frequently-asked-questions-students n.d.).

Do you ever worry that you might have the wrong motivations for becoming a genetic counselor? In our opinion, motivations, in and of themselves, are neither right nor wrong, good nor bad. Rather, *how* and *when* we try *to* satisfy our needs may lead to positive or negative outcomes. For example, you may be pursuing a career in genetic counseling because it allows you to feel competent or capable. One positive aspect of this motivation is it will likely prompt you to continually build your skills and knowledge. On the other hand, if your desire to be competent is excessive, that is, you believe you must be successful with every patient, the motivation may drive you to try to get patients and supervisors to say you did a great job even when you did not. Similarly, if you desire to be liked, one positive aspect is that you will probably be warm, nonthreatening, and encouraging with your patients. But an excessive need to be liked could also lead you to avoid confronting patients and/or keeping patients from expressing negative emotions toward you (e.g., anger). It is important that you recognize and periodically review your motivations so you can gauge their impact on your clinical practice. Staying aware of your motivations increases the likelihood that you will remain positive about your clinical work and act in patients' best interests.

Our motivations are strongly grounded in our cultural values. Davis and Voegtle (1994) identify four major cultural settings or affiliations that shape our values:

Religious Affiliation

- Affiliation of family of origin
- Religious group with which you identify
- Values or practices associated with the group with which you identify

Socioeconomic Class

- Socioeconomic class of family of origin (family into which you were born)
- Your own socioeconomic class
- Values or practices associated with the group in which you place yourself

Ethnic Group

(Note: Ethnic group may overlap with religious affiliation.)

- Ethnic group(s) of family of origin
- Ethnic group(s) with which you identify
- Values or practices associated with the group with which you identify

Other Group Identifications

(Note: Examples might include a community or neighborhood group, social action group, or group whose members share special interests such as music or sports.)

- Other Group Identifications of Family of Origin
- Other groups with which you identify (e.g., your professional genetic counseling group).
- Values or practices associated with the groups with which you identify.

We tend to think of cultural issues as those belonging to others. However, we all have cultures and therefore bring our unique cultural backgrounds to any relationship.

Pirzadeh et al. (2007) described personal values genetic counselors have identified as important. As part of their study, 292 genetic counselors completed the Schwartz Universal Values Questionnaire (SUVQ; Schwartz 1992). The SUVQ was developed based on extensive international research resulting in the identification of universal value types that exist across cultures. These values have been associated with career behaviors and career satisfaction in physicians (Eliason and Schubot

1995; Eliason et al. 2000). The four values rated most highly by the participants were benevolence (concern for others), self-direction (independence), achievement (personal success), and universalism (protecting the welfare of all).

13.2 Professional Values

The National Society of Genetic Counselors (NSGC) states its primary professional values in its Code of Ethics (found in Appendix B). The NSGC Code of Ethics provides an overview of counselors' obligations to themselves, patients, colleagues, and society. "Each section of this code begins with an explanation of the relevant relationship, along with the key values and characteristics of that relationship. These values are drawn from the ethical principles of autonomy, beneficence, nonmaleficence and justice, and they include the professional principles of fidelity, veracity, integrity, dignity and accountability" (Appendix B). It is important for all professionals to be able to identify their personal values, those of their profession, and those of the organizations in which they work. Knowing these values can help you decide what is an appropriate response in each situation and identify where there are conflicting expectations you must consider when choosing how to respond.

Ethical challenges are challenges to our personal and professional values. They are part of everyday practice for genetic counselors. As noted above, The NSGC Code of Ethics (Appendix B) provides an overview of counselors' obligations to patients, to society, and to themselves. Genetic counselors will face some ethical dilemmas because of these multiple, and at times conflicting, obligations. In some instances, what is best for a family or for the broader society is not what is best for an individual patient. Honoring one principle (such as respecting patient autonomy) might mean ignoring other obligations (like acting fairly). Value conflicts occur when counselors experience the tension of competing values or when patient expectations and counselor values conflict (Abad-Perotin et al. 2012; Alliman et al. 2009; Bower et al. 2002; Gschmeidler and Flatscher-Thoeni 2013; McCarthy Veach et al. 2001). In such instances, you will need to select the principle(s) most important to a particular situation to guide your actions.

In the following section, we describe six ethical principles that might be used as a basis for decision-making.

13.3 Guiding Ethical Principles for Health Professionals

Beauchamp and Childress (2012) describe principles from moral philosophy as a guide for health professional behaviors. These principles are based on respect for all persons as intrinsically valuable.

13.3.1 Respect for Patient Autonomy

This principle, which focuses on the patient's right to self-governance, has been a guiding value in health care since the late 1960s and early 1970s. Enhancing patient autonomy is a major goal of genetic counseling. The NSGC Code of Ethics (Appendix B) says that genetic counselors "enable their clients to make informed independent decisions, free of coercion, by providing or illuminating the necessary facts and clarifying the alternatives and anticipated consequences." Patient autonomy is also a major tenet of the Reciprocal-Engagement Model of genetic counseling, specifically, "patient autonomy must be supported" (McCarthy Veach et al. 2007, p. 719). As discussed in Chap. 10, the term "nondirective" that was historically used to describe the strategy by which genetic counselors *enhanced* patient autonomy is problematic; it is more appropriate to consider the skills genetic counselors employ to *protect* patient autonomy.

Bartels et al. (1997) investigated counselor descriptions of directive behaviors and found a distinction between directing the process and directing the outcome of genetic counseling. Process refers to conducting a genetic counseling session in ways that benefit the patients you see. For instance, you are responsible for orienting the patient to the session (describing the format, outlining the purpose, etc.). You also may need to help patients clarify the meaning of genetic information in their lives and help them identify their own values and decision strategies.

Directing the outcome means you influence a patient to act in concert with your values. This kind of influence violates the spirit of respecting the patient's right to self-governance. In a situation where you believe you must tell a patient what to do, for example, whether to have predictive testing for a late-onset disorder, you must carefully consider your reasons for taking this step. You might ask whether you are responding to the patient's needs/values or to your own needs/values. Situations where you direct the outcome should be the exception and not the rule in your counseling practice. As noted in Chap. 10, however, it is crucial to differentiate between clinical information and recommendations and other types of advice or influencing responses in genetic counseling. Patients who see genetic counselors usually expect the counselor to have clinical expertise that could be helpful to them.

Genetic counselors committed to protecting patient autonomy sometimes question whether they must always do what the patient prefers and whether they must sacrifice their own values in the name of enhancing patient autonomy. The answer to those questions is "no." As a professional, you also have an obligation to abide by your professional and personal values. Being clear about your own values and motivations, as well as patient motivations, can help clarify where value conflicts may occur. The NSGC Code of Ethics (Appendix B) indicates that genetic counselors may "refer clients to an alternate genetic counselor or other qualified professional when situations arise in which a genetic counselor's personal values, attitudes and beliefs may impede his or her ability to counsel a client." This may be an appropriate response in situations where you believe that providing assistance to a patient would mean supporting an action you regard as morally wrong. In most situations, good communication will allow patients and counselors to understand one another and respect each person's right to act in accordance with his or her own values.

13.3.2 Nonmaleficence

Nonmaleficence means doing no harm; it is considered by many to be a bottom-line bioethical principle. Yet, with newer technologies and the ability to provide information about the likelihood of illness in the future, counselors often find the potential for harm coincides with providing benefit. For example, predictive testing or sharing susceptibility information can support patients who want to plan for a future situation. At the same time, however, this information can create stress and sometimes even major crises in the lives of the people who receive this information. "Not only does the individual have to live with the knowledge for a long period of time, but they also have the choice to use or disregard that knowledge when making reproductive decisions" (Chapman 2002, p. 362).

As we can't guarantee we will not inflict harm, a more practical interpretation of nonmaleficence is to consider permitting harm only when harm is unavoidable and ensuring there is a corresponding benefit. An example might be encouraging a patient to participate in genetic research only when she/he understands fully the possible risks as well as the benefits to participation.

Keep in mind that harm can extend beyond the physical realm to include emotional and financial harm and harm to one's reputation or integrity. For instance, you might consider harm to a marital relationship, and even harm to employment or insurance status, as you assist patients with making decisions about genetic testing (Billings et al. 1992; Trepanier et al. 2004). Part of honoring autonomy and preventing harm is meeting a professional duty to provide informed consent about genetic tests. Given relevant information, patients will be more prepared to assess for themselves the harms and benefits of genetic testing or consequences of sharing test results.

Preventing harm requires that you have a lifelong commitment to ensuring patient safety, to keeping current with respect to professional standards and policies, to practicing within these standards, and to maintaining your competency to practice.

13.3.3 Beneficence

For health-care professionals, beneficence usually means considering a patient's medical best interests. For example, you might believe that most people would benefit by knowing whether they are highly susceptible to a familial cancer. Therefore, from your point of view, participating in genetic testing would be in their best interest. Some patients, or their family members, however, will refuse to participate in testing because they fear they could not handle receiving a positive test result. In this situation, beneficence (acting in a patient's best interest) is challenged by duty to respect patient autonomy. We act paternalistically or parentally when we assume we are in a better position than the patient's family to determine what is in their best interest. The NSGC Code of Ethics challenges paternalism by advocating respect for patient autonomy so that patients can act in accordance with their own values, even when you might disagree with their decisions. In the case above, you may want to first ensure the patient understands the risks and benefits of both testing and not testing. If you find the patient is making an informed, autonomous choice, your primary obligation would be to respect her or his decision.

13.3.4 Justice/Fairness

Justice is a principle that concerns the equitable distribution of burdens and benefits of health care. Justice includes preventing discrimination with respect to access to services. The NSGC Code of Ethics (Appendix B) addresses nondiscrimination by saying that counselors "provide genetic counseling services to their clients regardless of their clients' abilities, age, culture, religion, ethnicity, language, sexual orientation and gender identity." In terms of counselors and societal obligations, the Code of Ethics encourages counselors to "promote policies that aim to prevent genetic discrimination and oppose the use of genetic information as a basis for discrimination."

Many questions remain unresolved with respect to the types of genetic services that ought to be offered, what will be paid for, and how to balance cost with efficacy. For instance, you may consider, as other counselors sometimes do, whether you would offer a genetic test that insurance does not cover and the patient could not afford. Most counselors would tell people about all options. You may find that you need to help the patient seek funding and/or advocate for financial coverage of options they cannot afford.

Acting justly also means equitably serving all who seek services. Throughout this book we have highlighted cultural considerations in providing genetic counseling. "Increasing the cultural competence of genetic counselors may help ameliorate some ethnic/racial disparities experienced during genetic counseling clinical encounters. Culturally competent counselors may also be able to effect change in the clinic and in society at large; cultural competence may help in making policy choices that promote the health and well-being of persons affected by ethnic and racial disparities in genetic health care" (Lewis 2010, p. 202).

13.3.5 Fidelity and Veracity

Fidelity and veracity are principles that support patient autonomy. Fidelity, or faithfulness, includes promise-keeping, meeting contracts, and being trustworthy. Section II of the NSGC Code of Ethics encourages genetic counselors to "Clarify and define their professional role(s) and relationships with clients, disclose any real or perceived conflict of interest, and provide an accurate description of their services" (Appendix B).

The obligation to be faithful presumes that professionals have a duty to care for their patients. Patients generally assume their interests are a primary concern of the counselor's, and professionals generally focus solely on patients' best interests. Genetic counselors may encounter challenges to honoring a patient's wishes when they reflect on the impact genetic information could have on other family members (McCarthy Veach et al. 2001; Hodgson and Gaff 2013).

Fidelity also challenges counselors to watch what they promise and to let people know the limits and consequences of the genetic information they will receive. Concerning what you promise to patients, remember there are mandatory reporting requirements related to illegal substance use, child and vulnerable adult abuse and neglect, and threats of harm to self or others. Therefore, you should inform patients that in such situations, maintaining confidentiality would not be possible. With respect to consequences of genetic information, you will often give patients prenatal and presymptomatic test information and will need to tell them what that information might mean for future situations such as jobs and insurance.

Veracity, or truthfulness, concerns your duty to tell the truth, meaning you do not lie to or deceive patients. Truth telling supports patient autonomy because patients can only be empowered to make decisions when they receive accurate information. Veracity is closely related to fidelity and to sharing accurate information in the informed consent process.

13.3.6 Comments About Ethical Principles

Ethical principles can serve as guidelines for addressing ethical dilemmas. They provide a language you can use to think about and discuss challenging situations with colleagues. You will find, however, that an awareness of these principles does not automatically provide the answer to ethical questions. In fact, ethical dilemmas often consist of competing obligations, that is, a desire to do two mutually incompatible things. In some situations, you will want to maintain an individual's confidentiality, but will also be concerned with harm to family members if genetic information is not disclosed. For instance, you might see a parent affected with familial adenomatous polyposis (FAP) who refuses to disclose that fact to his or her children. You may be concerned the child will not have information about the importance of screening that could prevent the occurrence of this cancer. In instances such as this, you must weigh the relevant principles, consult with other professionals, and choose the most important principle as a basis for action. Increasingly, genetic technologies such as microarray testing and whole exome sequencing raise ethical issues with regard to informed consent and sharing of results (Blackburn et al. 2015; Lohn et al. 2014; Richardson and Ormond 2017).

Genetic counselors draw upon many resources to help them sort out what to do when facing ethical dilemmas. Strategies used by clinical genetic counselors (Bower et al. 2002) include:

- *Further discussion with patient*: to clarify possible implications of test results, the patient and/or family situation, and policies regarding testing.
- *Consulting with a health professional*: consulting with genetic counselors, other health-care professionals (depending on the expertise needed), and an institutional ethics committee for help with defining and resolving ethical challenges.
- *Referral to a professional*: recommending that the patient seek assistance from another professional (see Chap. 6 on referrals).
- *Informing/educating health professionals*: addressing situations where other professionals have made errors, for example, erroneously ordering or interpreting test results or, more generally, providing health professional education.
- *Defer to preestablished rules or guidelines*: following health-care facility policies, professional guidelines [e.g., from NSGC or the American Society of Human Genetics (ASHG)], and consent policies.
- *Advocate for the patient*: appealing to third parties to get medical care, genetic testing, or reimbursement.
- *Withholding information*: this strategy usually relates to situations involving requests for information from third parties. The counselor refrains from disclosing information, believing that it would be detrimental to the patient.
- *Disregarding personal beliefs and biases*: promote patient autonomy by refraining from expressing one's disagreement with the patient's decision.
- *Determine boundaries within a family*: when facing conflicting duties to family members, clarifying to whom one's professional obligation lies, with whom information should be shared, and which family member is responsible for decisions.

Groepper et al. (2015) found that laboratory genetic counselors use strategies similar to those found by Bower et al. (2002). Laboratory genetic counselors' strategies were characterized by communication and education (with providers and patients), consultation, adherence to professional guidelines and policies, and patient advocacy. Balcom et al. (2016) suggest a series of steps for managing ethical and professional challenges in the laboratory setting; we view these steps as equally appropriate in a clinical setting:

- Gathering the facts
- Identifying the parties involved and their responsibilities
- Defining the problem
- Determining course(s) of action
- Weighing potential ethical benefits and risks (especially ethics of care, justice, and beneficence/nonmaleficence)

It is important to learn about the available resources within the facility in which you practice (both as a student and later as a professional genetic counselor). These include peer resources, supervisory resources, legal resources, ethical resources, and referral resources. It is essential (particularly as a student and in early practice) that you identify both support and consultation resources for yourself. Peers tend to be the first recourse when genetic counselors meet a challenging situation. Sharing common experiences is important for reassurance, even when you have decided the best action in a particular situation. Ethics committees exist in most health-care facilities in the USA. Additionally, the NSGC has a committee that is available to assist with ethical dilemmas. These consultants provide recommendations, not imperatives, about available options.

13.4 MORAL Model for Ethical Decisions in Clinical Situations

Crisham (1985) created the MORAL model for clinical decision-making. In this model, Crisham explicitly identifies ethical principles as relevant factors. The moral model includes a grid (shown in Table 13.1) for identifying the *values* you wish to honor in making a particular decision and the *practical considerations* you need to take into account. Values might include the ethical principles previously described in this chapter, or the values might be implied in explicit behavioral outcomes such as maximizing coping ability or avoiding escalation of family conflict. Practical considerations may include legal issues, time constraints, reimbursement concerns, and other factors that influence decisions in a particular work setting.

Prior to decision-making, you need to describe the problem and the participants, including who makes the decision and what ethical value(s) or principle(s) is at stake. The steps in Crisham's decision-making model spell out the acronym MORAL:

- *Massage the dilemma*: This process includes recognizing whose interests are involved in a conflict and defining the dilemma from their perspectives. The patient's dilemma might result from a sense of conflicting loyalties. To formulate a goal for decision-making, consider beginning with a sentence, "I would like to act in such a way that…".

Table 13.1 MORAL model for ethical decision-making grid

Options	Values	Practical Considerations
–	–	–
–	–	–
–	–	–
–	–	–
–	–	–

Adapted from Crisham (1985)

- *Outline options*: List all alternatives in the column on the left side of the grid. In this step, it is important to identify as many options as possible. Brainstorming with other students or colleagues may reveal possibilities you might miss by completing the grid alone.
- *Review criteria and resolve*: Criteria are the values and practical considerations relevant to the situation. List these in the corresponding columns. Next, go through each option, placing a plus (+) where the criterion is met or a minus (−) in each column where that criterion is violated. You may decide in this process that one criterion is more important than the others. In that case, you would give the criterion more weight. Looking over the grid, you will find that some options meet more of your defined criteria than others do, and thus they are more viable options for action.
- *Affirm position and act:* Now that you have done the moral analysis and decided, based on that analysis, what you will do, you need to consider a strategy for acting on that moral commitment. Try to anticipate any obstacles to acting.
- *Look back*: After taking action, consider how successful you were and what worked and didn't work in the analysis of the ethical dilemma and the action taken. In this process, you will learn what works for you and which pieces of the model you will take with you into your daily counseling practice and ethical decision-making.

As you gain more experience, you will recognize commonly occurring ethical situations. Although you will still experience ethical dilemmas, you will become more comfortable knowing you have the tools and resources to address them.

13.5 Reflective Practice and Professional Development

Each chapter in this book presents multiple activities and exercises that challenge you to reflect on your experiences as you learn and practice skills. Self-reflection is a crucial component of professional growth and development. In this section, we further define and describe reflective practice and discuss its relationship to professional development.

13.5.1 Professional Development in Genetic Counseling

As students complete their genetic counseling training program, they are eager to embark on their post-degree professional journey. As you transition from training to practice, you will likely feel excitement, but perhaps some anxiety. You may be asking yourself "Am I really ready to see patients on my own?" or "Did I make the right decision about accepting this job offer?" This can be a good time to think about what it means to grow and develop *professionally* as a genetic counselor.

Genetic counseling is *never* a static profession. Discoveries in the field make it imperative that you engage in lifelong learning. It is also important to take care of your physical and emotional health and to reflect on the impact of professional and personal experiences on your practice. The NSGC Code of Ethics (Appendix B) and the ACGC Practice-Based Competencies (Appendix A) reflect the imperative to act in ways that enable your professional development (ACGC 2015; NSGC 2017).

Section 1 of the NSGC Code of Ethics encourages genetic counselors to "Continue their education and training to keep abreast of relevant guidelines, regulations, position statements, and standards of genetic counseling practice" and to "Be responsible for their own physical and emotional health as it impacts their professional judgment and performance, including seeking professional support, as needed" (NSGC 2017).

Domain IV of the ACGC Practice-Based Competencies describes competencies related to professional development, including "Demonstrate a self-reflective, evidenced based and current approach to genetic counseling practice" (ACGC 2015). Activities and skills that contribute to the development of this competency include the following:

- Display initiative for lifelong learning.
- Recognize one's limitations and capabilities in the context of genetic counseling practice.
- Seek feedback and respond appropriately to performance critique.
- Demonstrate a scholarly approach to genetic counseling, including using available evidence-based principles in the preparation and execution of a genetic counseling encounter.
- Identify appropriate individual and/or group opportunities for ongoing personal supervision and mentorship.
- Accept responsibility for one's physical and emotional health as it impacts on professional performance.

Although at first glance, this may all sound a bit daunting, you can take encouragement from the experience of your genetic counseling colleagues. Runyon et al. (2010) surveyed 184 genetic counselors, asking them two open-ended questions: "What is the most important thing you have learned about yourself in your practice as a genetic counselor"; and "What advice would you offer to genetic counseling students just starting their career?" (p. 373). Responses to the first question were coded into three themes: intrapersonal lessons, interpersonal lessons, and professional lessons.

Intrapersonal lessons included:

- Self-efficacy (e.g., how to more accurately assess their abilities and set realistic expectations for their professional performance; developed increased confidence because of how they handled difficult situations).
- Synergy between personal and professional life experiences (e.g., experiences in their personal life increased their ability to understand patient situations, and professional experiences helped clarify perspectives and appreciation of their own life experiences; importance of self-care; and setting boundaries to avoid burnout).

- Letting go of control (developed or became more aware of their open-mindedness about patients' views and decisions; learned not to direct patients to a certain outcome; learned to recognize and manage their hot-button issues; and learned to accept that some matters are uncontrollable).

Interpersonal lessons included:

- Meaningfulness of patient relationships (deepening of empathy and ability to relate to patients; learned how to manage patients' difficult emotions as well as their own).
- Managing uncertainty (it is okay not to know everything; developed ability to handle unknown or new situations as well as ambiguity).

Professional lessons included:

- Discovery that certain professional activities (e.g., teaching, clinical work, problem-solving, mentoring) were particularly enjoyable.
- Certain traits, behaviors, and attitudes facilitate optimal functioning in the workplace (e.g., taking ownership to get important work done, identifying priorities, advocating for positive change).
- Some reported learning lessons from handling undesirable aspects of the job, such as issues with colleagues.
- Energy and growth come from a commitment to ongoing learning from a variety of sources.

Responses to the second question about advice for genetic counseling students just starting their careers were coded into similar themes: intrapersonal advice, interpersonal advice, and professional advice. "Across the themes and domains of advice the major 'take home' points appear to be: (1) take care of one's self by learning coping behaviors, assertiveness in job settings, cultivation of non-work related interests, and creation of 'balance' in life and work; (2) approach the profession and one's work with an open mind about patients and ways of practicing genetic counseling, and by learning from a variety of sources; (3) cultivate self-confidence by learning to manage high expectations of self and others; (4) focus on becoming autonomous in one's professional functioning, including knowing when and how to seek support from others; (5) taking charge of one's professional and career development by seeking out responsibilities and additional roles, and participating in national organizations; and (6) learning to let go of one's agenda and information-driven approach in order to empathically attend to psychosocial aspects of cases" (Runyon et al. 2010, p. 383).

Zahm et al. (2016) interviewed novice, experienced, and seasoned genetic counselors about their professional development. Based on their findings, the researchers developed a model for genetic counselor professional development shown in Fig. 13.1.

Zahm et al. (2016) described professional development as "an on-going, non-linear, and gradual process, with 'defining moments' or key events providing additional 'bursts' of influence. Professional development processes, influences, and outcomes are reciprocal, suggesting changes in one area may promote changes in other areas" (p. 830). Study participants "continually identified self-reflection as critical to professional development. These findings align with literature suggesting optimal growth occurs when experience is accompanied by reflection in order to translate information from one's experiences into professional change…" (p. 830). The authors noted that although professional development processes, influences, and outcomes were similar across the three stages of professional development, seasoned practitioners reported "a wider range and depth of clinical experiences, more ways in which their personal lives had intertwined with and affected their professional work, and perceptions of the field as quite different from when they began" (p. 830).

Miranda et al. (2016) characterized "master genetic counselor clinicians" based on qualitative interviews with 15 peer-nominated genetic counselors. Their description, consistent with Zahm et al.'s (2016) proposed model of genetic counselor professional development, is as follows: "Master genetic counselors have deep empathy and are inspired by patients and colleagues, and they derive personal meaning from their work. They are affected emotionally by their work, but effectively manage the emotional impact. They view their professional development as ongoing, influenced by colleagues, patients, mentoring, multicultural considerations and their own family of origin. They also believe professional development of expertise occurs through critical reflection upon the experiences one accrues" (p. 767).

13.5.2 *Reflective Practice*

Throughout your training as a genetic counselor, you have most likely been exposed to more experienced genetic counselors who served as positive role models and mentors. Whether in the classroom, clinic, research, laboratory, or other settings, your interactions with genetic counselors and other genetics and health-care professionals have helped to shape your view of what it means to be a competent professional. While hopefully most of these experiences have been positive, you may have also had interactions with genetic counselors and others that you viewed more negatively, demonstrating attitudes and behaviors you would not wish to emulate in your own professional practice. One thing you probably realized is that years of experience alone do not ensure expertise or competence. While some of your most inspirational role models may have been "seasoned" genetic counselors, it's likely that you were also inspired by genetic counselors with just a few years of postgraduate experience. Indeed, some of the participants in Miranda et al.'s (2016) master genetic counselor study were individuals who had only a few years of experience.

Zahm (2010) comprehensively explored the role of reflective practice in professional development. She states, "Simply engaging in an experience or set of experiences – say, a 10-week clinical rotation- is not enough, necessarily to produce growth. Two genetic counselors with 5 years of postdegree experience, for example, may differ widely in their professional growth, due in part to their willingness

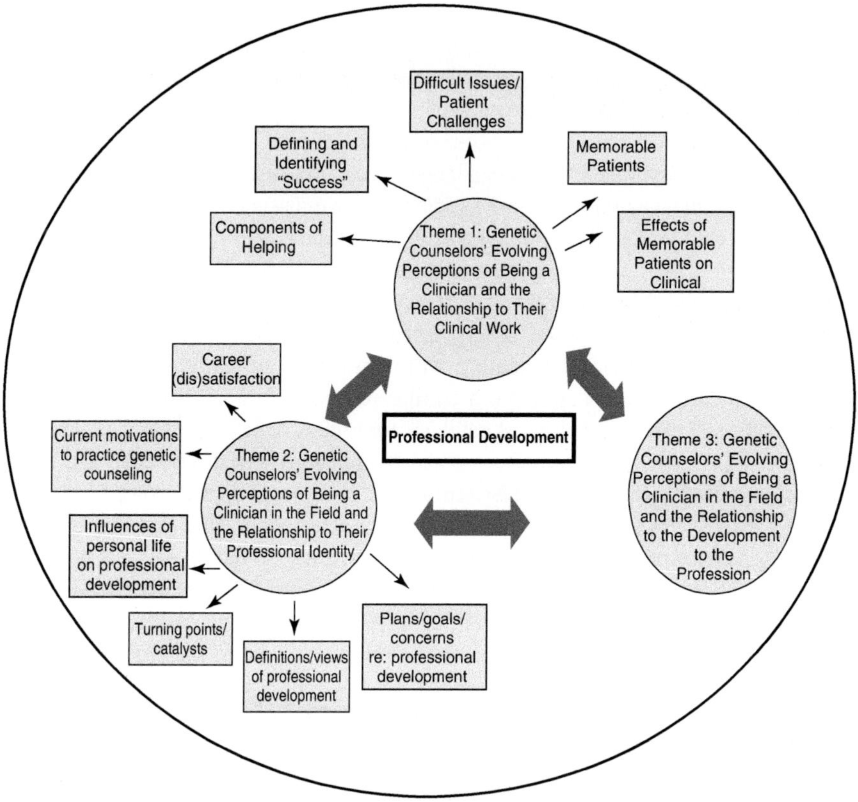

Fig. 13.1 Visual representation of proposed model of genetic counselor development. The *circles* represent the three themes. The *squares* represent the 11 domains. The *arrows* represent the mutual influences among the themes in genetic counselor professional development. Source: Zahm et al. (2016). Reprinted with permission from the *Journal of Genetic Counseling*

and ability to engage in reflective practice" (p. 355). Zahm describes reflective practice as "deliberate, necessitating a conscious effort to examine one's experiences and integrate the resulting reflections into one's approach to his or her practice" (p. 356). A key point here is not just thinking about a case or experience, but using the insights you gain from your reflections to change your practice (build skills). As discussed previously, other studies (Miranda et al. 2016; Runyon et al. 2010; Zahm, et al. 2016) have also emphasized the importance of reflection in the professional development of genetic counselors. Self-reflection can also be a useful strategy for preventing or managing burnout and/or compassion fatigue as discussed in Chap. 12.

Zahm (2010) offers several suggestions for optimizing reflective practice. These include engaging in peer-group supervision, informal interactions with colleagues, reading reflective literature, periodically taping and critiquing your own work, and making time for reflective practice (pp. 369–372).

You may wonder how you will find time for reflection in a busy clinical or other professional setting. Keep in mind that it is not the quantity but, rather, the quality of your reflection that matters. Take time to think about how your views about your patients' situations have changed over time or have been impacted by things happening in your own life. Do you find that you view your pregnant patients' concerns differently since becoming pregnant yourself? Has a challenge to your own health or the health of a close relative altered the way you approach patients when discussing their health concerns?

You may find yourself reflecting on clinical cases or other situations during your commute to and from work. Or you might informally discuss difficult cases or problematic situations with your colleagues. These types of discussions can provide valuable insights about your own reactions to those situations as well as helpful suggestions and strategies for dealing with similar situations in the future. More formal case conferences can serve a similar purpose. Zahm (2010) suggests you consider the following questions as catalysts for reflective practice: "Notice an experience, remember it, and think about it and the nuances. What happened and how? How did it affect me? What did I learn from this? How does/did this experience affect me personally? Professionally? How has my genetic counseling practice changed because of this experience? How do I want it to change? What do I wish I had done differently? What will I do differently in the future? How does this experience influence my view of humanity? My view of the practice of genetic counseling? Consider discussing your answers to these questions with trusted others" (p. 371).

13.6 Closing Comments

In this chapter, we discussed motivations for choosing a career in genetic counseling, professional values, and guiding ethical principles. We presented strategies for managing ethical challenges. We also discussed professional development and the importance of reflective practice.

As a practicing genetic counselor, you will continue to gain experience, develop your expertise, and expand your skills. You will have an impact on your patients, colleagues, and students, and they will have an impact on you. We encourage you to engage in activities that will enable you to remain enthusiastic about your work, regardless of where your professional journey leads you. Trust yourself, learn from your experiences, and be genuine and compassionate with others and with yourself.

13.7 Class Activities

Activity 1: Motivations to Be a Genetic Counselor (Think-Pair-Share Dyads)

Pairs of students discuss with a classmate the major reasons they decided to become a genetic counselor. Identify together the strengths and limitations these reasons may bring to their practice.

Estimated time: 20 min.

Activity 2: Culture and Helpers (Part I: Discussion, Think-Pair-Share Dyads)

Pairs of students discuss the following questions: (1) What is culture? (2) What is genetic counseling? (3) How does culture impact genetic counseling? (4) Pirzadeh et al. (2007) identified four values that are important to genetic counselors: benevolence (concern for others), self-direction (independence), achievement (personal success), and universalism (protecting the welfare of all). Which of these values are important to you? Are there other values that are important to you? (5) How might these values affect your work with patients? (6).

Estimated time: 30 min.

Activity 3: Culture and Helpers (Part II: Discussion, Think-Pair-Share Dyads)

Pairs of students discuss the following questions: (1) What kinds of differences in culture do I perceive in others? (2) How do I respond to the differences that I see in others? (3) What biases am I aware that I have?

Estimated time: 20 min.

Process: Activities 1 Through 3

Why do you think it is important to discuss motivations for being a counselor in relation to cultural differences? What did you learn from these exercises? What are your feelings about examining your cultural values, your motivations, and cultural differences?

Estimated time: 10–15 min.

Activity 4: Cultural Identities (Think-Pair Share Dyads)

Students work in pairs to complete this activity. The students should take turns interviewing each other for 10 min about their respective cultural identities. Questions can include the following:

1. Where were you born? Where did you grow up?
2. What do you consider to be your cultural/ethnic heritage?
3. What reactions or curiosities do you have about your own cultural programming?
4. What are your current cultural affiliations (e.g., religious, ethnic alliances)?
5. Does any aspect of your cultural identity come in conflict with other aspects?

Process

- Students should make notes as they complete their interviews.

- When the interviews have been completed, students take turns "introducing" the person they interview to the class. *Introductions should only include information the student being introduced is comfortable having disclosed to the whole class.*
- Students discuss what they learned about culture and identity in completing this exercise.

Estimated time: 20 min for interviews (if done in class); 10 min per dyad for introductions

Activity 5: Structured Controversy

The structured controversy activity gives you an opportunity to try on and evaluate alternative perspectives. Address the following situation using the steps and time allotments for each step as described in the structured controversy instructions.

Situation

A 16-year-old healthy patient with a family history of HD requests testing. The patient is at 50% risk. His father was affected and recently died. The patient's mother is adamant that he not be tested at this time. She is concerned that he will not be able to deal emotionally with a positive test result and that a positive result could have major negative effects on other decisions he is currently facing (e.g., going to college, employment, relationships, etc.). Although there are guidelines for testing minors, not everyone follows these, especially when the minor is an older adolescent. You need to decide whether you support the mother's position or the son's position. No matter which position you support, you will need to be able to discuss your reasoning behind your decision.

Structured Controversy Instructions

- Assign one person to be the timekeeper.
- Count off the participants; odd numbers will take one position, and even numbers will take an alternate position.
- Initially the odd-numbered people will take the mother's perspective, and the even-numbered people will take the patient's perspective.

Assigned Perspective

- Prepare presentation with partner(s) (20 min).
- Present arguments (5 min per side; 10 min total).
- Ask clarification questions when the opposite side finishes presenting (5 min total).
- General discussion (5 min).

Estimated time: 40 min.

Reverse Perspective

- Prepare presentation with partner(s) (10 min).

- Present arguments not included by alternative side (5 min).
- Present arguments (5 min per side).

 Estimated time: 20 min.

Open Discussion: Decision-Making
- Drop perspective.
- Seek and provide clarification, elaboration, justification, and rationale.
- Summarize arguments.
- Reach conclusions.

 Estimated time: 15 min.

Report Preparation (Optional)
- Prepare a written response to the question (your group's conclusion, the data/arguments supporting your conclusion, the counterarguments to your conclusion, and the weaknesses of those counterarguments).

 Estimated time: 20 min.

Small Groups Discuss Conclusions/Rationale with Large Group
Estimated time: 15 min.

13.8 Written Exercises

Exercise 1: Cultural Impact on Motivations to Be a Genetic Counselor

Prepare a three- to four-page, double-spaced, paper discussing the following:

- How do you define culture?
- Did your personal definition of culture change because of the class discussion? If so, how?
- Describe your own ethnocultural background.
- Identify *four* of your personal motivations (desires, needs), and discuss how they are potentially beneficial and potentially harmful in your practice of genetic counseling. For each motivation, describe (a) how it might affect your counseling in ways that are *beneficial* to the patient and to you and (b) how it might affect your counseling in ways that are *harmful* to the patient and to you.
 [*Hint*: Motivations are not the same thing as traits. For example, it is not sufficient to say that one of your motivations is that you are empathic. Why or how does this trait lead to a desire to be a genetic counselor?]
- What impact has your culture had on your motivations to be a genetic counselor?

Exercise 2: Promoting Patient Autonomy (Informed Consent)

The purpose of providing consent is to enhance patient autonomy. Ideally, the counselor-patient relationship is a collaborative one in which the counselor attempts to understand patient expectations and explain how the counseling session will proceed.

Consider the following questions:

- What three things might patients want to know about the purpose of genetic counseling?
- What might they want to know about the process and outcome of genetic counseling?
- What might they want to know about you (assume you are still in a student role)?
- What would you tell them about the limits to confidentiality?
- What would you want to know if you were the patient?

Create a checklist of items you will discuss with patients so that they are informed about genetic counseling. Next, compare your checklist with that of another student, and then create a combined list of items to describe genetic counseling.

Exercise 3: Addressing an Ethical Dilemma

Using the MORAL model grid in Table 13.1, list every option you might have to define and address for the ethical dilemma described in the case example below. At the top of the grid, list the ethical principles you would like to address in your response: For example: "I want to act in such a way that to ensure that I am not doing harm to my patient…" Then list practical considerations, such as the availability of a test, reimbursement, or legal concerns that also must be considered. Work through the MORAL model grid. Select the option you would choose, and the rationale, based on ethical principles and practical considerations, for your decision.

Case Example

A 4-year-old girl, Emily, is evaluated in your genetics clinic. Emily has unexplained developmental deficits. Previous evaluation included a normal karyotype and negative fragile X testing. Emily's mother, Sue, is 31 years old, and her father, John, is 32 years old. This is the couple's first child. In reviewing the family history, you obtain the following information: Sue has two sisters, ages 28 and 26. Her mother died at age 49 of breast cancer. Her sisters each have two children with no growth or developmental problems. John's parents are both alive and well. He was an only child, but his mother experienced two early miscarriages. Sue is eager to learn the cause of Emily's developmental deficits. She is also interested in learning if they have an increased risk for having other children with similar developmental problems. Sue has heard about whole exome sequencing (WES) and is specifically requesting this testing for Emily. Sue mentions that her family is not supportive of this testing. Her sisters have expressed that Sue should just "accept Emily's problems" and move on with her plans to have additional pregnancies. Sue tells you she does not agree with her sisters and that she believes "knowledge is power." She wants to learn as much as she can about Emily's developmental problems in hopes that this may lead to interventions which will be helpful to her. You notice that John has been very quiet throughout this discussion and ask him directly what his thoughts are about proceeding with the WES study. John responds that he will go along with whatever Sue wants, but he is personally "worn out" by the multiple evaluations and visits to doctors and developmental specialists. He tends to agree with Sue's sisters that they should go ahead with their plans to have more children and "hope for the best." Whole exome sequencing (WES) performed on a blood sample obtained from Emily reveals nothing relevant to her developmental deficits, but it does reveal a mutation in BRCA1. Should this result be shared with Sue and John?

Instructor Note

- Students can be asked to redo the grid for an alternative WES result which reveals a mutation in the PSEN1 gene (early-onset Alzheimer disease). Should this result be shared with Sue and John?
- You could use the students' grids as the basis for an in-class activity in which they share their responses to the following questions: What option did each of you select? What is your rationale for selecting that option? After discussing their responses, students consider together which elements of the model explain the similarities, or differences, in their choices.
- Students should also discuss pre-counseling strategies that would be helpful in addressing situations such as these.

Exercise 4: Role-Play

Engage in a 20-min role-play of a genetic counseling session with a classmate. The role-play can be based on a patient you saw in the clinic, or it can be a made-up patient situation. Focus on an ethical dilemma that arises during the interaction. Audio record the role-play. Next transcribe the role-play and critique your work. Use the following method for transcribing the session:

Counselor	Patient	Self-critique	Instructor
Key phrases of dialogue	Key phrases	Comment on your own response	Will provide feedback on your responses

Create a brief summary:

1. Briefly describe patient *demographics* (e.g., age, gender, ethnicity, socioeconomic status, relationship status), *reason* for seeking genetic counseling, and the *nature of the ethical dilemma* that arose.
2. Identify *two* things you said/did during the role play that were effective, and *two* things you could have done differently:

Give the recording, transcript, and self-critique to the instructor who will provide feedback.

[*Hint*: This assignment encourages self-reflective practice regarding your clinical performance. The goal is not to do a perfect session. Rather the goal is to assess the extent to which you can accurately assess your psychosocial counseling skills. You will gain more from this exercise if you refrain from scripting what you plan to say as the counselor.]

References

Abad-Perotín R, Asúnsolo-Del Barco Á, Silva-Mato A. A survey of ethical and professional challenges experienced by Spanish health-care professionals that provide genetic counseling services. J Genet Couns. 2012;21:85–100.

Accreditation Council for Genetic Counseling. Practice based competencies for genetic counselors. 2015. http://gceducation.org/Documents/ACGC%20Core%20Competencies%20Brochure_15_Web.pdf. Accessed 18 Aug 2017.

Alliman S, Veach PM, Bartels DM, Lian F, James C, LeRoy BS. A comparative analysis of ethical and professional challenges experienced by Australian and US genetic counselors. J Genet Couns. 2009;18:379–94.

Balcom JR, Kotzer KE, Waltman LA, Kemppainen JL, Thomas BC. The genetic counselor's role in managing ethical dilemmas arising in the laboratory setting. J Genet Couns. 2016;25:838–54.

Bartels DM, LeRoy BS, McCarthy PR, Caplan AL. Nondirectiveness in genetic counseling: a survey of practitioners. Am J Med Genet A. 1997;72:172–9.

Beauchamp TL, Childress JF. Principles of biomedical ethics. 7th ed. London: Oxford University Press; 2012.

Billings PR, Kohn MA, de Cuevas M, Beckwith J, Alper JS, Natowicz M. Discrimination as a consequence of genetic testing. Am J Hum Genet. 1992;50:476–82.

Blackburn HL, Schroeder B, Turner C, Shriver CD, Ellsworth DL, Ellsworth RE. Management of incidental findings in the era of next-generation sequencing. Curr Genomics. 2015;16:159–74.

Bower MA, Veach PM, Bartels DM, LeRoy BS. A survey of genetic counselors' strategies for addressing ethical and professional challenges in practice. J Genet Couns. 2002;11:163–86.

Cavanagh M, Levitov JE. The counseling experience a theoretical and practical approach. 2nd ed. Prospect Heights IL: Waveland Press; 2002.

Chapman E. Ethical dilemmas in testing for late onset conditions: reactions to testing and perceived impact on other family members. J Genet Couns. 2002;11:351–67.

Crisham P. How can I do what's right? Nurs Manag. 1985;16:42A–N.

Davis BJ, Voegtle KH. Culturally competent health care for adolescents. Chicago: Department of Adolescent Health, American Medical Association; 1994. p. 19–24.

Eliason BC, Guse C, Gottlieb MS. Personal values of family physicians, practice satisfaction, and service to the underserved. Arch Fam Med. 2000;9:228–32.

Eliason BC, Schubot DB. Personal values of exemplary family physicians: implications for professional satisfaction in family medicine. J Fam Pract. 1995;41:251–6.

Groepper D, McCarthy Veach P, LeRoy BS, Bower M. Who are laboratory genetic counselors and what ethical and professional challenges do they encounter? J Genet Couns. 2015;24:580–96.

Gschmeidler B, Flatscher-Thoeni M. Ethical and professional challenges of genetic counseling–the case of Austria. J Genet Couns. 2013;22:741–52.

Hodgson J, Gaff C. Enhancing family communication about genetics: ethical and professional dilemmas. J Genet Couns. 2013;22:16–21.

Lewis L. Honoring diversity: cultural competence in genetic counseling. In: LeRoy BS, McCarthy Veach P, Bartels DM, editors. Genetic counseling practice. Hoboken: Wiley-Blackwell; 2010. p. 201–34.

Lohn Z, Adam S, Birch PH, Friedman JM. Incidental findings from clinical genome-wide sequencing: a review. J Genet Couns. 2014;23:463–73.
McCarthy Veach P, Bartels DM, LeRoy BS. Ethical and professional challenges posed by patients with genetic concerns: a report of focus group discussions with genetic counselors, physicians, and nurses. J Genet Couns. 2001;10:97–119.
McCarthy Veach P, Bartels DM, LeRoy BS. Coming full circle: a Reciprocal-Engagement Model of genetic counseling practice. J Genet Couns. 2007;16:713–28.
Miranda C, Veach PM, Martyr MA, LeRoy BS. Portrait of the master genetic counselor clinician: a qualitative investigation of expertise in genetic counseling. J Genet Couns. 2016;25:767–85.
National Society of Genetic Counselors. National society of genetic counselors code of ethics. J Genet Couns. 2017. https://doi.org/10.1007/s10897-017-0166-8. [Epub ahead of print].
National Society of Genetic Counselors. n.d.. http://www.nsgc.org/page/frequently-asked-questions-students. Accessed 1 Nov 2017.
Pirzadeh S, McCarthy Veach P, Bartels DM, Kao J, LeRoy BS. A national survey of genetic counselor personal values. J Genet Couns. 2007;16:763–73.
Richardson A, Ormond KE. Ethical considerations in prenatal testing: genomic testing and medical uncertainty. Semin Fetal Neonatal Med. 2017. https://doi.org/10.1016/j.siny.2017.10.001. [Epub ahead of print].
Runyon M, Zahm KW, Veach PM, MacFarlane IM, LeRoy BS. What do genetic counselors learn on the job? A qualitative assessment of professional development outcomes. J Genet Couns. 2010;19:371–86.
Schwartz SH. Universals in the content and structure of values: theoretical advances and empirical tests in 20 countries. Adv Exp Soc Psychol. 1992;25:1–65.
Trepanier A, Ahrens M, McKinnon W, Peters J, Stopfer J, Campbell Grumet S, et al. Genetic cancer risk assessment and counseling: recommendations of the National Society of Genetic Counselors. J Genet Couns. 2004;13:83–114.
Wells DM, Veach PM, Martyr MA, LeRoy BS. Development, experience, and expression of meaning in genetic counselors' lives: an exploratory analysis. J Genet Couns. 2016;25:799–817.
Zahm KW, Veach PM, Martyr MA, LeRoy BS. From novice to seasoned practitioner: a qualitative investigation of genetic counselor professional development. J Genet Couns. 2016;25:818–34.
Zahm KW. Professional development: reflective genetic counseling practice. In: LeRoy BS, McCarthy Veach P, Bartels DM, editors. Genetic counseling practice. Hoboken: Wiley-Blackwell; 2010. p. 353–80.

Appendix A: Accreditation Council for Genetic Counseling (ACGC) Practice-Based Competencies

This document defines and describes the 22 practice-based competencies that an entry-level provider must demonstrate to successfully practice as a genetic counselor. It provides guidance for the training of genetic counselors and an assessment for maintenance of competency of practicing genetic counselors. The didactic and experiential components of a genetic counseling training curriculum and maintenance of competency for providers must support the development of competencies categorized in the following domains: **(1) genetics expertise and analysis; (2) interpersonal, psychosocial, and counseling skills; (3) education; and (4) professional development and practice.** These domains describe the minimal skill set of a genetic counselor, which should be applied across practice settings. Some competencies may be relevant to more than one domain. *Italicized words are defined in the glossary.*

Domain 1: Genetics Expertise and Analysis

1. Demonstrate and utilize a depth and breadth of understanding and knowledge of *genetics* and *genomics* core concepts and principles.
2. Integrate knowledge of psychosocial aspects of conditions with a genetic component to promote *client* well-being.
3. Construct relevant, targeted, and comprehensive personal and family histories and pedigrees.
4. Identify, assess, facilitate, and integrate genetic testing options in genetic counseling practice.
5. Assess individuals' and their relatives' *probability of conditions with a genetic component* or carrier status based on their pedigree, test result(s), and other pertinent information.
6. Demonstrate the skills necessary to successfully manage a genetic counseling case.
7. Critically assess genetic/genomic, medical, and social science literature and information.

P. McCarthy Veach et al., *Facilitating the Genetic Counseling Process*,
https://doi.org/10.1007/978-3-319-74799-6

Domain 2: Interpersonal, Psychosocial, and Counseling Skills

1. Establish a mutually agreed-upon genetic counseling agenda with the client.
2. Employ active listening and interviewing skills to identify, assess, and empathically respond to stated and emerging concerns.
3. Use a range of genetic counseling skills and models to facilitate informed decision- making and adaptation to genetic risks or conditions.
4. Promote client-centered, informed, noncoercive, and value-based decision-making.
5. Understand how to adapt genetic counseling skills for varied service delivery models.
6. Apply genetic counseling skills in a culturally responsive and respectful manner to all clients.

Domain 3: Education

1. Effectively educate clients about a wide range of genetics and genomics information based on their needs, their characteristics, and the circumstances of the encounter.
2. Write concise and understandable clinical and scientific information for audiences of varying educational backgrounds.
3. Effectively give a presentation on genetics, genomics, and genetic counseling issues.

Domain 4: Professional Development and Practice

1. Act in accordance with the ethical, legal, and philosophical principles and values of the genetic counseling profession and the policies of one's institution or organization.
2. Demonstrate understanding of the research process.
3. Advocate for individuals, families, *communities*, and the genetic counseling profession.
4. Demonstrate a self-reflective, evidenced-based, and current approach to genetic counseling practice.
5. Understand the methods, roles, and responsibilities of the process of clinical supervision of trainees.
6. Establish and maintain professional *interdisciplinary relationships* in both team and one-on-one settings, and recognize one's role in the larger health-care system.

Appendix: Samples of Activities and Skills That May Assist in Meeting Practice-Based Competencies

These samples may assist in curriculum planning, development, implementation, and program and counselor evaluation. They are not intended to be exhaustive nor mandatory, as competencies can be achieved in multiple ways.

Domain 1: Genetics Expertise and Analysis

1. Demonstrate and utilize a depth and breadth of understanding and knowledge of *genetics* and *genomics* core concepts and principles.

   a. Demonstrate knowledge of principles of human, medical, and public health genetics and genomics and their related sciences. These include:

      Mendelian and non-Mendelian inheritance
      Population and quantitative genetics
      Human variation and disease susceptibility
      Family history and *pedigree* analysis
      Normal/abnormal physical and psychological development
      Human reproduction
      Prenatal genetics
      Pediatric genetics
      Adult genetics
      Personalized genomic medicine
      Cytogenetics
      Biochemical genetics
      Molecular genetics
      Embryology/teratology/developmental genetics
      Cancer genetics
      Cardiovascular genetics
      Neurogenetics
      Pharmacogenetics
      Psychiatric genetics

   b. Apply knowledge of genetic principles, and understand how they contribute to etiology, clinical features and disease expression, natural history, differential diagnoses, genetic testing and test report interpretation, pathophysiology, recurrence risk, management and prevention, and *population screening*.

2. Integrate knowledge of psychosocial aspects of conditions with a genetic component to promote *client* well-being.

   a. Demonstrate an understanding of psychosocial, ethical, and legal issues related to genetic counseling encounters.
   b. Describe common emotional and/or behavioral responses that may commonly occur in the genetic counseling context.
   c. Recognize the importance of understanding the lived experiences of people with various genetic/genomic conditions.
   d. Evaluate the potential impact of psychosocial issues on client decision-making and adherence to medical management.

3. Construct relevant, targeted, and comprehensive personal and family histories and pedigrees.

    a. Demonstrate proficiency in the use of pedigree symbols, standard notation, and nomenclature.
    b. Utilize interviewing skills to elicit a family history and pursue a relevant path of inquiry.
    c. Use active listening skills to formulate structured questions for the individual case depending on the reason for taking the family history and/or potential diagnoses.
    d. Elicit and assess pertinent information relating to medical, developmental, pregnancy, and psychosocial histories.
    e. Extract pertinent information from available medical records.

4. Identify, assess, facilitate, and integrate genetic testing options in genetic counseling practice.

    a. Investigate the availability, analytic validity, clinical validity, and clinical utility of screening, diagnostic, and predictive genetic/genomic tests.
    b. Evaluate and assess laboratories, and select the most appropriate laboratory and test based on the clinical situation.
    c. Identify and discuss the potential benefits, risks, limitations, and costs of genetic testing.
    d. Coordinate and facilitate the ordering of appropriate genetic testing for the client.
    e. Interpret the clinical implications of genetic test reports.
    f. Recognize and differentiate specific considerations relevant to genetic versus genomic and clinical versus research testing in terms of the informed consent process, results disclosure, Institutional Review Board (IRB) guidelines, and clinical decision-making.

5. Assess individuals' and their relatives' *probability of conditions with a genetic component* or carrier status based on their pedigree, test result(s), and other pertinent information.

    a. Assess probability of conditions with a genetic component or carrier status using relevant knowledge and data based on pedigree analysis, inheritance patterns, genetic epidemiology, quantitative genetics principles, and mathematical calculations.
    b. Incorporate the results of screening, diagnostic, and predictive genetic/genomic tests to provide accurate risk assessment for clients.
    c. Evaluate familial implications of genetic/genomic test results.
    d. Identify and integrate relevant information about environmental and lifestyle factors into the risk assessment.

6. Demonstrate the skills necessary to successfully manage a genetic counseling case.

    a. Develop and execute a *case management* plan that includes case preparation and follow-up.
    b. Assess and modify the case management plan as needed to incorporate changes in management and surveillance recommendations.

c. Document and present the genetic counseling encounter information clearly and concisely, orally and in writing, in a manner that is understandable to the audience and in accordance with professional and institutional guidelines and standards.
d. Identify and introduce research options when indicated and requested in compliance with applicable privacy, human subjects, and regional and institutional standards.
e. Identify, access, and present information to clients on local, regional, national, and international resources, services, and support.

7. Critically assess genetic/genomic, medical, and social science literature and information.

a. Plan and execute a thorough search and review of the literature.
b. Evaluate and critique scientific papers, and identify appropriate conclusions by applying knowledge of relevant *research methodologies* and statistical analyses.
c. Synthesize information obtained from a literature review to utilize in genetic counseling encounters.
d. Incorporate medical and scientific literature into evidenced-based practice recognizing that there are limitations and gaps in knowledge and data.

Domain 2: Interpersonal, Psychosocial, and Counseling Skills

8. Establish a mutually agreed-upon genetic counseling agenda with the client.

a. Describe the genetic counseling process to clients.
b. Elicit client expectations, perceptions, knowledge, and concerns regarding the genetic counseling encounter and the reason for referral or contact.
c. Apply client expectations, perceptions, knowledge, and concerns toward the development of a mutually agreed-upon agenda.
d. Modify the genetic counseling agenda, as appropriate by continually *contracting* to address emerging concerns.

9. Employ active listening and interviewing skills to identify, assess, and empathically respond to stated and emerging concerns.

a. Elicit and evaluate client emotions, individual and family experiences, beliefs, behaviors, values, coping mechanisms, and adaptive capabilities.
b. Engage in relationship-building with the client by establishing rapport, employing active listening skills, and demonstrating empathy.
c. Assess and respond to client emotional and behavioral cues, expressed both verbally and nonverbally, including emotions affecting understanding, retention, perception, and decision-making.

10. Use a range of genetic counseling skills and models to facilitate informed decision-making and adaptation to genetic risks or conditions.

a. Demonstrate knowledge of psychological defenses, family dynamics, family systems theory, coping models, the grief process, and reactions to illness.

b. Utilize a range of basic counseling skills, such as open-ended questions, reflection, and normalization.
c. Employ a variety of advanced genetic counseling skills, such as anticipatory guidance and in-depth exploration of client responses to risks and options.
d. Assess clients' psychosocial needs, and evaluate the need for intervention and referral.
e. Apply evidence-based models to guide genetic counseling practice, such as short-term *client-centered* counseling, grief counseling, and crisis counseling.
f. Develop an appropriate follow-up plan to address psychosocial concerns that have emerged in the encounter, including referrals for psychological services when indicated.

11. Promote client-centered, informed, noncoercive, and value-based decision-making.

    a. Recognize one's own values and biases as they relate to genetic counseling.
    b. Actively facilitate client decision-making that is consistent with the client's values.
    c. Recognize and respond to client-counselor relationship dynamics, such as transference and countertransference, which may affect the genetic counseling interaction.
    d. Describe the continuum of nondirectiveness to directiveness, and effectively utilize an appropriate degree of guidance for specific genetic counseling encounters.
    e. Maintain professional boundaries by ensuring directive statements, self-disclosure, and self-involving responses are in the best interest of the client.

12. Understand how to adapt genetic counseling skills for varied service delivery models.

    a. Tailor communication to a range of service delivery models to meet the needs of various audiences.
    b. Compare strengths and limitations of different service delivery models given the genetic counseling indication.
    c. Describe the benefits and limitations of *distance encounters*.
    d. Tailor genetic counseling to a range of service delivery models using relevant verbal and nonverbal forms of communication.
    e. Recognize psychosocial concerns unique to distance genetic counseling encounters.

13. Apply genetic counseling skills in a culturally responsive and respectful manner to all clients.

    a. Describe how aspects of culture including language, ethnicity, lifestyle, socioeconomic status, disability, sexuality, age, and gender affect the genetic counseling encounter.

b. Assess and respond to client cultural beliefs relevant to the genetic counseling encounter.
c. Utilize multicultural genetic counseling resources to plan and tailor genetic counseling agendas, and assess and counsel clients.
d. Identify how the genetic counselor's personal cultural characteristics and biases may impact encounters, and use this knowledge to maintain effective client-focused services.

Domain 3: Education

14. Effectively educate clients about a wide range of genetics and genomics information based on their needs, their characteristics, and the circumstances of the encounter.

    a. Identify factors that affect the learning process such as intellectual ability, emotional state, socioeconomic factors, physical abilities, religious and cultural beliefs, motivation, language, and educational background.
    b. Recognize and apply risk communication principles and theory to maximize client understanding.
    c. Communicate relevant genetic and genomic information to help clients understand and adapt to conditions or the risk of conditions and to engage in informed decision-making.
    d. Utilize a range of tools to enhance the learning encounter such as handouts, visual aids, and other educational technologies.
    e. Communicate both orally and in writing using a style and method that is clear and unambiguous.
    f. Present balanced descriptions of lived experiences of people with various conditions.
    g. Explain and address client concerns regarding genetic privacy and related protections.
    h. Employ strategies for successful communication when working with interpreters.

15. Write concise and understandable clinical and scientific information for audiences of varying educational backgrounds.

    a. Develop written educational materials tailored to the intended audience.
    b. Recognize the professional and legal importance of medical documentation and confidentiality.
    c. Assess the challenges faced by clients with low literacy, and modify the presentation of information to reduce the literacy burden.

16. Effectively give a presentation on genetics, genomics, and genetic counseling issues.

    a. Assess and determine the educational goals and learning objectives based on the needs and characteristics of the audience.
    b. Develop an educational method or approach that best facilitates the educational goals of the presentation and considers the characteristics of the audience.

c. Present using a delivery style that results in effective communication to the intended audience that is clear and unambiguous.
d. Assess one's own teaching style, and use feedback and other outcome data to refine future educational encounters.

Domain 4: Professional Development and Practice

17. Act in accordance with the ethical, legal, and philosophical principles and values of the genetic counseling profession and the policies of one's institution or organization.

    a. Follow the guidance of the National Society of Genetic Counselors Code of Ethics.
    b. Recognize and respond to ethical and moral dilemmas arising in genetic counseling practice, and seek outside consultation when needed.
    c. Identify and utilize factors that promote client autonomy.
    d. Ascertain and comply with current professional credentialing requirements, at the institutional, state, regional, and national level.
    e. Recognize and acknowledge situations that may result in a real or perceived conflict of interest.

18. Demonstrate understanding of the research process.

    a. Articulate the value of research to enhance the practice of genetic counseling.
    b. Demonstrate an ability to formulate a research question.
    c. Recognize the various roles a genetic counselor can play on a research team, and identify opportunities to participate in and/or lead research studies.
    d. Identify available research-related resources.
    e. Apply knowledge of research methodology and *study design* to critically evaluate research outcomes.
    f. Apply knowledge of research methodology and study designs to educate clients about research studies relevant to them/their family.
    g. Describe the importance of human subjects' protection and the role of the Institutional Review Board (IRB) process.

19. Advocate for individuals, families, communities, and the genetic counseling profession.

    a. Recognize the potential tension between the values of clients, families, communities, and the genetic counseling profession.
    b. Support client and community interests in accessing, or declining, social and health services and clinical research.
    c. Identify genetic professional organizations, and describe opportunities for participation and leadership.
    d. Employ strategies that increase/promote access to genetic counseling services.

20. Demonstrate a self-reflective, evidenced-based, and current approach to genetic counseling practice.

    a. Display initiative for lifelong learning.
    b. Recognize one's limitations and capabilities in the context of genetic counseling practice.
    c. Seek feedback and respond appropriately to performance critique.
    d. Demonstrate a scholarly approach to genetic counseling, including using available evidence-based principles in the preparation and execution of a genetic counseling encounter.
    e. Identify appropriate individual and/or group opportunities for ongoing personal supervision and mentorship.
    f. Accept responsibility for one's physical and emotional health as it impacts on professional performance.
    g. Recognize and respect professional boundaries between clients, colleagues, and supervisors.

21. Understand the methods, roles, and responsibilities of the process of clinical supervision of trainees.

    a. Engage in active reflection of one's own clinical supervision experiences.
    b. Identify resources to acquire skills to appropriately supervise trainees.
    c. Demonstrate understanding of the dynamics and responsibilities of the supervisor/supervisee relationship.

22. Establish and maintain professional *interdisciplinary relationships* in both team and one-on-one settings, and recognize one's role in the larger health-care system.

    a. Distinguish the genetic counseling *scope of practice* in relation to the roles of other health professionals.
    b. Develop positive relationships with professionals across different disciplines.
    c. Demonstrate familiarity with the *health-care system* as it relates to genetic counseling practice including relevant privacy regulations, referral, and payment systems.
    d. Demonstrate effective interaction with other professionals within the health-care infrastructure to promote appropriate and equitable delivery of genetic services.
    e. Assist nongenetic health-care providers in utilizing genetic information to improve patient care in a cost-effective manner.
    f. Promote responsible use of genetic/genomic technologies and information to enhance the health of individuals, communities, and the public.

Glossary

Case management: The planning and coordination of health-care services appropriate to achieve a desired medical and/or psychological outcome. In the context of genetic counseling, case management requires the evaluation of a medical condition and/or risk of a medical condition in the client or family, evaluating psychological needs, developing and implementing a plan of care, coordinating medical resources and advocating for the client, communicating health-care needs to the individual, monitoring an individual's progress, and promoting client-centered decision-making and cost-effective care.

Client centered: A nondirective form of talk therapy that was developed by Carl Rogers during the 1940s and 1950s. The goal of client-centered counseling is to provide clients with an opportunity to realize how their attitudes, feelings, and behavior are being negatively affected and to make an effort to find their true positive potential. The counselor is expected to employ genuineness, empathy, and unconditional positive regard, with the aim of clients finding their own. (This is also known as person-centered or Rogerian therapy.)

Client: Anyone seeking the expertise of a genetic counselor. Clients include anyone seeking the expertise of a genetic counselor such as individuals seeking personal health information, risk assessment, genetic counseling, testing and case management, health-care professionals, research subjects, and the public.

Contracting: The two-way communication process between the genetic counselor and the patient/client which aims to clarify both parties' expectations and goals for the session.

Distance encounters: At present, and even more so in the future, clinical genetic services will be provided to patients/clients by providers who are not physically in the same location as the patient/client. These encounters can be called distance encounters, even if the provider and patient are not physically located at great distances from each other. Ways in which this care can be provided include interactive two-way video sessions in real time; asynchronous virtual consultations by store-and-forward digital transmission of patient images, data, and clinical questions from the patient/client's health-care provider to the genetic services provider; telephone consultation between genetic provider and patient/client; and perhaps additional forms of interaction between providers and patients/clients unimagined at present.

Family history: The systematic research and narrative of past and current events relating to a specific family that often include medical and social information.

Genetics: The branch of biologic science which investigates and describes the molecular structure and function of genes, how gene function produces effects in the organism (phenotype), how genes are transmitted from parent to offspring, and the distribution of gene variations in populations.

Genetic counseling: The process of helping people understand and adapt to the medical, psychological, and familial implications of genetic contributions to disease. Genetic counselors work in various settings and provide services to diverse clients.

Genomics: The branch of biology which studies the aggregate of genes in an organism. The main difference between genomics and genetics is that genetics generally studies the structure, variation, function, and expression of single genes, whereas genomics studies the large number of genes in an organism and their interrelationship.

Health-care system: The organization of people, institutions, and resources to deliver health-care services to meet the health needs of target populations. The laws, regulations, and policies governing health-care systems differ depending on the country, state/province, and institution.

Interdisciplinary relationships: Connections and interactions among members of a team of health-care staff from different areas of practice.

Pedigree: A diagram of family relationships that uses symbols to represent people and lines to represent relationships. These diagrams make it easier to visualize relationships within families, particularly large extended families.

Population screening: Testing of individuals in an identified, asymptomatic, target population who may be at risk for a particular disease or may be at risk to have a child with a particular disease. Population screening may allow for the provision of information important for decision-making, early diagnosis, and improved treatment or disease prevention.

Probability of conditions with a genetic component: The chance, typically expressed as a fraction or a percentage, for an individual or a specific population to experience a condition that has a genetic component. This terminology is used intentionally rather than "genetic risk" because the concept of "risk" is not synonymous with "probability." The origin of a probability can come from principles of Mendelian inheritance or from epidemiology. The probability of genetic disease is differentiated from risk of genetic disease in that probability conveys the numerical estimate for an individual patient or a specific population, while risk includes additional elements including the burden of disease.

Population genetics: The study of allele frequency distribution and change under evolutionary processes and includes concepts such as the Hardy-Weinberg principle and the study of quantitative genetic traits.

Research methodologies: The process to define the activity (how, when, where, etc.) of gathering data.

Scope of practice: Genetic counselors work as members of a health-care team in a medical genetics program or other specialty/subspecialty, including oncology, neurology, cardiology, obstetrics, and gynecology, among others. They are uniquely trained to provide information, counseling, and support to individuals and families whose members have genetic disorders or who may be at risk for these conditions. The genetic counseling scope of practice is carried out through collaborative relationships with clinical geneticists and other physicians, as well as other allied health-care professionals such as nurses, physicians, and social workers.

Study design: The formulation of trials and experiments in medical and epidemiological research. Study designs can be qualitative, quantitative, descriptive (e.g., case report, case series, survey), analytic-observational (e.g., cross sectional, case-control, cohort), and/or analytic-experimental (randomized controlled trials).

Source Accreditation Council for Genetic Counseling. Practice based competencies for genetic counselors; 2015. Accessed November 22, 2017 at http://gceducation.org/Documents/ACGC%20Core%20Competencies%20Brochure_15_Web.pdf.

Appendix B: NSGC Code of Ethics

A Code of Ethics is a document which attempts to clarify and guide the conduct of a professional so that the goals and values of the profession might best be served.

Preamble

Genetic counselors are health professionals with specialized education, training, and experience in medical genetics and counseling. The National Society of Genetic Counselors (NSGC) is the leading voice, authority, and advocate for the genetic counseling profession. Through this code of ethics, the NSGC affirms the ethical responsibilities of its members. NSGC members are expected to be aware of the ethical implications of their professional actions and work to uphold and adhere to the guidelines and principles set forth in this code.

Introduction

A code of ethics is a document that attempts to clarify and guide the conduct of a professional so that the goals and values of the profession are best served. The NSGC Code of Ethics is based upon the distinct relationships genetic counselors have with (1) themselves, (2) their clients, (3) their colleagues, and (4) society. Each section of this code begins with an explanation of the relevant relationship, along with the key values and characteristics of that relationship. These values are drawn from the ethical principles of autonomy, beneficence, nonmaleficence, and justice, and they include the professional principles of fidelity, veracity, integrity, dignity, and accountability.

No set of guidelines can provide all the assistance needed in every situation, especially when different values appear to conflict. In certain areas, some ambiguity remains, allowing for the judgement of the genetic counselor(s) involved to determine how best to respond to difficult situations.

Section 1: Genetic Counselors Themselves

Genetic counselors value professionalism, competence, integrity, objectivity, veracity, dignity, accountability, and self-respect in themselves as well as in each other. Therefore, genetic counselors work to:

1. Seek out and acquire balanced, accurate, and relevant information required for a given situation.
2. Continue their education and training to keep abreast of relevant guidelines, regulations, position statements, and standards of genetic counseling practice.
3. Work within their scope of professional practice and recognize the limits of their own knowledge, expertise, and competence.
4. Accurately represent their experience, competence, and credentials, including academic degrees, certification, licensure, and relevant training.
5. Identify and adhere to institutional and professional conflict of interest guidelines and develop mechanisms for avoiding or managing real or perceived conflict of interest when it arises.
6. Acknowledge and disclose to relevant parties the circumstances that may interfere with or influence professional judgment or objectivity, or may otherwise result in a real or perceived conflict of interest.
7. Assure that institutional or professional privilege is not used for personal gain.
8. Be responsible for their own physical and emotional health as it impacts their professional judgment and performance, including seeking professional support, as needed.

Section 2: Genetic Counselors and Their Clients

The counselor-client relationship is based on values of care and respect for the client's autonomy, individuality, welfare, and freedom in clinical and research interactions. Therefore, genetic counselors work to:

1. Provide genetic counseling services to their clients within their scope of practice regardless of personal interests or biases, and refer clients, as needed, to appropriately qualified professionals.
2. Clarify and define their professional role(s) and relationships with clients, disclose any real or perceived conflict of interest, and provide an accurate description of their services.
3. Provide genetic counseling services to their clients regardless of their clients' abilities, age, culture, religion, ethnicity, language, sexual orientation, and gender identity.

4. Enable their clients to make informed decisions, free of coercion, by providing or illuminating the necessary facts, and clarifying the alternatives and anticipated consequences.
5. Respect their clients' beliefs, inclinations, circumstances, feelings, family relationships, sexual orientation, religion, gender identity, and cultural traditions.
6. Refer clients to an alternate genetic counselor or other qualified professional when situations arise in which a genetic counselor's personal values, attitudes, and beliefs may impede his or her ability to counsel a client.
7. Maintain the privacy and security of their client's confidential information and individually identifiable health information, unless released by the client or disclosure is required by law.
8. Avoid the exploitation of their clients for personal, professional, or institutional advantage, profit, or interest.

Section 3: Genetic Counselors and Their Colleagues

The genetic counselors' professional relationships with other genetic counselors, trainees, employees, employers, and other professionals are based on mutual respect, caring, collaboration, fidelity, veracity, and support. Therefore, genetic counselors work to:

1. Share their knowledge and provide mentorship and guidance for the professional development of other genetic counselors, employees, trainees, and colleagues.
2. Respect and value the knowledge, perspectives, contributions, and areas of competence of colleagues, trainees, and other professionals.
3. Encourage ethical behavior of colleagues.
4. Assure that individuals under their supervision undertake responsibilities that are commensurate with their knowledge, experience, and training.
5. Maintain appropriate boundaries to avoid exploitation in their relationships with trainees, employees, employers, and colleagues.
6. Take responsibility and credit only for work they have actually performed and to which they have contributed
7. Appropriately acknowledge the work and contributions of others.
8. Make employers aware of genetic counselors' ethical obligations as set forth in the NSGC Code of Ethics.

Section 4: Genetic Counselors and Society

The relationships of genetic counselors with society include interest and participation in activities that have the purpose of promoting the well-being of society and access to genetic services and health care. These relationships are based on the principles of veracity, objectivity, and integrity. Therefore, genetic counselors, individually or through their professional organizations, work to:

1. Promote policies that aim to prevent genetic discrimination and oppose the use of genetic information as a basis for discrimination.
2. Serve as a source of reliable information and expert opinion on genetic counseling to employers, policymakers, payers, and public officials. When speaking publicly on such matters, a genetic counselor should be careful to separate their personal statements and opinions made as private individuals from statements made on behalf of their employers or professional societies.
3. Participate in educating the public about the development and application of technological and scientific advances in genetics and the potential societal impact of these advances.
4. Promote policies that assure ethically responsible research in the context of genetics.
5. Adhere to applicable laws and regulations. However, when such laws are in conflict with the principles of the profession, genetic counselors work toward change that will benefit the public interest.

Source Adopted 1/92 by the National Society of Genetic Counselors, Inc.; Revised 12/04, 1/06, 4/17. https://www.nsgc.org/p/cm/ld/fid=12.

Index

P. McCarthy Veach et al., *Facilitating the Genetic Counseling Process*,
https://doi.org/10.1007/978-3-319-74799-6